Cancer Treatment and Research

Volume 195

This book series provides detailed updates on the state of the art in the treatment of different forms of cancer and also covers a wide spectrum of topics of current research interest. Clinicians will benefit from expert analysis of both standard treatment options and the latest therapeutic innovations and from provision of clear guidance on the management of clinical challenges in daily practice. The research-oriented volumes focus on aspects ranging from advances in basic science through to new treatment tools and evaluation of treatment safety and efficacy. Each volume is edited and authored by leading authorities in the topic under consideration. In providing cutting-edge information on cancer treatment and research, the series will appeal to a wide and interdisciplinary readership. The series is listed in PubMed/Index Medicus.

Sumel Ashique
Farzad Taghizadeh-Hesary
Biplab Debnath • Ayush Madan
Editors

Cancer Metabolism

Molecular Mechanisms and Therapeutic Strategies

Springer

Editors
Sumel Ashique
Pharmaceutical Technology
Bharat Technology
Howrah, West Bengal, India

Biplab Debnath
Pharmaceutical Technology
Bharat Technology
Howrah, West Bengal, India

Farzad Taghizadeh-Hesary
Breast Cancer Research Center
Iran University of Medical Sciences
Tehran, Iran

Ayush Madan
Biotechnology Department, School of Research and Technology
People's University
Bhopal, Madhya Pradesh, India

ISSN 0927-3042 ISSN 2509-8497 (electronic)
Cancer Treatment and Research
ISBN 978-3-032-21860-5 ISBN 978-3-032-21861-2 (eBook)
https://doi.org/10.1007/978-3-032-21861-2

This Springer imprint is published by the registered company Springer Nature Switzerland AG
The registered company address is: Gewerbestrasse 11, 6330 Cham, Switzerland

Contents

Contributors

Hamed Afkhami Cellular and Molecular Research Center, Qom University of Medical Sciences, Qom, Iran

Sumel Ashique Department of Pharmaceutical Technology, Bharat Technology, Uluberia, West Bengal, India

Ramyar Azar Iran University of Medical Sciences, Tehran, Iran

Aganta Chakraborty Department of Pharmaceutical Technology, Bharat Technology, Uluberia, West Bengal, India

Soukat Chandra Department of Pharmaceutical Technology, Bharat Technology, Uluberia, West Bengal, India

Subhajit Chatterjee Laboratory of Cellular Oncology, National Cancer Institute, National Institute of Health (NIH), Bethesda, MD, USA

Priya Chaudhary Centre for Herbal Pharmacology and Environmental Sustainability, Chettinad Hospital and Research Institute, Chettinad Academy of Research and Education, Chennai, Tamil Nadu, India

Biswajit Das Department of Molecular, Cell and Developmental Biology, University of California, Santa Cruz, CA, USA

Chinmay Das School of Biotechnology, Kalinga Institute of Industrial Technology Deemed to be University, Bhubaneswar, Odisha, India

Joy Das School of Pharmaceutical Sciences, Lovely Professional University, Phagwara, Punjab, India

Srijani Dasgupta Department of Pharmaceutical Sciences, Jharkhand Rai University, Rajaulatu, Namkum, Ranchi, India

Bangmayee Dash School of Allied and Health Care Sciences, DRIEMS University, Cuttack, Odisha, India

Somya Ranjan Dash Cancer Metastasis & Therapeutics Lab, Department of Biological Sciences, Indian Institute of Science Education and Research (IISER), Berhampur, Odisha, India

Biplab Debnath Department of Pharmaceutical Technology, Bharat Technology, Uluberia, West Bengal, India

Sunaina Demiwal Department of Pharmaceutical Sciences, Lord Shiva College of Pharmacy, Sirsa, Haryana, India

Mohamed Dkhi Department of Zoology and Entomology, Faculty of Science, Helwan University, Helwan, Egypt

Amir Hossein Esfandiari Antimicrobial Resistance Research Center, Basic Science Research Institute, Mashhad University of Medical Sciences, Mashhad, Iran

Pedram Fadavi Breast Cancer Research Center, Iran University of Medical Sciences, Tehran, Iran
Department of Radiation Oncology, School of Medicine, Iran University of Medical Sciences, Tehran, Iran

Ali Ahmadizad Firouzjaei Bioinformatics Research Center, Basic Sciences Research Institute, Mashhad University of Medical Sciences, Mashhad, Iran

Fatemeh Forouzanfar Neuroscience Research Center, Mashhad University of Medical Sciences, Mashhad, Iran

Mirunalini Gobinath Department of Pharmacognosy & Phytopharmacy, JSS College of Pharmacy, JSS Academy of Higher Education & Research, Ooty, Tamil Nadu, India

Mohammad Habeeb Department of Pharmaceutics, Crescent School of Pharmacy, B.S. Abdur Rahman Crescent Institute of Science and Technology, Chennai, India

Nafiseh Izadi Antimicrobial Resistance Research Center, Basic Science Research Institute, Mashhad University of Medical Sciences, Mashhad, Iran

Mayukh Jana Department of Pharmaceutical Technology, Bharat Technology, Uluberia, West Bengal, India

Pracheta Janmeda Department of Bioscience and Biotechnology, Banasthali Vidyapith, Banasthali, Rajasthan, India

Rishabh Kasnia Department of Pharmaceutical Sciences, Lord Shiva College of Pharmacy, Sirsa, Haryana, India

Ayush Madan Department of Biotechnology, School of Research and Technology, People's University, Bhopal, Madhya Pradesh, India

Hanie Mahaki Vascular and Endovascular Surgery Research Center, Mashhad University of Medical Sciences, Mashhad, Iran

Naina Mohamed Pakkir Maideen Clinical Associate Professor of Pharmacology, College of Medicine, Mohammed Bin Rashid, University of Medicine and Health Sciences, Dubai, UAE
Dubai Health, Dubai, UAE

Mona Mansourian Metabolic Syndrome Research Center, Mashhad University of Medical Sciences, Mashhad, Iran

Mukesh Meena Laboratory of Phytopathology and Microbial Biotechnology, Department of Botany, Mohanlal Sukhadia University, Udaipur, Rajasthan, India

Uttam Kumar Mishra Department of Chemistry, Birla Institute of Technology, Mesra, Ranchi, India

Gomathi Mohan Centre for Herbal Pharmacology and Environmental Sustainability, Chettinad Hospital and Research Institute, Chettinad Academy of Research and Education, Chennai, Tamil Nadu, India

Naheed Mojgani Razi Vaccine and Serum Research Institute- Agricultural Research, Education and Extension Organization, Karaj, Iran

Khatere Mokhtari Department of Cell and Molecular Biology and Microbiology, Faculty of Biological Science and Technology, University of Isfahan, Isfahan, Iran

Mohini Mondal Department of Pharmaceutical Technology, Bharat Technology, Uluberia, West Bengal, India

Subhajit Mandal Department of Pharmaceutical Sciences, Faculty of Science and Engineering, Dibrugarh University, Dibrugarh, Assam, India

Shrabasti Mullick Department of Pharmaceutical Technology, Bharat Technology, Uluberia, West Bengal, India

Nahid Nafissi Breast Cancer Research Center, Iran University of Medical Sciences, Tehran, Iran

Sisir Nandi Global Institute of Pharmaceutical Education & Research (GIPER), Kashipur, Uttarakhand, India

Rajarshi Nath Department of Pharmaceutical Technology, Bharat Technology, Uluberia, West Bengal, India

Bhabani Shankar Nayak KIIT School of Pharmacy, KIMS, KIIT Deemed to be University, Bhubaneswar, Odisha, India

Bhupender Nehra Department of Pharmaceutical Sciences, Guru Jambheshwar University of Science & Technology, Hisar, Haryana, India

Radheshyam Pal Department of Pharmacology, Bengal College of Pharmaceutical Technology, Phagwara, West Bengal, India

Tithi Parija School of Biotechnology, Kalinga Institute of Industrial Technology Deemed to be University, Bhubaneswar, Odisha, India

Shakti Prasad Pattanayak Department of Biochemistry, School of Medicine, Case Western Reserve University, Euclid Ave, Cleveland, OH, USA

Nebojša Pavlović Department of Pharmacy, Faculty of Medicine, University of Novi Sad, Novi Sad, Serbia

Pratik Phalke Department of Pharmaceutics, JSS College of Pharmacy, JSS Academy of Higher Education & Research, Ooty, Tamil Nadu, India

Sam Pournezhad Marcus Stroke and Neuroscience Center, Grady Memorial Hospital, Atlanta, GA, USA
Department of Clinical Sciences, Touro University California College of Pharmacy, Vallejo, CA, USA

Sanket Pramanik Department of Pharmaceutical Technology, Bharat Technology, Uluberia, West Bengal, India

Gaurav Ranjan Department of Pharmacy, School of Health Science, Central University of South Bihar, Gaya, Bihar, India

Gaurav Raturi Institute of Genomics for Crop Abiotic Stress Tolerance, Texas Tech University, Lubbock, TX, USA

Ciniraj Raveendran Department of Radiation Oncology, Government Medical College Thiruvananthapuram, Thiruvananthapuram, India

Mahdieh Ameri Shah Reza Cellular and Molecular Research Center, Qom University of Medical Sciences, Qom, Iran

Parikshit Roychowdhury Department of Pharmaceutics, JSS College of Pharmacy, JSS Academy of Higher Education & Research, Ooty, Tamil Nadu, India

Himanshu Sharma Teerthanker Mahaveer College of Pharmacy, Teerthanker Mahaveer University, Moradabad, India

Mohsen Sheykhhasan Cellular and Molecular Research Center, Qom University of Medical Sciences, Qom, Iran

Manzer H. Siddiqui Department of Botany and Microbiology, College of Science, King Saud University, Riyadh, Saudi Arabia

Priyashree Sunita Department of Surgery, Case Comprehensive Cancer Centre, Case Western Reserve University, Wolstein Research Building, Cleveland, OH, USA

Sourabh Suthar Department of Pharmaceutical Sciences, Lord Shiva College of Pharmacy, Sirsa, Haryana, India

Farzad Taghizadeh-Hesary Breast Cancer Research Center, Iran University of Medical Sciences, Tehran, Iran
ENT and Head and Neck Research Center and Department, The Five Senses Health Institute, School of Medicine, Iran University of Medical Sciences, Tehran, Iran

Hamid Tanzadehpanah Antimicrobial Resistance Research Center, Basic Science Research Institute, Mashhad University of Medical Sciences, Mashhad, Iran

Hariharan Thirumalai Vengateswaran Department of Pharmaceutics, Crescent School of Pharmacy, B.S. Abdur Rahman Crescent Institute of Science and Technology, Chennai, India

Alberto Ouro Villasante NeuroAging Laboratory (NEURAL) Group, Clinical Neurosciences Research Laboratory (LINC), Health Research Institute of Santiago de Compostela (IDIS), Hospital Clínico Universitario, Santiago de Compostela, Spain
Centro de Investigación Biomédica en Red en Enfermedades Neurodegenerativas (CIBERNED), Instituto de Salud Carlos III, Madrid, Spain

Huay Woon You Pusat PERMATA@Pintar Negara, Universiti Kebangsaan Malaysia, Bangi, Malaysia

Introduction to Cancer Metabolism

1

Gomathi Mohan, Mukesh Meena, Manzer H. Siddiqui, Gaurav Raturi, Pracheta Janmeda, and Priya Chaudhary

1.1 Introduction

Cancer is a group of intricate genetic disorders that are distinguished by the uncontrolled and autonomous cell growth, primarily due to complex genomic changes involving mutations in tumor suppressor and oncogene genes. The corresponding changes make it easier for healthy cells to develop malignant characteristics [1]. Normal and malignant cells have different microenvironments. Oxygen deprivation and dietary shortage force malignant cells to change biochemical pathways to meet energy, biosynthetic, and redox needs [2]. The

G. Mohan · P. Chaudhary (✉)
Centre for Herbal Pharmacology and Environmental Sustainability, Chettinad Hospital and Research Institute, Chettinad Academy of Research and Education, Chennai, Tamil Nadu, India
e-mail: priyachaudhary@care.edu.in

M. Meena
Laboratory of Phytopathology and Microbial Biotechnology, Department of Botany, Mohanlal Sukhadia University, Udaipur, Rajasthan, India

M. H. Siddiqui
Department of Botany and Microbiology, College of Science, King Saud University, Riyadh, Saudi Arabia
e-mail: mhsiddqui@ksu.edu.sa

G. Raturi
Institute of Genomics for Crop Abiotic Stress Tolerance, Texas Tech University, Lubbock, TX, USA

P. Janmeda
Department of Bioscience and Biotechnology, Banasthali Vidyapith, Banasthali, Rajasthan, India
e-mail: pracheta@banasthali.in

S. Ashique et al. (eds.), *Cancer Metabolism*, Cancer Treatment and Research 195, https://doi.org/10.1007/978-3-032-21861-2_1

"Warburg effect" in cancer is presently one of the most extensively examined metabolic reprogramming mechanisms in cells. Despite the availability of adequate oxygen, malignant cells predominantly utilize glycolysis for adenosine triphosphate (ATP) production [3]. Furthermore, fluctuations in external nutrient levels and adverse conditions induce tumor cells to modify their metabolic pathways. The cross talk between malignant cells and host cells, as well as gene and protein expression, influences two and three metabolic reprogramming, which leads to modifications such as an increase in glucose utilization in cancer. It is involved in the regulation of numerous metabolic pathways, such as the metabolism of glucose, lipids, and amino acids [4]. Tumor cells produce ATP with the help of the pentose phosphate pathway (PPP), aerobic glycolysis, glutaminase (GLS) degradation, and one-carbon metabolization, leading to the generation of various biological macromolecules that support proliferation [5]. Enzymes, signaling molecules, and proteins, such as AMP-activated protein kinase (AMPK) and the mTOR signaling cascade, work together to reorganize metabolic pathways. Furthermore, intricate systems are utilized [6].

Tumor therapy aimed at regulating metabolism is currently classified into pharmacological therapy and nutritional intervention therapy, reflecting the distinct methods of intervention utilized [7]. Various pharmacological agents focused on metabolic remodeling have been studied and are expected to develop into therapeutic strategies for the regulation of tumor metabolism, specifically targeting critical proteins within pertinent signaling pathways to tackle metabolic complexity [8]. One common alternative therapy strategy for tumors is nutritional intervention. Dietary control modifies the pace at which nutrients are used by the cellular milieu, including by tumor cells, which impacts a number of physiological functions related to these cells. At the same time, an increasing amount of data indicates that combining several treatments could be a practical therapeutic approach [9].

This chapter analyzes the metabolic mechanisms that facilitate tumor cell adaptation to their distinctive growth requirements and investigates their growth characteristics. It focuses on three main areas: the metabolism of lipids, glucose, and amino acids. It also provides an overview of the settings that influence alterations in these three metabolic pathways, the variables that drive tumor metabolism reprogramming, and the possible targets for metabolic reprogramming treatment. The elements affecting reprogramming are summarized in this work from the perspective of cell-cell interactions, protein, and gene. Additionally, it offers a thorough summary of certain medications that target every metabolic route linked to tumor metabolism reprogramming, providing a potential option for cancer treatment in the future.

1.2 Insights into Cellular Energy Metabolism in Normal and Tumor Cells

In healthy cells, mitochondrial oxidative phosphorylation is the primary process for producing energy. The production of acetyl-CoA requires the conversion of carbohydrates, primarily glucose, into pyruvate. The tricarboxylic acid (TCA) cycle is supported by intermediates generated during the catabolism of proteins and lipids [10].

Although all cells require energy for homeostasis, malignant cells have an increased energy demand due to their continuous division and expansion. The multiplication of tumor cells necessitates significant amounts of energy and nutrients. The fundamental components include ribonucleic acid (RNA), lipids, deoxyribonucleic acid (DNA), and proteins [11]. The Warburg effect is the term for the fact that, even under an aerobic environment and with fully functional mitochondrial metabolism, the rate of glucose uptake increases substantially, along with lactate generation rather than pyruvate [12].

The Warburg effect is a prime example of inefficient energy generation. Under aerobic conditions, one glucose molecule produces 36 adenosine triphosphate (ATP) molecules. Since cancer cells proliferate continuously, it is necessary to regulate high amounts of glycolytic metabolites, such as glyceraldehyde-3-phosphate, and fructose-6-phosphate, to produce ribose-5-phosphate, which is necessary for the generation of NADPH and nucleotides [13]. Reactive oxygen species (ROS) are reduced when glutathione reductase (GR) uses NADPH as a cofactor to reduce glutathione (GSH). It also plays a vital function in the generation of acetate for fatty acid formation and the de novo generation of nonessential amino acids [14].

The buildup of tumor-associated metabolites, including succinate, glutamate, lactate, and fumarate, has a significant impact on the metabolization of cancer cells, increasing their survival and ability for proliferation [15]. Glycolytic enzyme overexpression, glutaminolysis, and a high concentration of metabolic transporters are all related to increased lactate generation, which promotes angiogenesis through a number of pathways [16]. Lactate promotes angiogenesis by activating the NF-κB-mediated IL-8 signaling in endothelial cells. The expression of the LDH isoform correlates with the production of HIF-2α and HIF-1α, as well as Vascular endothelial growth factor (VEGF), vital mediators of the angiogenic process. Tumor-associated macrophages (TAMs) promote abnormal angiogenesis by activating mTORC1, ERK1, and STAT3 mediated by HIF-1α ubiquitination, up-regulating CA9 gene expression, and responding to genome instability [17].

In some cancer situations, ROS-induced glycolysis causes cancer-associated fibroblasts (CAFs) to produce lactate in addition to cancer cells [18]. The excessive lactate generated can pass through the malignant cell via monocarboxylate transporter 1 (MCT-1). The reverse Warburg effect enables cells to operate independently, utilizing alternative energy sources beyond glucose [19].

On the other hand, α-ketoglutarate is produced from glutamate, a consequence of glutamine metabolism, and then incorporated into the TCA cycle [20]. When pyruvate dehydrogenase (PDH) and pyruvate carboxylase (PC) are inhibited in cancer cells, high lactate levels and HIF1 activation cause a metabolic reprogramming in the Krebs cycle toward glutamate dependence. Tumors metabolize glutamine as an energy source, resulting in increased levels of malate and citrate, thereby promoting nucleotide biosynthesis essential for neoplastic cell proliferation [21].

In the reductive carboxylation pathway mediated by IDH1, glutamine is converted to 2-hydroxyglutarate through alpha-ketoglutarate; thereafter, citrate, which also derives from glutamine, promotes fatty acid synthesis. This phenomenon facilitates the removal of reactive oxygen species (ROS) generated in malignant cells by producing NADH via IDH1-dependent glutamine reductive metabolism [22].

Similarly, lipids play a vital role in carcinogenesis by facilitating the absorption of fatty acids through the specialized transport proteins. Enhanced lipogenesis, fatty acid β-oxidation, and modified lipid storage are associated with a more prometastatic phenotype, leading to enhanced cell motility and resistance to programmed cell death [23].

1.3 Tumor Microenvironment (TME) and Metabolic Cross Talk

In solid tumors with hypoxia, Hypoxia-Inducible Factor-1α (HIF-1α) is stabilized because the normal prolyl hydroxylases (PHDs) stop working. This stops HIF-1α from being hydroxylated, which would typically indicate it for VHL-mediated ubiquitination and proteasomal destruction. HIF-1α enhances glycolysis by promoting the production of glucose transporters and several glycolytic protein isoforms [24]. Cancer upregulates the glucose-related PPP. The PPP utilizes glucose 6-phosphate to make fructose 6-phosphate, and glyceraldehyde 3-phosphate, unlike glycolysis. The nonoxidative PPP generates ribose 5-phosphate (R5P) and provides reducing equivalents for sterol, amino acid biosynthesis, nucleotide, and fatty acid [25]. These alterations modify the functionality of tumor and stromal cells, enabling them to adapt to hypoxia and nutrition levels, alter mitochondrial activity, manage ROS, and influence the accumulation of metabolites such as lactate and succinate. This subsequently alters the functionality of HIF signaling [26].

The state of equilibrium of the tumor microenvironment (TME) is significantly impacted by cancer-associated fibroblasts (CAFs). Cancer cells engage with adjacent cancer-associated fibroblasts, influencing growth, metabolism, metastasis, and progression. This analysis suggests a "dual-chamber" model called the "Reverse Warburg effect" [27]. Cancer cells release H_2O_2 into the tumor microenvironment, causing oxidative stress in surrounding stromal cells. CAFs perform aerobic glycolysis, generating high amounts of energy-rich metabolites, including fatty acids, lactic acid, ketone bodies, and pyruvate. These substances provide nourishment to cancer cells [28].

Research indicates that cancer-associated fibroblasts (CAFs) affect cancer progression via multiple mechanisms, such as inducing chemoresistance, altering tumor invasion and metastatic progression, and promoting angiogenesis. CAFs possess the ability to remodel the tumor immune microenvironment (TIME), leading to tumor immune escape. The TIME comprises cells from both the innate and adaptive immune systems, also secretes cytokines, and includes various other immune cell populations [29]. Tumor-associated macrophages (TAMs) undergo analogous reprogramming, particularly in hypoxic conditions: Stabilization of HIF-1α in TAMs results in a shift from oxidative metabolism to increased glucose metabolism and lactate regulation. The expression of M2-like (protumoral) genes is also increased, along with the production of immunosuppressive cytokines, the release of angiogenic factors, and resistance to therapy [30].

Tumor-infiltrating lymphocytes (TILs), similar to cancer cells, require nutrients from the tumor microenvironment (TME) for growth and differentiation. Naïve T cells are based on oxidative phosphorylation, whereas activated T cells necessitate aerobic glycolysis for their activation and effector functions [31]. Glucose deprivation in T cells leads to a decrease in calcium signaling, interferon-gamma production, and cytotoxic activity. T lymphocytes and tumor cells necessitate glutamine for growth. Tumor cells need glutaminolysis to synthesize nucleotides, amino acids, fatty acids, and glutathione and replenish metabolites via anaplerotic processes [32]. Cancer cells produce extracellular vesicles (EVs) with donor cell proteins, lipids, RNAs, and metabolites that alter recipient metabolism. Cancer therapy may target exosomes. Exosomal miR-210 and miR-155 induce glycolysis and premetastatic conditions in human adult dermal fibroblasts (HADF). FasL-positive exosomes from activated T cells can transport melanoma cells to the lung [33]. In rats, exosomes from marrow stromal cells released MiR-146b to reduce malignant glioma [34]. Dietary competition and exosome-mediated metabolite exchange affect immunotherapy, tumor growth, and immune suppression [35]. As depicted in Fig. 1.1, the tumor microenvironment is characterized by metabolic coupling between cancer cells, CAFs, TAMs, and TILs, leading to enhanced glycolysis, lactate export, and immune suppression.

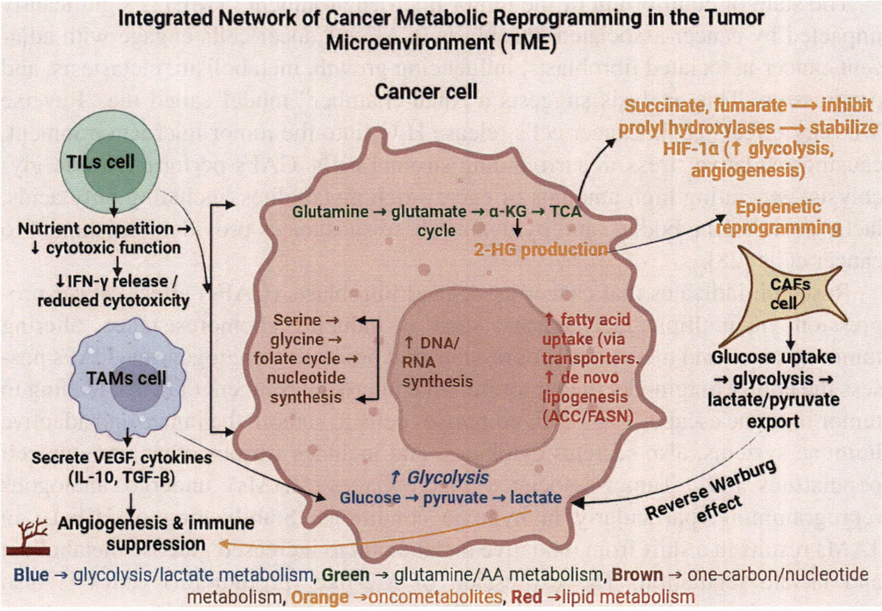

Fig. 1.1 In this schematic, cancer cells undergo significant metabolic alterations and interact with stromal and immune cells. Cancer cells switch pyruvate from mitochondrial oxidation to lactate synthesis due to the Warburg effect. This lowers immunity and promotes angiogenesis. CAFs support the metabolic needs of cancer cells by increasing glycolysis and providing lactate and pyruvate. The reverse Warburg effect occurs. Hypoxic circumstances cause tumor-associated macrophages (TAMs) to undergo glycolytic reprogramming, resulting in the production of VEGF and immunosuppressive cytokines such as TGF-β and IL-10, which promote angiogenesis. IFN-γ secretion and cytotoxicity decrease due to nutrient competition in tumor-infiltrating lymphocytes (TILS). The oncometabolites succinate and fumarate block prolyl hydroxylases, stabilizing HIF-1α and encouraging glycolysis and angiogenesis. Glutamine metabolism enhances the TCA cycle, supports nucleotide synthesis, and facilitates the reduction of carboxylation to produce 2-hydroxyglutarate, resulting in epigenetic reprogramming. Fatty acid absorption and de novo lipogenesis boost cell growth. These pathways show the tumor microenvironment's metabolic plasticity, supporting cancer development, immune evasion, and therapeutic resistance [5, 10, 31, 36–38]

1.4 Key Metabolic Pathways in Cancer Progression

1.4.1 One-Carbon Metabolism and Nucleotide Biosynthesis

One-carbon metabolism (1C metabolism), also known as folate metabolism since the single carbon unit is connected to tetrahydrofolate, which is generated from folate, is crucial for various metabolic functions. Essential syntheses, especially purine and thymidylate, depend on it [39]. 5,10-methylene tetrahydrofolate dehydrogenase 2 (MTHFD2) and Serine hydroxymethyltransferase 2 (SHMT2) serve as independent prognostic molecules and potent therapeutic targets within the mitochondrial serine catabolic pathway in various cancers [40]. There are several ways that cells produce one-carbon units. The glycine cleavage system (GCS), serine metabolism to glycine, choline metabolism, and other amino acid metabolism are included. The cytoplasmic and mitochondrial methyltransferases SHMT1 and SHMT2 convert serine to glycine. The one-carbon group of serine is added to THF to make methylene-THF [41]. Dietary sources are converted into molecules needed for protein, nucleotide, methylation, and antioxidant production. Studies suggest that elevated blood folate levels may increase lung disorders, breast cancer, and colorectal cancer [42]. The Hoffman effect links methionine dependence to cancer cell aggression. Methionine-dependent and methionine-independent osteosarcoma cells were studied. In mouse experiments, methionine-addicted cells showed increased motility, invasion, tumor growth, and metastatic potential [43].

1.4.2 Pentose Phosphate Pathway (PPP) and Redox Balance

The pentose phosphate pathway (PPP), also referred to as the phosphogluconate pathway or hexose monophosphate shunt, initiates the metabolization of glucose in parallel to glycolysis. Cancer cells need the PPP to synthesize pentose phosphate for the generation of nucleic acids and NADPH for the synthesis of fatty acids to survive and proliferate [44]. PPP involves two irreversible oxidative reactions followed by reversible interconversions, which occur in the cytosol. Thus, the PPP has two metabolic pathways: the oxidative pathway and the nonoxidative pathway. Through the oxidative mechanism, G6P is changed to Ru5P, CO2, and NADPH [45]. Sugars like F6P, G3P, and sedoheptulose are made by the nonoxidative mechanism, which also makes sugar phosphate precursors to synthesize amino acids and nucleic acids [46]. The tumor suppressor p53 interacts with G6PD to prevent the active dimer from forming, thereby blocking NADPH generation, glucose utilization, and biosynthesis, and the pentose phosphate pathway [47]. The free-radical hypothesis of cancer suggests that oxidative stress, resulting from reactive species, leads to DNA damage and promotes genetic instability. ROS and RNS are presently thought to have roles in both direct DNA damage and the modification of redox-regulated signaling pathways, which can have either positive or negative consequences in cancer [48].

1.4.3 Amino Acid Metabolism in Tumor Growth and Immune Evasion

Cancer cell metabolism studies have found several common traits, including increased nitrogen demand for biosynthetic reactions, increased amino acid consumption and transporter upregulation, insufficient intracellular supply of specific unnecessary amino acids, which require external sources, and altered enzyme levels that synthesize and/or catabolize amino acids [49]. Tumors often modify amino acid metabolism, making nonessential amino acids essential. Thus, targeting specific amino acids may help treat certain types of cancer. Clinical trials target asparaginase to cure leukemia [50]. Tryptophan metabolism involves three key processes: (i) synthesizing indole and its derivatives; (ii) forming serotonin (5-HT) via tryptophan hydroxylase 1 (TPH); and (iii) producing kynurenine from over 95% of free tryptophan through three rate-limiting steps. These enzymes create kynurenine, which may induce cancer by affecting oncogenic signaling or immune surveillance [51]. Human arginine (Arg) comes from nutrition and endogenous synthesis in two stages. Ornithine and citrulline are produced by intestinal epithelial cells from dietary glutamine, glutamate, and proline. Citrulline is converted into arginine in kidney proximal tubules and immune cells to produce nitric oxide (NO), an immunological signaling chemical [52].

1.4.4 Fatty Acid Oxidation (FAO) and Metastasis

Metastatic breast cancer cells had higher mitochondrial lipid levels, which facilitated fatty acid oxidation. Elevated FAO increased mitochondrial fission. Overexpression of DEAD-box polypeptide 3, X-linked (DDX3), increased mitochondrial fission and FAO [53]. FAO and Mitochondrial energy metabolism play a crucial function in enhancing cancer survival and chemotherapy resistance in breast cancer patients. Citrate, a vital carbon source for fatty acid oxidation and cholesterol production, is also required for cellular metabolism [54]. The Metabolic adaptability of cancer cells enables flexibility and dependence primarily on mitochondrial fatty acid oxidation for sustained energy production, even under physiological stress [55]. Metabolic reprogramming serves as a significant indicator of tumor cells, with a growing body of research indicating a correlation between cancer drug resistance and metabolic reprogramming, particularly in the context of FAO [56]. Conversely, modifications in FAO redirect fatty acid transport and sustain an epithelial cell identity, hence preventing EMT-associated metastatic progression in breast cancer in animal models [57].

1.4.5 Mitochondrial Metabolism and Metabolic Plasticity

Mitochondrial reactive oxygen species (ROS) facilitate the aggregation of potentially carcinogenic DNA mutations and the activation of tumorigenic signaling pathways; abnormal accumulation of mitochondria-derived oncometabolites such as 2-hydroxyglutarate (2-HG), fumarate, and succinate exerts significant transforming effects (at least in specific models); and functional impairments in the mitochondrial outer membrane occur [58]. Cancer carcinogenesis depends on mitochondrial regulation of various cellular processes. Altered metabolism enables tumor cells to utilize aerobic glycolysis, alterations in lipid metabolism, and glutamine metabolism for unregulated growth, survival, and resistance to therapy. Different cancer types have different mitochondrial dysfunction, which affects disease symptoms and therapy responses [59]. The metabolic adaptability of malignant cells' mitochondria offers a substantial opportunity for effective antineoplastic treatment, as transformed cells exhibit unique metabolic needs relative to nontransformed cells, with inhibitors like PDH, IDH1/2, and glutaminase currently in clinical trials [60].

1.5 A Brief Overview of Interventions Modulating Metabolic Pathways

Given the significance of metabolic remodeling in tumor proliferation and survival, it constitutes a compelling molecular target that must be considered in the development of potential anticancer therapy. Various pharmacological agents have been investigated over the years for their potential to modify the tumor cell metabolism, as shown in Table 1.1, and assist in combating the disease [61].

1.5.1 mTOR Inhibitors

The mechanistic target of rapamycin (mTOR) functions as a threonine/serine kinase, and it has two protein complexes: mTORC2 and mTORC1. mTORC1 is modulated by Nutrients, growth factors, and stressors, also facilitates the production of proteins, lipids, and nucleotides, promotes glycolysis and PPP, modulates gene expression, and suppresses autophagy, among other functions. The enzymatic phosphorylation of mTORC1 promotes cell proliferation and survival by binding to its primary substrate, AKT, while PI3K/Akt upregulates mTORC2. mTORC1 inhibits mTORC2 [86].

mTORC1 is the most commonly hyperactive protein in cancer, and mTORC2 can be abnormally activated in various cancers due to mutations in its encoding genes or in associated cascades, such as Akt or PI3K. Consequently, it is a key player in cancer progression. Therefore, mTOR-targeting medicines are an innovative treatment strategy that shows potential for cancer treatment [87].

1.5.2 ATP-Competitive Inhibition of mTOR

Many drugs, including AZD8055, AZD2014, and sapanisertib (INK128, TAK-228, MLN0128), compete with ATP to inhibit mTOR. These medications selectively kill cancer cells by blocking their mTORC1 and mTORC2 enzymes, rather than only rapalogs, which leads to a more severe restriction of protein generation, cell cycle arrest, and selective death [88].

Table 1.1 Summarizes essential clinical evidence supporting metabolic remodeling as a therapeutic target for cancer

Inhibitors	Drug	Application	Effect	References
mTOR inhibitors	Rapamycin	Modulates cell growth and division by restricting mTOR, particularly mTORC1, to modify the tumor cell metabolization	Everolimus, temsirolimus, and ridaforolimus are examples of rapalogs, which are similar to rapamycin but have enhanced pharmacological properties. This is because rapamycin's solubility and pharmacokinetics are inadequate	[62]
	Temsirolimus	Management of advanced kidney carcinoma and refractory/relapsed mantle cell lymphoma	Nevertheless, the administration of these medications is certainly not an ideal substitute, and adverse effects are frequently noted in monotherapy	[63, 64]
	Everolimus	Treatment of certain nonfunctional neuroendocrine tumors along with breast cancer		[65, 66]
mTOR ATP-Competitive Blockers	TAK-228 and AZD8055	Some solid tumors exhibit promising antitumor properties	Additionally, in a Phase II clinical study conducted in subjects with various cancer types, AZD2014 demonstrated promising clinical efficacy and tolerability as a single agent	[67, 68]
	MLN0128	In metastatic prostate carcinoma	The effects of MLN0128 appeared to be constrained, potentially due to dose reductions in specific individuals resulting from medication toxicity	[69]
	AZD2014	In a phase II trial involving subjects with recurrent or resistant diffuse large B-cell lymphoma (DLBCL)	Did not produce a satisfactory outcome compared to rapalog therapy	[70]

Dual PI3K/ mTOR Inhibitors	PF-502	Demonstrated significant antitumor efficacy in case of cutaneous T-cell lymphoma	Animal models and in vitro studies in cells derived from patients, particularly those with downregulated PTEN levels	[71]
	PKI-402	Induction of apoptosis, changes in mitochondrial function, and inhibition of cell growth in PIK3CA-mutant human ovarian cancer epithelial cells	Some of these medications have demonstrated tolerable safety profiles with moderate anticancer effectiveness for some cancer types; however, a phase II clinical trial showed that they were no better than rapalogs	[72]
	BEZ235	Enhanced the efficacy of cisplatin treatment while inhibiting tumor development in lung cancer in both laboratory and animal models		[73]
Glutaminase Inhibition	CB-839	Prevent osteosarcoma cell lines from growing	Similarly, phase I clinical research has demonstrated that other compounds, such as CB-839, are less hazardous	[74]
HER2 Inhibitor	KU004	Strongly block cGAS-STING signaling to stop cancer cells from releasing cytokines	It should be mentioned that drug resistance is one potential adverse effect	[75]
Ion Channels as Drug Targets	Ranolazine ("Ranexa") and Riluzole ("Rilutex")	Antimetastatic agents	Adverse effects, including prolonged QT syndrome, significant cardiac arrhythmias, and the risk of sudden cardiac arrest, restrict the use of channel inhibitors	[76]

(continued)

Table 1.1 (continued)

Inhibitors	Drug	Application	Effect	References
ALK inhibitors	Alectinib	ALK-positive lung cancer	This medicine was explicitly designed to help individuals with ALK receptor-positive NSCLC who have progressed in their disease and have shown intolerance to crizotinib. In contrast to crizotinib, Alectinib is effective against mutations that make the ALK inhibitor less selective	[77]
	Crizotinib	First-line and later-line treatment of ALK+ NSCLC	Crizotinib demonstrated more favorable results in terms of partial response (PR) and progression-free survival (PFS) when contrasted with chemotherapy in individuals with ALK-positive non-small cell lung cancer (NSCLC). The mechanism of action of crizotinib in non-NSCLC tumors remains unclear. Thyroid cancers and inflammatory myofibroblastic tumors (IMT) exhibited favorable responses	[77]
	Lorlatinib / Brigatinib / Ceritinib	Later-generation ALK inhibitors in ALK+ NSCLC	Overcome resistance mutations; enhance central nervous system activity; prolong progression-free survival in second- or first-line treatment, contingent upon the context	[77]
MET inhibitors	Capmatinib	Metastatic NSCLC with MET exon 14 mutation	Capmatinib (INC280) is an orally administered ATP-competitive MET inhibitor. In MET-driven murine tumor models, capmatinib has demonstrated remarkable efficacy and selectivity against MET, preventing MET-dependent tumor cell proliferation and tumor growth	[78]
	Tepotinib	MET exon 14 skipping NSCLC	In MET-driven neoplasms, oral MET inhibitor tepotinib has demonstrated significant therapeutic effectiveness when administered once daily. Tepotinib showed potential in treating advanced NSCLC in patients who possessed MET exon 14 skipping mutations	[79]
CDK9 inhibitors	AZD4573	Relapsed/refractory lymphomas / hematologic malignancies	The CDK9 inhibitor AZD4573 inhibited the growth of DLBCL cells. AZD4573, a therapeutic derivative of AZ5576, inhibited Mcl-1 and Bfl-1/A1 transcription in lymphoid malignancies and showed antitumor activity in vivo in AML models through a Mcl-1-dependent mechanism. It also stimulates apoptosis and epigenetic modification	[80]
	CDKI-73	Prostate cancer (including therapy-resistant subtypes)	Specifically, CDKI-73 decreases transcription and oncogenic proteins, such as MYC, BCL-2 family prosurvival proteins, and the Androgen Receptor (AR), by decreasing Ser2-RNAPII phosphorylation. Second, a significant post-translational alteration mediated by CDK9 is suppressed by CDKI-73	[81]
	MC180295	AML and colon cancer (preclinical models)	MC180295 demonstrated efficacy against many malignancies. MC180295 showed greater efficacy against acute myeloid leukaemia than against solid tumors	[82]

Epigenetic inhibitors	Tazemetostat (EZH2 inhibitor)	Follicular lymphoma; epithelioid sarcoma; other EZH2-mutant or overexpressed cancers	The FDA has approved Tazemetostat (Tazverik), a pioneering oral EZH2 inhibitor, for the treatment of follicular lymphoma (FL) and epithelioid sarcoma. Tazemetostat suppresses EZH2 gain-of-function mutations Y646X and A687V	[83]
	Mevrometostat (PF-06821497, EZH2 inhibitor)	Metastatic castration-resistant prostate cancer (mCRPC) in combination with enzalutamide	A small-molecule inhibitor of EZH2 that is both powerful and selective is mevrometostat (PF-06821497). There were no side effects from the M dose study that included enzalutamide (E) and androgen deprivation treatment. Safety, dose-dependent target modulation, and radiographic progression-free survival (rPFS) are good in preliminary trials	[84]
	Other EZH2 / epigenetic agents (e.g., in trials: SHR2554, PF-06821497, etc.)	Relapsed/refractory lymphomas; solid tumors; combinations with HDAC, DNMT inhibitors	EZH2 highly selective inhibitor SHR2554. Pharmacokinetic studies show that co-administration of itraconazole, a CYP3A4 enzyme inhibitor, with SHR2554 increases plasma levels while maintaining safety. PF-06821497 is a lactam EZH2 inhibitor. When used with HDAC inhibitors, it suppresses cancer cell proliferation and induces apoptosis	[85]

1.5.3 Dual Blockade of the PI3K–mTOR Pathway

This class of medications has a dual action on the mTOR catalytic site and the p110α subunit of PI3K. Unlike rapalogs, they can enhance the PI3K pathway's activity by minimizing negative feedback through the mTOR-ribosomal protein, S6 kinase beta-1 (S6K1), and Insulin receptor substrate 1 (IRS-1) loop. Medications like NVP-BEZ235, PF-04691502, PKI-402, WJD008, PF-502, and PI-103 are examples of medications that fall under this category [89].

1.5.4 Glutaminase Inhibition

GLS controls the conversion of glutamine into glutamate; its blockage can lead to a reduction in GSH and a rise in oxidative stress, both of which might compromise cancer cells' antioxidant defenses and perhaps cause their death. Consequently, this represents a potentially practical therapeutic approach, leading to the development of several agents designed to inhibit GLS, such as Bis-2-Sulfide (5-phenylacetamido-1,3,4-thiadiazol-2-yl) ethyl (BPTES), JHU-083, 968, fisapubescin, 6-Diazo-5-oxo-L-norleucine (DON), and CB-839, among others [90].

1.5.5 HER2 Inhibitor

Some cancers have abnormally high levels of the oncogenic receptor tyrosine kinase HER2. By successfully inhibiting cGAS-STING signaling, HER-2 has shown the ability to limit the production of cytokines by cancer cells. Hence, new methods targeting HER2, such as KU004, are currently being researched [75]. The HER2 gene, present on chromosome 17q21, is responsible for the 185 kDa transmembrane protein also known as ERBB2 and HER-2/neu. T-DM1, the new HER2-targeted antibody-drug conjugate, received FDA approval as a monotherapy for individuals with HER2-positive metastatic breast cancer [91]. DS-8201a, a new anti-HER2 antibody-drug combination, contains a derivative of topoisomerase I inhibitor DX-8951 (DXd). DS-8201a showed promising potential in preclinical research using a HER2-positive patient-derived xenograft model that was unresponsive to T-DM1.

1.5.6 ALK Inhibitors

Anaplastic lymphoma kinase 1 (ALK-1) belongs to the insulin receptor tyrosine kinase family. Crizotinib and ceritinib have received FDA approval for the treatment of locally progressed and metastatic non-small cell lung cancer (NSCLC). Novel, very effective ALK inhibitors with a tolerable toxicity profile have recently been developed due to recent advances. Below is a list of some medications, including examples: Entrectinib (RXDX-101, NMS-E628), CEP-28122/CEP-37440, brigatinib (AP26113), TSR-011, ASP3026, ceritinib (LDK378), PF-06463922, X-376/X-396, and alectinib (RG7853/AF 802/RO5424802/CH5424802). Patients with ALK+ NSCLC have also demonstrated clinical effectiveness with inhibitors of HSP90, a 90 kDa heat shock protein [92].

1.5.7 MET Inhibitor

5-((4-((2-amino-3-chloropyridin-4-yl)oxy)-3-fluorophenyl)amino)-3-(4-fluorophenyl) -1,6-naphthyridin-4(1H)-ones is a potent and innovative MET inhibitor, which was developed and produced by a scaffold-hopping technique derived from a 2,7-naphthyridinone MET kinase inhibitor. The major compound exhibited significant efficacy with an IC50 of 9.8 nM [93]. EMD1214063 and EMD1204831, indoline-2-one core MET kinase domain inhibitors, are selective, reversible, and potent oral ATP-competitive inhibitors. Targeting sensitive MET mutations with EMD1214063 reduced cellular proliferation, cell-cycle distribution, motility, and tumor cell growth independent of anchoring in an in vivo xenograft model [94].

1.5.8 CDK9 Inhibitors

CDKs regulate transcription, metabolism, cell cycle, and proliferation. However, second-generation inhibitors like AZD4573 and BAY1251152 have increased selectivity for other CDK kinases and are being tested in patients with solid tumor and hematological malignancies with improved safety [95]. A new, effective, and selective inhibitor of both wild-type CDK9 and the L156F mutant, which suppresses p-Ser2 RNA Pol II, cMYC, and MCL-1, ultimately inducing death in hematological cancer cells [96].

1.5.9 Epigenetic Inhibitors

Azacytidine and decitabine are two traditional DNMTi that can repair DNA hypermethylation through covalent binding to DNA and degrading the DNMTs [97]. There are now six epigenetic medications approved for clinical use by the FDA. These include DNMT inhibitors, EZH2 inhibitors, and HDAC inhibitors [98]. These epigenetic modifier drugs have the ability to upregulate E-cadherin, which reduces the tumorigenic properties of epithelial-derived hepatoma cell lines with diverse genetic and epigenetic backgrounds, thus influencing the canonical Wnt/E--catenin pathway [99].

1.6 Future Perspectives and Conclusion

Using metabolomics in precision oncology enables doctors to track tumor metabolism in real-time and identify patient-specific weaknesses. Advances in liquid biopsies and metabolic imaging, such as glucose and lactate analysis, provide dynamic biomarkers that help pick the best treatment options. Combining metabolic inhibitors with chemotherapy or immunotherapy may overcome resistance and improve treatment effectiveness. Personalized metabolomic profiles can support adaptive treatment plans that maximize results while reducing side effects. In summary, cancer metabolism influences tumor growth and resistance, presenting new therapeutic targets. Incorporating metabolic profiles alongside traditional and innovative therapies may help bypass resistance and enhance outcomes; however, challenges such as heterogeneity, toxicity, and clinical application still exist. Despite these hurdles, metabolomics-based approaches hold considerable promise for future cancer treatments.

References

1. Mullen AR, DeBerardinis RJ. Genetically-defined metabolic reprogramming in cancer. Trends Endocrinol Metab. 2012;23(11):552–9.
2. Nicolini A, Ferrari P. Involvement of tumor immune microenvironment metabolic reprogramming in colorectal cancer progression, immune escape, and response to immunotherapy. Front Immunol. 2024;15:1353787.
3. Epstein T, Gatenby RA, Brown JS. The Warburg effect as an adaptation of cancer cells to rapid fluctuations in energy demand. PLoS One. 2017;12(9):e0185085.
4. Ashique S, Debnath B, Ramzan M, Taj T, Islam A, Chaudhary P, et al. A critical review of the synergistic potential of targeting p53 and CAR T cell therapy in cancer treatment. Biomed Pharmacother. 2025;189:118308.
5. DeBerardinis RJ, Chandel NS. Fundamentals of cancer metabolism. Sci Adv. 2016;2(5):e1600200.
6. Shaw RJ. LKB1 and AMP-activated protein kinase control of mTOR signalling and growth. Acta Physiol. 2009;196(1):65–80.
7. Vernieri C, Casola S, Foiani M, Pietrantonio F, de Braud F, Longo V. Targeting cancer metabolism: dietary and pharmacologic interventions. Cancer Discov. 2016;6(12):1315–33.
8. Nong S, Han X, Xiang Y, Qian Y, Wei Y, Zhang T, et al. Metabolic reprogramming in cancer: mechanisms and therapeutics. MedComm. 2023;4(2):e218.
9. Roy S, Deka D, Kondaveeti SB, Ayyadurai P, Siripragada S, Philip N, et al. An overview of potential of natural compounds to regulate epigenetic modifications in colorectal cancer: a recent update. Epigenetics. 2025;20(1):2491316.
10. Vander Heiden MG, Cantley LC, Thompson CB. Understanding the Warburg effect: the metabolic requirements of cell proliferation. Science. 2009;324(5930):1029–33.
11. Tufail M, Jiang C-H, Li N. Altered metabolism in cancer: insights into energy pathways and therapeutic targets. Mol Cancer. 2024;23(1):203.
12. Vaupel P, Multhoff G. Revisiting the Warburg effect: historical dogma versus current understanding. J Physiol. 2021;599(6):1745–57.
13. Liberti MV, Locasale JW. The Warburg effect: how does it benefit cancer cells? Trends Biochem Sci. 2016;41(3):211–8.
14. Mullarky E, Cantley LC. Diverting glycolysis to combat oxidative stress. In: Innovative medicine: basic research and development; 2015. p. 3–23.

15. Baryła M, Semeniuk-Wojtaś A, Róg L, Kraj L, Małyszko M, Stec R. Oncometabolites—a link between cancer cells and tumor microenvironment. Biology. 2022;11(2):270.
16. Lanzetti L. Oncometabolites at the crossroads of genetic, epigenetic and ecological alterations in cancer. Cell Death Differ. 2024;31(12):1582–94.
17. Rastogi S, Aldosary S, Saeedan AS, Ansari MN, Singh M, Kaithwas G. NF-κB mediated regulation of tumor cell proliferation in hypoxic microenvironment. Front Pharmacol. 2023;14:1108915.
18. Tan S, Zhou F, Wu X. Lactate-mediated crosstalk between tumor cells and cancer-associated fibroblasts: mechanisms and therapeutic opportunities. Int J Mol Sci. 2025;26(12):5583.
19. Xu Z, Wang X, Cheng H, Li J, Zhang X, Wang X. The role of MCT1 in tumor progression and targeted therapy: a comprehensive review. Front Immunol. 2025;16:1610466.
20. Altman BJ, Stine ZE, Dang CV. From Krebs to clinic: glutamine metabolism to cancer therapy. Nat Rev Cancer. 2016;16(10):619–34.
21. Navarro C, Ortega Á, Santeliz R, Garrido B, Chacín M, Galban N, et al. Metabolic reprogramming in cancer cells: emerging molecular mechanisms and novel therapeutic approaches. Pharmaceutics. 2022;14(6):1303.
22. Mullen AR, Wheaton WW, Jin ES, Chen P-H, Sullivan LB, Cheng T, et al. Reductive carboxylation supports growth in tumour cells with defective mitochondria. Nature. 2012;481(7381):385–8.
23. Fu Y, Zou T, Shen X, Nelson PJ, Li J, Wu C, et al. Lipid metabolism in cancer progression and therapeutic strategies. MedComm. 2021;2(1):27–59.
24. Missiaen R, Lesner NP, Simon MC. HIF: a master regulator of nutrient availability and metabolic cross-talk in the tumor microenvironment. EMBO J. 2023;42(6):e112067.
25. Ge T, Yang J, Zhou S, Wang Y, Li Y, Tong X. The role of the pentose phosphate pathway in diabetes and cancer. Front Endocrinol. 2020;11:365.
26. Srinivasan D, Balakrishnan R, Chauhan A, Kumar J, Girija DM, Shrestha R, et al. Epithelial–Mesenchymal transition in cancer: insights into therapeutic targets and clinical implications. MedComm. 2025;6(9):e70333.
27. Liang L, Li W, Li X, Jin X, Liao Q, Li Y, et al. 'Reverse Warburg effect'of cancer-associated fibroblasts. Int J Oncol. 2022;60(6):1–13.
28. Chaudhary P, Janmeda P, Setzer WN, Aldahish AA, Sharifi-Rad J, Calina D. Breaking free from free radicals: harnessing the power of natural antioxidants for health and disease prevention. Chem Pap. 2024;78(4):2061–77.
29. Zhang F, Ma Y, Li D, Wei J, Chen K, Zhang E, et al. Cancer associated fibroblasts and metabolic reprogramming: unraveling the intricate crosstalk in tumor evolution. J Hematol Oncol. 2024;17(1):80.
30. Chaudhary P, Janmeda P, Pareek A, Chuturgoon AA, Sharma R, Pareek A. Etiology of lung carcinoma and treatment through medicinal plants, marine plants and green synthesized nanoparticles: a comprehensive review. Biomed Pharmacother. 2024;173:116294.
31. Huang K, Han Y, Chen Y, Shen H, Zeng S, Cai C. Tumor metabolic regulators: key drivers of metabolic reprogramming and the promising targets in cancer therapy. Mol Cancer. 2025;24(1):7.
32. Zhang H, Li S, Wang D, Liu S, Xiao T, Gu W, et al. Metabolic reprogramming and immune evasion: the interplay in the tumor microenvironment. Biomark Res. 2024;12(1):96.
33. Shu SL, Yang Y, Allen CL, Maguire O, Minderman H, Sen A, et al. Metabolic reprogramming of stromal fibroblasts by melanoma exosome microRNA favours a pre-metastatic microenvironment. Sci Rep. 2018;8(1):12905.
34. Dekhne AS, Hou Z, Gangjee A, Matherly LH. Therapeutic targeting of mitochondrial one-carbon metabolism in cancer. Mol Cancer Ther. 2020;19(11):2245–55.
35. Newman AC, Maddocks OD. One-carbon metabolism in cancer. Br J Cancer. 2017;116(12):1499–504.
36. Pavlova NN, Thompson CB. The emerging hallmarks of cancer metabolism. Cell Metab. 2016;23(1):27–47.

37. Lyssiotis CA, Kimmelman AC. Metabolic interactions in the tumor microenvironment. Trends Cell Biol. 2017;27(11):863–75.
38. O'Neill LA, Kishton RJ, Rathmell J. A guide to immunometabolism for immunologists. Nat Rev Immunol. 2016;16(9):553–65.
39. Mazat J-P. One-carbon metabolism in cancer cells: a critical review based on a core model of central metabolism. Biochem Soc Trans. 2021;49(1):1–15.
40. Lee SE, Park S, Yi S, Choi NR, Lim MA, Chang JW, et al. Unraveling the role of the mitochondrial one-carbon pathway in undifferentiated thyroid cancer by multi-omics analyses. Nat Commun. 2024;15(1):1163.
41. Pan S, Fan M, Liu Z, Li X, Wang H. Serine, glycine and one-carbon metabolism in cancer. Int J Oncol. 2020;58(2):158–70.
42. Banerjee A, Deka D, Muralikumar M, Sun-Zhang A, Bisgin A, Christopher C, et al. A concise review on miRNAs as regulators of colon cancer stem cells and associated signalling pathways. Clin Transl Oncol. 2023;25(12):3345–56.
43. Aoki Y, Han Q, Tome Y, Yamamoto J, Kubota Y, Masaki N, et al. Reversion of methionine addiction of osteosarcoma cells to methionine independence results in loss of malignancy, modulation of the epithelial-mesenchymal phenotype and alteration of histone-H3 lysine-methylation. Front Oncol. 2022;12:1009548.
44. Jin L, Zhou Y. Crucial role of the pentose phosphate pathway in malignant tumors. Oncol Lett. 2019;17(5):4213–21.
45. Patra KC, Hay N. The pentose phosphate pathway and cancer. Trends Biochem Sci. 2014;39(8):347–54.
46. Stincone A, Prigione A, Cramer T, Wamelink MM, Campbell K, Cheung E, et al. The return of metabolism: biochemistry and physiology of the pentose phosphate pathway. Biol Rev. 2015;90(3):927–63.
47. Jiang P, Du W, Wang X, Mancuso A, Gao X, Wu M, et al. p53 regulates biosynthesis through direct inactivation of glucose-6-phosphate dehydrogenase. Nat Cell Biol. 2011;13(3):310–6.
48. Chaudhary P, Janmeda P, Docea AO, Yeskaliyeva B, Abdull Razis AF, Modu B, et al. Oxidative stress, free radicals and antioxidants: potential crosstalk in the pathophysiology of human diseases. Front Chem. 2023;11:1158198.
49. Lukey MJ, Katt WP, Cerione RA. Targeting amino acid metabolism for cancer therapy. Drug Discov Today. 2017;22(5):796–804.
50. Chen J, Cui L, Lu S, Xu S. Amino acid metabolism in tumor biology and therapy. Cell Death Dis. 2024;15(1):42.
51. Liu Y, Zong X, Altea-Manzano P, Fu J. Amino acid metabolism in breast cancer: pathogenic drivers and therapeutic opportunities. Protein Cell. 2025;16:pwaf011.
52. Tomé D. Amino acid metabolism and signalling pathways: potential targets in the control of infection and immunity. Eur J Clin Nutr. 2021;75(9):1319–27.
53. Hsu W-J, Hsu M-C, Chu C-Y, Lee Y-C, Yang CC, Liu Z-W, et al. Metastatic breast cancer cells are vulnerable to fatty acid oxidation inhibition through DDX3-DRP1-mediated mitochondrial plasticity. Redox Biol. 2025;86:103845.
54. Ruidas B. Mitochondrial lipid metabolism in metastatic breast cancer. Mitochondrial Commun. 2024;2:58–66.
55. De Oliveira MP, Liesa M. The role of mitochondrial fat oxidation in cancer cell proliferation and survival. Cells. 2020;9(12):2600.
56. Lei Y, Cai S, Zhang J-K, Ding S-Q, Zhang Z-H, Zhang C-D, et al. The role and mechanism of fatty acid oxidation in cancer drug resistance. Cell Death Discov. 2025;11(1):277.
57. Loo SY, Toh LP, Xie WH, Pathak E, Tan W, Ma S, et al. Fatty acid oxidation is a druggable gateway regulating cellular plasticity for driving metastasis in breast cancer. Sci Adv. 2021;7(41):eabh2443.
58. Porporato PE, Filigheddu N, Pedro JMB-S, Kroemer G, Galluzzi L. Mitochondrial metabolism and cancer. Cell Res. 2018;28(3):265–80.
59. Dey A, Mitra A, Pathak S, Prasad S, Zhang AS, Zhang H, et al. Recent advancements, limitations, and future perspectives of the use of personalized medicine in treatment of colon cancer. Technol Cancer Res Treat. 2023;22:15330338231178403.

60. Cannino G, Ciscato F, Masgras I, Sánchez-Martín C, Rasola A. Metabolic plasticity of tumor cell mitochondria. Front Oncol. 2018;8:333.
61. Ngoi NY, Eu JQ, Hirpara J, Wang L, Lim JS, Lee S-C, et al. Targeting cell metabolism as cancer therapy. Antioxid Redox Signal. 2020;32(5):285–308.
62. Hua H, Kong Q, Zhang H, Wang J, Luo T, Jiang Y. Targeting mTOR for cancer therapy. J Hematol Oncol. 2019;12(1):71.
63. Hess G, Smith SM, Berkenblit A, Coiffier B, editors. Temsirolimus in mantle cell lymphoma and other non-Hodgkin lymphoma subtypes. Seminars in oncology. Elsevier; 2009.
64. Dancey JE, editor. Temsirolimus, a novel mTOR inhibitor: its clinical development for renal cell carcinoma and other tumors. Seminars in oncology; 2009.
65. Yao JC, Shah MH, Ito T, Bohas CL, Wolin EM, Cutsem EV, et al. Everolimus for advanced pancreatic neuroendocrine tumors. N Engl J Med. 2011;364(6):514–23.
66. Baselga J, Campone M, Piccart M, Burris HA, Rugo HS, Sahmoud T, et al. Everolimus in postmenopausal hormone-receptor–positive advanced breast cancer. N Engl J Med. 2012;366(6):520–9.
67. Voss MH, Gordon MS, Mita M, Rini B, Makker V, Macarulla T, et al. Phase 1 study of mTORC1/2 inhibitor sapanisertib (TAK-228) in advanced solid tumours, with an expansion phase in renal, endometrial or bladder cancer. Br J Cancer. 2020;123(11):1590–8.
68. Basu B, Dean E, Puglisi M, Greystoke A, Ong M, Burke W, et al. First-in-human pharmacokinetic and pharmacodynamic study of the dual m-TORC 1/2 inhibitor AZD2014. Clin Cancer Res. 2015;21(15):3412–9.
69. Graham L, Banda K, Torres A, Carver BS, Chen Y, Pisano K, et al. A phase II study of the dual mTOR inhibitor MLN0128 in patients with metastatic castration resistant prostate cancer. Investig New Drugs. 2018;36(3):458–67.
70. Eyre TA, Hildyard C, Hamblin A, Ali AS, Houlton A, Hopkins L, et al. A phase II study to assess the safety and efficacy of the dual mTORC1/2 inhibitor vistusertib in relapsed, refractory DLBCL. Hematol Oncol. 2019;37(4):352–9.
71. Bresin A, Cristofoletti C, Caprini E, Cantonetti M, Monopoli A, Russo G, et al. Preclinical evidence for targeting PI3K/mTOR signaling with dual-inhibitors as a therapeutic strategy against cutaneous T-cell lymphoma. J Invest Dermatol. 2020;140(5):1045–53. e6
72. Hu X, Xia M, Wang J, Yu H, Chai J, Zhang Z, et al. Dual PI3K/mTOR inhibitor PKI-402 suppresses the growth of ovarian cancer cells by degradation of Mcl-1 through autophagy. Biomed Pharmacother. 2020;129:110397.
73. Wu Y-Y, Wu H-C, Wu J-E, Huang K-Y, Yang S-C, Chen S-X, et al. The dual PI3K/mTOR inhibitor BEZ235 restricts the growth of lung cancer tumors regardless of EGFR status, as a potent accompanist in combined therapeutic regimens. J Exp Clin Cancer Res. 2019;38(1):282.
74. Harding JJ, Telli M, Munster P, Voss MH, Infante JR, DeMichele A, et al. A phase I dose-escalation and expansion study of telaglenastat in patients with advanced or metastatic solid tumors. Clin Cancer Res. 2021;27(18):4994–5003.
75. Wu S, Zhang Q, Zhang F, Meng F, Liu S, Zhou R, et al. HER2 recruits AKT1 to disrupt STING signalling and suppress antiviral defence and antitumour immunity. Nat Cell Biol. 2019;21(8):1027–40.
76. Mestre M, Djellas Y, Carriot T, Cavero I. Frequency-independent blockade of cardiac Na+ channels by riluzole: comparison with established anticonvulsants and class I anti-arrhythmics. Fundam Clin Pharmacol. 2000;14(2):107–17.
77. Kiełbowski K, Żychowska J, Becht R. Anaplastic lymphoma kinase inhibitors—a review of anticancer properties, clinical efficacy, and resistance mechanisms. Front Pharmacol. 2023;14:1285374.
78. Santarpia M, Massafra M, Gebbia V, D'Aquino A, Garipoli C, Altavilla G, et al. A narrative review of MET inhibitors in non-small cell lung cancer with MET exon 14 skipping mutations. Transl Lung Cancer Res. 2021;10(3):1536.
79. Paik PK, Felip E, Veillon R, Sakai H, Cortot AB, Garassino MC, et al. Tepotinib in non–small-cell lung cancer with MET exon 14 skipping mutations. N Engl J Med. 2020;383(10):931–43.

80. Thieme E, Bruss N, Sun D, Dominguez EC, Coleman D, Liu T, et al. CDK9 inhibition induces epigenetic reprogramming revealing strategies to circumvent resistance in lymphoma. Mol Cancer. 2023;22(1):64.
81. Rahman R, Rahaman MH, Hanson AR, Choo N, Xie J, Townley SL, et al. CDK9 inhibition constrains multiple oncogenic transcriptional and epigenetic pathways in prostate cancer. Br J Cancer. 2024;131(6):1092–105.
82. Zhang H, Huang C, Gordon J, Yu S, Morton G, Childers W, et al. MC180295 is a highly potent and selective CDK9 inhibitor with preclinical in vitro and in vivo efficacy in cancer. Clin Epigenetics. 2024;16(1):3.
83. Straining R, Eighmy W. Tazemetostat: EZH2 inhibitor. J Adv Pract Oncol. 2022;13(2):158.
84. Schweizer MT, Penkov K, Choudhury AD, Calvo E, Frank RC, Liu L, et al. Phase 1 trial of mevrometostat (PF-06821497), a potent and selective inhibitor of enhancer of zeste homolog 2 (EZH2), in castration-resistant prostate cancer (CRPC). Am Soc Clin Oncol. 2024;42:5061.
85. Dai W, Qiao X, Fang Y, Guo R, Bai P, Liu S, et al. Epigenetics-targeted drugs: current paradigms and future challenges. Signal Transduct Target Ther. 2024;9(1):332.
86. Ragupathi A, Kim C, Jacinto E. The mTORC2 signaling network: targets and cross-talks. Biochem J. 2024;481(2):45–91.
87. Bouyahya A, El Allam A, Aboulaghras S, Bakrim S, El Menyiy N, Alshahrani MM, et al. Targeting mTOR as a cancer therapy: recent advances in natural bioactive compounds and immunotherapy. Cancer. 2022;14(22):5520.
88. Sini P, James D, Chresta C, Guichard S. Simultaneous inhibition of mTORC1 and mTORC2 by mTOR kinase inhibitor AZD8055 induces autophagy and cell death in cancer cells. Autophagy. 2010;6(4):553–4.
89. Chow Z, Johnson J, Chauhan A, Izumi T, Cavnar M, Weiss H, et al. PI3K/mTOR dual inhibitor PF-04691502 is a schedule-dependent radiosensitizer for gastroenteropancreatic neuroendocrine tumors. Cells. 2021;10(5):1261.
90. Wang Z, Liu F, Fan N, Zhou C, Li D, Macvicar T, et al. Targeting glutaminolysis: new perspectives to understand cancer development and novel strategies for potential target therapies. Front Oncol. 2020;10:589508.
91. Xia X, Gong C, Zhang Y, Xiong H. The history and development of HER2 inhibitors. Pharmaceuticals. 2023;16(10):1450.
92. Sullivan I, Planchard D. ALK inhibitors in non-small cell lung cancer: the latest evidence and developments. Ther Adv Med Oncol. 2016;8(1):32–47.
93. Wang M-S, Zhuo L-S, Yang F-P, Wang W-J, Huang W, Yang G-F. Synthesis and biological evaluation of new MET inhibitors with 1, 6-naphthyridinone scaffold. Eur J Med Chem. 2020;185:111803.
94. Medová M, Pochon B, Streit B, Blank-Liss W, Francica P, Stroka D, et al. The novel ATP-competitive inhibitor of the MET hepatocyte growth factor receptor EMD1214063 displays inhibitory activity against selected MET-mutated variants. Mol Cancer Ther. 2013;12(11):2415–24.
95. Hu C, Shen L, Zou F, Wu Y, Wang B, Wang A, et al. Predicting and overcoming resistance to CDK9 inhibitors for cancer therapy. Acta Pharm Sin B. 2023;13(9):3694–707.
96. Shi C, Wu Y, Zou F, Yuan Y, Hu C, Liu Q, et al. Discovery of a novel Dihydroisoquinolinone derivative as a potent CDK9 inhibitor capable of overcoming L156F mutant for the treatment of hematologic malignancies. J Med Chem. 2025;68(8):8106–23.
97. Jain SM, Nagainallur Ravichandran S, Murali Kumar M, Banerjee A, Sun-Zhang A, Zhang H, et al. Understanding the molecular mechanism responsible for developing therapeutic radiation-induced radioresistance of rectal cancer and improving the clinical outcomes of radiotherapy-a review. Cancer Biol Ther. 2024;25(1):2317999.
98. Yang T, Yang Y, Wang Y. Predictive biomarkers and potential drug combinations of epi-drugs in cancer therapy. Clin Epigenetics. 2021;13(1):113.
99. Uribe D, Cardona A, Degli Esposti D, Cros M-P, Cuenin C, Herceg Z, et al. Antiproliferative effects of epigenetic modifier drugs through E-cadherin up-regulation in liver cancer cell lines. Ann Hepatol. 2018;17(3):444–60.

The Warburg Effect and Aerobic Glycolysis in Tumors

2

Bhupender Nehra, Sourabh Suthar, Rishabh Kasnia, Sunaina Demiwal, Mohini Mondal, Himanshu Sharma, and Naheed Mojgani

2.1 Introduction

In the last few decades, the field concerning cancer metabolism has experienced a paradigm shift, i.e., moving from a descriptive study of altered energy generation to a profoundly mechanistic perspective on metabolic reprogramming as a cause of cancer. Otto Warburg, who found in the 1920s that tumor tissues absorb glucose at very fast rates and convert a significant amount thereof into lactate in spite of normoxic conditions, which was then recognized as the Warburg effect [1]. One of the main theories that describes this metabolic cascade is represented by it. Despite oxygen supply, cancer cells redirect glucose metabolism toward glycolysis, which appears to be an inefficient process from an energetic standpoint, in contrast with normally proliferated cells that primarily rely on mitochondrial oxidative phosphorylation (OXPHOS) for ATP synthesis [2]. However, this change offers a number of adaptive benefits that promote tumor development, survival, and advancement. The traditional theory that this metabolic shift is caused by mitochondrial dysfunction is

B. Nehra
Department of Pharmaceutical Sciences, Guru Jambheshwar University of Science & Technology, Hisar, Haryana, India

S. Suthar · R. Kasnia · S. Demiwal
Department of Pharmaceutical Sciences, Lord Shiva College of Pharmacy, Sirsa, Haryana, India

M. Mondal
Department of Pharmaceutical Technology, Bharat Technology, Uluberia, West Bengal, India

H. Sharma
Teerthanker Mahaveer College of Pharmacy, Teerthanker Mahaveer University, Moradabad, India

N. Mojgani (✉)
Razi Vaccine and Serum Research Institute- Agricultural Research, Education and Extension Organization, Karaj, Iran

S. Ashique et al. (eds.), *Cancer Metabolism*, Cancer Treatment and Research 195, https://doi.org/10.1007/978-3-032-21861-2_2

challenged by the Warburg effect. According to recent research, the majority of cancer cells still include mitochondria, which are even necessary for anabolic and bioenergetic requirements [3, 4]. In fact, aerobic glycolysis is a controlled and beneficial metabolic approach that allows cancer cells to maintain high glucose flux rates (see Fig. 2.1) in order to guarantee a steady supply of glycolytic intermediates for biosynthesis of nucleotides, amino acids, and lipids, followed by rapid cell division [5]. Additionally, glycolytic adjustment helps to maintain redox equilibrium, generates NADPH, and offers metabolic flexibility through auxiliary shunts like the pentose phosphate route under varying microenvironmental conditions [6].

The preference for aerobic glycolysis is closely related to carcinogenic signaling pathways at the cellular level. Furthermore, expression of glucose transporters (like GLUT1) and glycolytic enzymes, including hexokinase II, phosphofructokinase-1,

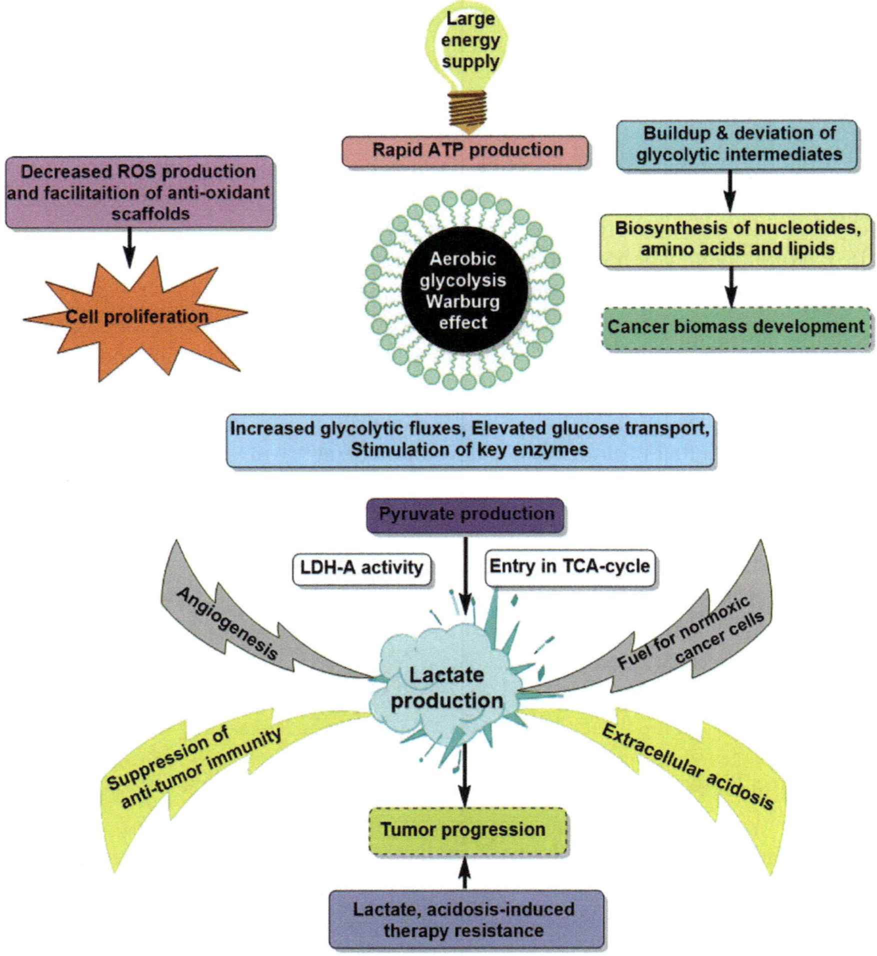

Fig. 2.1 The metabolic changes through the Warburg effect to accelerate the growth of tumors

pyruvate kinase M2, lactate dehydrogenase-A, and others, is increased via activation of PI3K/AKT/mTOR, MYC amplification, and stabilization of HIF-1α [7]. Additionally, coordinated activity of these enzymes facilitates the distraction of carbon skeletons into biosynthetic pathways and enhances glycolytic flux. By stimulating mitochondrial respiration and inhibiting glycolysis, tumor suppressors, particularly p53 and LKB1, have contrary effects, and their absence solidifies the Warburg phenotype. The Warburg effect has physiological significance that goes beyond the metabolism of individual cells [8]. In this case, resultant lactate buildup causes the tumor microenvironment to become more acidic, hinders the ability of cytotoxic lymphocytes and natural killer (NK) cells to monitor the immune system, and increases the function of proteolytic enzymes that break down extracellular matrix to encourage invasion and metastasis. Additionally, lactate serves as a signaling molecule that promotes angiogenesis by inducing the production of vascular endothelial growth factor (VEGF) in both stromal and tumor cells [9]. As a result, the Warburg effect is a biochemical mystery linked to a complex strategy that combines environmental remodeling, oncogenic signaling, metabolic adaptation, and immunological evasion. Understanding the Warburg effect offers a theoretical foundation to focus on tumor metabolism as a treatment strategy. LDH-A blockers, pyruvate dehydrogenase kinase (PDK) modulators, and inhibitors of glycolytic enzymes are being researched as effective options to reduce tumor metabolic flexibility. Furthermore, this modified glucose metabolism is used for tumor monitoring and detection by metabolic imaging methods such as ^{18}F-fluorodeoxyglucose positron emission tomography (FDG-PET). As a result, the Warburg effect has evolved beyond its historical roots to become a fundamental concept in cancer biology, diagnosis, and treatment [10, 11].

2.2 Biochemical Principles of Warburg Effect

Even in aerobic settings, the Warburg effect is defined as a metabolic change from OXPHOS to glycolysis as the primary driver of ATP synthesis. Through the mitochondrial electron transport chain (ETC) and tricarboxylic acid (TCA) cycle, one glucose molecule typically produces 36–38 ATP molecules. In contrast, glycolysis produces only 2 ATP molecules per glucose molecule [12]. Despite this inefficiency, cancer cells compensate by a dramatic increase in glucose uptake and glycolytic flux via enabling sufficient energy production alongside anabolic substrate generation. The biochemical architecture underlying this metabolic reprogramming involves alteration of the route for pyruvate metabolism. Under normal oxygen tension, pyruvate is transported into mitochondria through mitochondrial pyruvate carrier and converted by pyruvate dehydrogenase into acetyl-CoA, which enters the TCA cycle [13]. In cancer cells, PDH activity is inhibited by pyruvate dehydrogenase kinase to prevent pyruvate oxidation and promote its conversion to lactate by LDH-A. This diversion sustains glycolytic cycling and also regenerates NAD^+ in order to ensure continuous glycolytic flux. Elevated expression of LDH-A and suppression of mitochondrial PDH are therefore biochemical markers of the Warburg phenotype [14]. The glycolytic pathway itself becomes reprogrammed through transcriptional and post-translational modulation of key enzymes, as given in Table 2.1, Hexokinase II, which catalyzes the phosphorylation of glucose to glucose-6-phosphate, exhibits mitochondrial localization in cancer cells, in which it binds to the voltage-dependent anion channel on the outer mitochondrial membrane [15]. This association confers protection from apoptosis while ensuring preferential access to ATP generated by mitochondria to effectively couple energy generation with glucose utilization. In addition, phosphofructokinase-1 (PFK1), i.e., a rate-limiting enzyme of glycolysis, is activated by the allosteric modulator fructose-2,6-bisphosphate (synthesized by PFKFB3) frequently upregulated in tumors. Similarly, PKM2 is an isoform of pyruvate kinase predominantly expressed in proliferating cells, which exhibits regulated enzymatic activity to favors accumulation of upstream intermediates for biosynthesis instead of complete glycolytic throughput [16].

Additional metabolic control is exerted through the interplay between glycolysis and ancillary biosynthetic pathways. Hereby, diversion of glucose-6-phosphate into the pentose phosphate pathway generates ribose-5-phosphate for nucleotide synthesis and NADPH for reductive biosynthesis as well as oxidative stress defense. Similarly, methylation processes and nucleotide metabolism are aided by the serine-glycine-one-carbon network that emerges from glycolytic intermediates. Glycolysis is changed from a straightforward energy-inducing activity to a biosynthetic core via these interconnected pathways [17]. According to systems

Table 2.1 Key enzymatic adaptations underlying the Warburg effect

Entry	Enzyme/transporter	Function	Regulatory mechanism	Impact on tumor metabolism
1.	Hexokinase II (HK-II)	Phosphorylates glucose to G6P	Overexpressed, binds mitochondria (VDAC)	Promotes glycolysis and inhibits apoptosis
2.	Phosphofructokinase-1 (PFK1)	Rate-limiting glycolytic enzyme	Activated by F-2,6-BP via PFKFB3	Increases glycolytic throughput
3.	Pyruvate kinase M2 (PKM2)	Converts PEP to pyruvate	Exists in dimer/ tetramer forms Allosterically regulated	Supports anabolic metabolism
4.	Lactate dehydrogenase-A (LDH-A)	Converts pyruvate to lactate	Upregulated by HIF-1α, MYC	Regenerates NAD^+, maintains glycolytic flux
5.	Pyruvate dehydrogenase kinase (PDK1–4)	Inhibits PDH complex	Induced by HIF-1α	Blocks pyruvate oxidation, promotes lactate formation
6.	GLUT1/GLUT3	Glucose transporters	Upregulated by MYC, HIF-1α	Enhances glucose uptake
7.	MCT1/MCT4	Lactate transporters	Controlled by HIF-1α	Regulates lactate export and pH balance

biology, the Warburg effect is a reorganization of metabolic fluxes controlled by substrate supply, enzyme kinetics, and feedback regulation. Although monocarboxylate transporters (MCT1 and MCT4) mediate lactate export, greater expression of glucose transporters like GLUT1 and GLUT3 assures increased glucose input. This export-import equilibrium preserves intracellular pH homeostasis and promotes metabolic symbiosis in the tumor microenvironment, in which hypoxic and oxygenated cancer cells employ the "lactate shuttle" phenomenon to swap lactate as a carbon source. Therefore, the Warburg effect functions even beyond glycolysis through networked adaptability that maintains cellular energetics and biosynthetic requirements [18, 19].

2.3 Biochemical Control of Aerobic Glycolysis

By rearrangement of cellular metabolism, an intricate framework of oncogenes, tumor suppressors, transcription factors, and signaling cascades enables cancer cells to continue aerobic glycolysis. There are three master regulators that are key to this mechanism, viz. PI3K/AKT/mTOR signaling, MYC oncogene, and HIF-1α transcription factor, which synergistically drive the expression of glycolytic enzymes and transporters to inhibit mitochondrial oxidative metabolism and promote anabolic growth. Herein, the PI3K/AKT/mTOR axis is one of the most frequently dysregulated pathways in human cancers [20, 21]. Activation of AKT enhances glucose uptake by upregulation of GLUT1 and triggers phosphorylation of HK-II in order to increase its catalytic efficiency and mitochondrial association. Further, AKT signaling also activates mTOR complex 1 (mTORC1), which drives translation of glycolytic as well as anabolic enzymes through S6K and 4E-BP1. Moreover, mTORC1 induces HIF-1α under normoxic conditions and thereby links nutrient sensing to glycolytic adjustments. The PI3K/AKT/mTOR axis establishes a metabolic environment through these mechanisms, i.e., conducive to sustained glycolysis and biosynthesis [22]. In contrast, the MYC oncogene exerts a multifaceted control over cellular metabolism by transcriptionally upregulating genes involved in glycolysis, glutaminolysis, and mitochondrial biogenesis. MYC enhances expression of LDH-A, PKM2, and PDK1 in order to encourage glycolytic phenotype while simultaneously driving glutamine metabolism to replenish TCA intermediates (anaplerosis) [23]. This dual regulation ensures that cancer cells can maintain both energy and biosynthetic precursors even when oxidative metabolism is attenuated. MYC also cooperates with HIF-1α to amplify glycolytic gene expression under hypoxic or pseudo-hypoxic conditions that further entrench the Warburg phenotype. Moreover, transcription factor HIF-1α (hypoxia-inducible factor 1-α) serves as a key coordinator of glycolytic adaptation under both hypoxia and normoxic circumstances. Additionally, HIF-1α dimerizes with HIF-1β and binds hypoxia-responsive elements (HREs) in promoters of glycolytic genes, including GLUT1, HK-II, PFKFB3, LDH-A, and PDK1, i.e., stabilized under low oxygen conditions [24]. In normoxic conditions, oncogenic activation of PI3K or loss of the VHL tumor suppressor can stabilize HIF-1α to stimulate aerobic glycolysis. Also,

HIF-1α enhances lactate production while repressing mitochondrial respiration through PDK-mediated inhibition of PDH and hence, reinforces the glycolytic cycle. Other regulatory elements further refine this metabolic control. In this context, AMP-activated protein kinase (AMPK) acts as an energy sensor by normally suppressing anabolic metabolism and activating catabolic pathways in order to restore ATP levels [25]. In cancer, some tumors adapt by co-opting AMPK for survival under metabolic stress, but chronic mTOR activation often overrides the inhibitory effects of AMPK. Tumor suppressors such as p53, PTEN, and LKB1 counterbalance glycolytic signaling through stimulation of oxidative phosphorylation, reducing glucose transporter expression, and maintaining mitochondrial function. In contrast, loss of these suppressors removes key metabolic checkpoints to allow unrestricted glycolysis [26].

2.4 Mitochondrial Function and Metabolic Flexibility in Cancer Cells

The early interpretation of the Warburg effect suggested that mitochondrial dysfunction was the root cause of aerobic glycolysis in tumors. Meanwhile, modern research has firmly refuted this idea. The majority of cancer cells have mitochondria that are both physically as well as functionally competent and actively involved in apoptotic signaling, redox control, and biosynthetic metabolism. By viewing a smooth run of glycolysis even when mitochondria are intact, the Warburg effect could function as a purposefully reprogrammed mechanism that allows for metabolic adaptation and flexibility to vary microenvironmental conditions rather than a sign of metabolic failure. Because they provide anabolic precursors through the TCA cycle, mitochondria continue to be crucial for sustaining the growth of cancer cells. For the production of lipids, amino acids, and nucleotides, intermediates like citrate, α-ketoglutarate, and oxaloacetate are frequently syphoned off [27]. Tumor cells use anaplerotic processes, most notably glutaminolysis, in order to preserve TCA cycle function in spite of decreased pyruvate oxidation. Glutaminase transforms glutamine, i.e., a significant C- and N-donor, into glutamate and afterward into α-ketoglutarate. By promoting macromolecular synthesis and preserving the equilibrium of $NADH/NAD^+$ and $FADH_2/FAD$ for redox stability, this restores TCA intermediates. Hereby, dynamic control of pyruvate dehydrogenase kinase toward the pyruvate dehydrogenase complex is another essential adaptation (Table 2.2) [28]. In hypoxic or carcinogenic environments, PDK phosphorylates and inhibits PDC, thereby reducing the entry of acetyl-CoA into the TCA cycle. By preventing overproduction of Reactive Oxygen Species (ROS), this regulated restriction of oxidative metabolism shields cancer cells from oxidative damage. In order to highlight their exceptional metabolic flexibility, cancer cells tend to temporarily reactivate mitochondrial metabolism in response to dietary restriction or treatment intervention. The metabolic switch (required for survival in a variety of

Table 2.2 Major mitochondrial adaptations to support the Warburg effect

S. No.	Mitochondrial mechanism	Adaptation in tumor cells	Functional impact
1.	Pyruvate dehydrogenase regulation	PDK-mediated PDH inhibition	Shifts pyruvate from oxidation to lactate production
2.	Glutaminolysis	Upregulated GLS and GDH activity	Maintains TCA anaplerosis and biosynthesis
3.	HK-II-VDAC interaction	Enhanced binding of HK-II to mitochondria	Prevents apoptosis and enhances glycolytic coupling
4.	Mitochondrial dynamics	Altered fission-fusion via DRP1/MFN1	Supports rapid adaptation and proliferation
5.	ROS modulation	Controlled mitochondrial respiration	Limits oxidative damage, maintains signaling ROS
6.	Anaplerotic reactions	Pyruvate carboxylase and malic enzyme activation	Replenishes TCA intermediates, supports biosynthetic needs

tumor microenvironments) is the capacity to toggle between glycolysis and oxidative phosphorylation [29, 30].

Additionally, mitochondria are involved in signaling processes that control metabolic reprogramming. Glycolysis is anchored to mitochondrial ATP synthesis by the outer membrane-bound HK-II, which also limits cytochrome c release. This is followed by a combination of bioenergetic activity and antiapoptotic defence. Moreover, mitochondrial biogenesis and dynamics are rearranged by oncogenic signaling through c-MYC, Rat Sarcoma (RAS), and mTOR [31]. To ensure that mitochondria can maintain biosynthetic demands even though oxidative ATP production is reduced, MYC upregulates transcription of nuclear-encoded mitochondrial genes through PGC-1β. It is notable that new metabolomic and isotope-tracing research has explored the common engagement of cancer cells in hybrid metabolism by concurrently exploiting both glycolysis and OXPHOS. Whereas, some tumor subpopulations primarily rely on glycolysis in hypoxic environments, while pt. preferentially use oxidative metabolism, particularly in nutrient-poor or oxygen-deprived niches. This metabolic variability assists in treatment resistance, which assures that tumors can tolerate variations in oxygen and food supplies [32]. Malate-aspartate and glycerol phosphate shuttles, which connect cytosolic glycolysis with mitochondrial redox cycles, are two further ways that involve mitochondrial metabolism in order to promote NAD^+ regeneration. The functional robustness of mitochondria presents a major problem from a therapeutic standpoint. While inhibitors of mitochondrial respiration may cause compensatory glycolytic activation, some medicines that target glycolysis may push cancer cells to return to oxidative metabolism. In order to collapse metabolic plasticity, combined strategies that target both mitochondrial and glycolytic pathways are being investigated. Therefore, comprehending the relationship between aerobic glycolysis and mitochondrial activity is still crucial to assess the metabolic resilience of cancer [33].

2.5 Tumor Microenvironment and Glycolytic Reprogramming

The Warburg effect is an emerging characteristic influenced by the tumor microenvironment rather than a singular intracellular occurrence. Cancer cells, stromal fibroblasts, endothelial cells, immunological infiltrates, and extracellular matrix components are all part of the tumor microenvironment, which is embedded to change gradients of oxygen, nutrients, and metabolites. Figure 2.2 illustrates the function of lactate in the tumor microenvironment. The metabolic interactions between these elements have a significant impact on immunological escape, tumor growth, and treatment response [34]. Acidification of the extracellular environment is one of the most noticeable effects of glycolytic metabolism. Instead of physiological pH (7.4), extracellular pH is lowered to 6.5–6.8 by high lactate synthesis and proton efflux via monocarboxylate transporters (MCT1 and MCT4). By activating proteases like cathepsins and matrix metalloproteinases, this acidic environment weakens the integrity of the extracellular matrix and promotes tumor invasion and metastasis. Acidification also affects immune effector function. For example, cytotoxic T lymphocytes and NK cells are less active at low pH levels, although regulatory T cells, which support immunological tolerance in tumors, are mostly unaffected

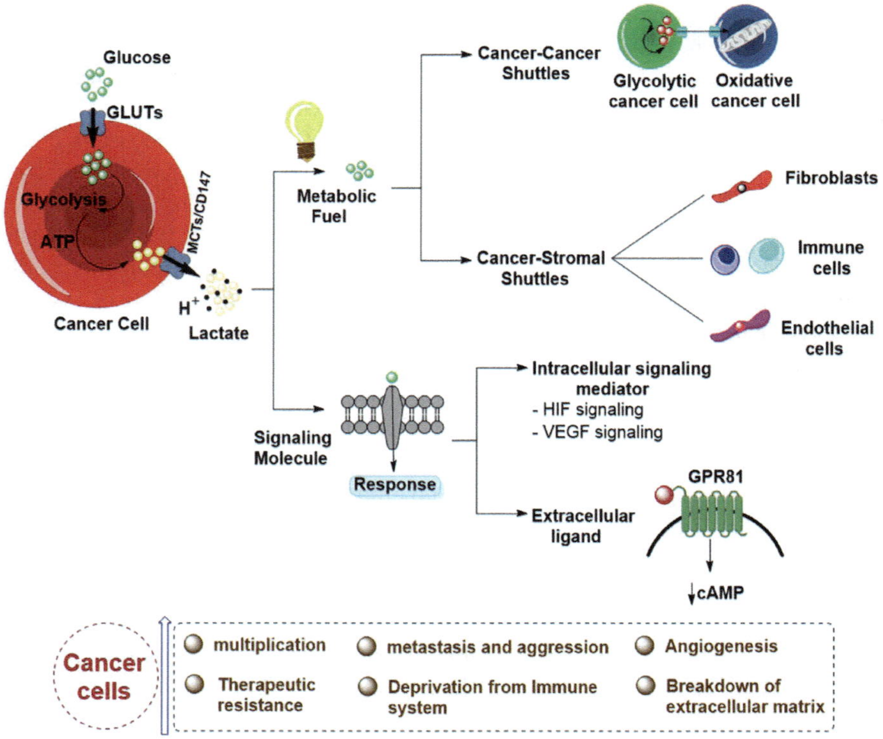

Fig. 2.2 Role of lactate in tumor microenvironment to trigger tumor aggressiveness

[35]. The metabolic symbiosis of various cellular compartments of the tumor gives rise to an additional aspect of metabolic cross talk. Hypoxic core cells rely heavily on glycolysis to produce lactate that diffuses outward and is taken up by oxygenated peripheral cells through MCT1. These cells oxidize lactate in their mitochondria as a fuel source to conserve glucose for central tumor regions. This cooperative metabolic relationship optimizes resource utilization and sustains growth under spatial metabolic heterogeneity. Furthermore, tumor-associated fibroblasts and immune cells undergo metabolic reprogramming in response to tumor-derived signals [36]. Cancer cells secrete transforming growth factor-β and reactive oxygen species to induce glycolysis in adjacent fibroblasts, i.e., also termed as reverse Warburg effect. In turn, these stromal cells release lactate, pyruvate, and other metabolites that feed cancer cell mitochondrial metabolism to illustrate a reciprocal metabolic dependency. Similarly, macrophages polarized toward an M2-like phenotype rely on oxidative metabolism and contribute to immunosuppressive cytokine production and hence, reinforce tumor progression [37].

Hypoxia is a key driver of glycolytic reprogramming in the tumor microenvironment. Additionally, reduced oxygen availability stabilizes HIF-1α, which enhances glycolytic enzyme expression along with angiogenesis advancement through the induction of VEGF and angiopoietins. However, tumor vasculature remains abnormal and leaky, which perpetuates hypoxia and reinforces a metabolic feedback loop in order to sustain glycolytic dependency. Further, competition for glucose and amino acids between cancer and immune cells imposes a metabolic challenge on antitumor immunity [38]. Activated T cells require robust glycolysis for proliferation and effector function, but they become functionally exhausted to allow immune evasion in a glucose-depleted tumor microenvironment. Emerging evidence suggests that lactate serves as a metabolic signaling molecule beyond its energetic role. Lactate can activate G-protein-coupled receptor GPR81, which leads to downstream signaling for modulation of angiogenesis, migration, and immune regulation. It also contributes to epigenetic reprogramming through lactylation of histones and thereby influences gene expression patterns to encourage tumor aggressiveness. Thus, lactate acts as both a metabolic by-product and a signaling hub to connect metabolism with gene regulation and microenvironmental adaptation. Various microenvironmental factors that have an influence on the Warburg effect are listed in Table 2.3, along with their mechanisms and role in tumor metabolism [38, 39].

2.6 Clinical Applications and Therapeutic Targeting of the Warburg Effect

The unique importance of glycolytic reprogramming to cancer biology makes the Warburg effect an attractive therapeutic target. However, the challenge lies in the selective disruption of tumor metabolism without impairment of normal proliferative tissues such as immune cells or intestinal epithelium. Multiple strategies have been developed to target glycolysis at different nodes to encompass direct enzyme inhibitors, metabolic modulators, and combinational regimens that exploit

Table 2.3 Microenvironmental factors that modulate the Warburg effect

Entry	Microenvironmental factor	Mechanism of influence	Outcome on tumor metabolism
1.	Hypoxia	Stabilizes HIF-1α, induces glycolytic enzymes	Enhances glycolysis, suppresses OXPHOS
2.	Lactate accumulation	Activates GPR81, histone lactylation	Promotes angiogenesis, invasion, and immune evasion
3.	Acidic pH	Alters enzyme kinetics, suppresses immune activity	Facilitates metastasis and immune tolerance
4.	Nutrient competition	Glucose and amino acid depletion by tumor cells	Limits T-cell activity, promotes immune escape
5.	Cancer-associated fibroblasts	Induced glycolysis by ROS/ TGF-β	Provide metabolic substrates to tumor cells
6.	Abnormal vasculature	Fluctuates oxygen/nutrient gradients	Creates metabolic heterogeneity, therapy resistance

metabolic vulnerabilities [40]. In this context, one of the most investigated agents is 2-deoxy-D-glucose, i.e., a glucose analog phosphorylated by hexokinase but unable to undergo further glycolytic processes. Also, accumulation of 2-DG-6-phosphate inhibits glycolysis and induces energy stress to activate AMPK and mTOR signaling suppression. Despite promising preclinical results, systemic toxicity and limited selectivity have restricted its clinical efficacy [41]. Herein, targeting HK-II directly offers greater specificity because this enzyme is overexpressed and mitochondrially bound in cancer cells. Compounds such as 3-bromopyruvate disrupt HKII-VDAC interactions to endorse apoptosis and metabolic collapse [42]. Another promising approach involves inhibition of LDH-A, which is the enzyme responsible for pyruvate-to-lactate conversion. LDH-A inhibitors such as FX11 and GNE-140 reduce NAD^+ regeneration to force reliance on mitochondrial respiration and enhance oxidative stress. In a similar pattern, blocking PDK with dichloroacetate reactivates PDH in order to restore pyruvate oxidation and reverse the Warburg phenotype [43]. DCA also enhances ROS-mediated apoptosis, particularly in tumors with mitochondrial reserve capacity. In addition, targeting glucose transporters (GLUT1 and GLUT3) and PFKFB3 has also gained traction. GLUT1 inhibitors reduce glucose uptake while PFKFB3 inhibitors limit synthesis of fructose-2,6-bisphosphate followed by diminished PFK1 activation and glycolytic throughput. Inhibition of PKM2, especially its dimeric form, may redirect carbon flux away from biosynthesis toward oxidative metabolism to attenuate tumor growth [44]. Due to the complexity of cancer metabolism, combination strategies hold the greatest therapeutic promise. Additionally, concurrent inhibition of glycolysis and OXPHOS can overcome metabolic compensation. Moreover, integration of metabolic inhibitors with immunotherapy has shown synergistic potential. In this regard, tumor glycolysis suppression can normalize tumor microenvironment acidity and restore immune cell functionality. For example, LDH-A inhibition enhances T-cell cytotoxicity by increasing intratumoral glucose availability. Furthermore, metabolic synthetic lethality is another emerging concept through which specific metabolic vulnerabilities are targeted in genetically defined tumors. For instance, tumors with LKB1 or p53 loss exhibit dependency on glycolysis for survival, making them particularly sensitive to glycolytic inhibitors [45]. Furthermore, metabolic coupling between hypoxic and normoxic cells can be disrupted by lactate transporters (MCT1/4) modulators, which results in the collapse of tumor metabolic symbiosis. Therapeutic approaches will be further guided in the future by developments in metabolic imaging and biomarker discovery. Thus, metabolomic profiling aids in identifying patient subgroups with elevated glycolytic dependence while FDG-PET imaging offers quantitative measurements of glycolytic flux and therapy response. A precision oncology strategy to selectively and successfully take advantage of the Warburg effect is promised by further integration of metabolic, genetic, and epigenomic data. The diagnostic value of the Warburg effect in positron emission tomography (PET) imaging is only one aspect of its clinical significance. Aerobic glycolysis presents a number of promising targets for cancer treatment, but there are drawbacks due to its importance for both tumor and healthy cell metabolism. Furthermore, a sophisticated understanding of metabolic relationships is essential in order to create targeted and successful therapies [46].

2.6.1 Applications in Diagnosis and Prognosis

The Warburg effect was first used in clinical settings in ^{18}F-fluorodeoxyglucose-PET imaging, which takes advantage of increased consumption of glucose in tumor cells. The intensity of FDG uptake correlates with tumor aggressiveness, metastatic potential, and therapeutic response. Moreover, metabolic gene signatures such as overexpression of HK-II, LDHA, and MCT4 are increasingly used as prognostic biomarkers for poor clinical outcomes. Beyond imaging, circulating metabolites like lactate, pyruvate, and 2-hydroxyglutarate (in IDH-mutant tumors) are being investigated as potential noninvasive biomarkers for early detection and disease monitoring [47, 48].

2.6.2 Targeting Glycolytic Enzymes

Direct inhibition of glycolytic enzymes has gained traction as a therapeutic strategy. For instance, 2-deoxyglucose is a glucose analog that competitively inhibits hexokinase and thereby causes disruption of glycolysis and induces energetic stress. Further, PFKFB3 inhibitors effectively suppress tumor angiogenesis and proliferation. Similarly, LDHA inhibitors aim to block lactate production and, hence, reverse the acidic tumor microenvironment and restore immune function. However, systemic toxicity and compensatory metabolic activation limit the efficacy of these inhibitors. Thus, selective delivery systems (e.g., nanoparticle formulations) and combinatorial approaches are being explored to enhance therapeutic specificity [49, 50].

2.6.3 Targeting Lactate Transport and pH Regulation

Monocarboxylate transporters (MCT1 and MCT4) are key regulators of lactate dynamics. Inhibition of MCT1 disrupts the lactate shuttle in order to starve oxidative tumor cells of substrates. Conversely, MCT4 inhibition leads to intracellular lactate accumulation and cytotoxicity in glycolytic cells. Dual inhibition of both MCT isoforms has shown potent antitumor effects in preclinical models. Additionally, targeting CAIX, i.e., a pH-regulating enzyme induced by HIF-1α, represents an innovative strategy to disrupt acid-base balance in tumors. These approaches impair tumor metabolism along with re-sensitizing immune cells to acidic environments [51, 52].

2.6.4 Oncogenic Signaling Modulation

As glycolysis is often driven by oncogenic signaling, targeting upstream regulators provides an indirect but effective route. For example, PI3K/AKT/mTOR inhibitors simultaneously attenuate glycolysis, protein synthesis, and cell proliferation. Similarly, HIF-1α inhibitors prevent transcriptional activation of glycolytic genes under hypoxia [53]. Although MYC inhibition remains challenging but still being approached through synthetic lethality and downstream pathway targeting. Therapeutic strategies through combining metabolic inhibitors with targeted or immune-based therapies hold significant promise. For instance, dual inhibition of glycolysis and immune checkpoints (e.g., PD-1/PD-L1 blockade) can overcome metabolic immunosuppression and improve antitumor efficacy [54, 55].

2.6.5 Immunometabolic Interventions and Overcoming Metabolic Plasticity and Resistance

Due to the relationship between metabolism and immune function, reprogramming tumor metabolism to restore immune activity is an emerging frontier. Inhibition of lactate production or export reactivates cytotoxic T cells, while controlling glucose availability can modulate macrophage polarization. Metabolic checkpoint blockade via targeting enzymes like IDO1, ARG1, and LDHA represents a hybrid approach that integrates metabolic and immunological control [56, 57]. A major limitation of metabolic therapies is tumor adaptability. When glycolysis is inhibited, cancer cells can reroute metabolic flux through compensatory pathways such as glutaminolysis or FAO. Therefore, rational combination therapies that target multiple nodes, including glycolysis, mitochondrial metabolism, and redox systems, are essential to overcome resistance. By enabling physicians to customize metabolic therapies according to unique tumor profiles, real-time metabolic imaging and flux analysis (such as hyperpolarized MRI) contribute to improved precision oncology [58].

2.7 Attention Toward Metabolic Vulnerabilities and Novel Therapies

Cancer metabolism has evolved from a descriptive phenomenon to a therapeutic target having enormous potential as a result of the discovery about ability of cancer cells to undergo significant metabolic changes for malignant growth. The Warburg effect is one of these metabolic markers that sheds light on the underlying mechanisms of tumor cells in metabolic pathways, i.e., different from those of healthy tissues [59]. Awareness of complex metabolic circuits that support cancer survival and growth while simultaneously being in command of tumor heterogeneity and metabolic adaptability is necessary to attack these dependencies. Therapeutic strategies aimed at exploiting glycolytic addiction have focused on the inhibition of rate-limiting enzymes (see Table 2.4) within the glycolytic pathway [60]. In this context, Hexokinase II (HK2) is an enzyme that catalyzes the first step of glycolysis and is overexpressed in multiple tumors and anchored to the outer mitochondrial membrane to afford metabolic coupling between glycolysis and OXPHOS. Pharmacological disruption of HK2 by using agents like 2-deoxy-D-glucose has demonstrated antiproliferative effects through competitive inhibition of glucose phosphorylation that leads to ATP depletion and impaired biosynthetic flux. However, limited specificity and systemic toxicity of 2-DG have necessitated more refined approaches [61, 62]. Novel HK2 inhibitors capable of disrupting its mitochondrial binding domain without affecting normal isoforms are under exploration to selectively target tumor cells. Another crucial therapeutic target is phosphofructokinase-1 (PFK1) and its regulatory kinase, viz. PFKFB3, which amplifies glycolytic flux in response to oncogenic signaling. For instance, inhibition of PFKFB3 can suppress tumor angiogenesis and proliferation by limiting the availability of fructose-2,6-bisphosphate (a potent activator of PFK1) [63]. Similarly, pyruvate

Table 2.4 Therapeutic targets in aerobic glycolysis

S. No.	Target pathway	Molecular target	Therapeutic agent/approach	Mechanism of action	Clinical potential
1.	Glycolysis	Hexokinase II	2-Deoxyglucose, lonidamine	Blocks glucose phosphorylation	Metabolic stress induction
2.	Glycolysis	PFKFB3	3PO, PFK15	Inhibits glycolytic flux and angiogenesis	Antiproliferative
3.	Lactate metabolism	LDHA, MCT1/MCT4	FX11, AZD3965	Blocks lactate production/export	Reverses acidosis
4.	Hypoxia signaling	HIF-1α	PX-478	Downregulates glycolytic genes	Suppresses tumor survival
5.	Oncogenic signaling	PI3K/AKT/mTOR	Rapamycin, alpelisib	Attenuates glycolysis and biosynthesis	Broad-spectrum efficacy
6.	pH regulation	CAIX	SLC-0111	Disrupts extracellular acidification	Reduces invasion/metastasis

kinase M2 (PKM2) is a tumor-specific isoform that favors lactate production over mitochondrial oxidation and has emerged as a key metabolic checkpoint. Furthermore, PKM2 can be locked in its highly active tetrameric form by small compounds that change metabolism to OXPHOS. It ultimately inhibits anabolic growth and increases reactive oxygen species to cause cytotoxicity [64]. Targeting lactate metabolism is another crucial tactic in addition to glycolysis. It is now known that lactate (a consequence of glycolysis, see Fig. 2.3) is a signaling molecule that influences angiogenesis, immunological evasion, and metastasis. Oxamate and galloflavin are examples of inhibitors of lactate dehydrogenase A (LDH-A) that decrease pyruvate-to-lactate conversion and restore mitochondrial respiration, rendering tumors more sensitive to chemotherapy and radiation [65]. Furthermore, primary targets to halt metabolic symbiosis of the tumor microenvironment are monocarboxylate transporters (MCT1 and MCT4) that mediate lactate movement between tumor and stromal cells. In glycolytic tumors, dual inhibition of MCTs causes intracellular acidification and cell death by interfering with lactate export and reuptake. Additionally, the Warburg effect is closely linked to oncogenic signaling pathways that coordinate metabolic reprogramming, including PI3K/Akt/mTOR, c-Myc, and HIF-1α [66]. Thus, there has been evidence of synergistic potential when metabolic inhibitors and targeted molecular therapies are combined. For instance, Akt inhibition restricts glucose uptake and transporter expression, while mTOR inhibitors such as rapamycin can lower glycolytic flow by suppressing HIF-1α translation. Moreover, transcriptional regulation of enzymes, such as LDH-A and PKM2 (strikes at the core of metabolic phenotype), can be broken down by dual targeting of c-Myc and glycolysis [67].

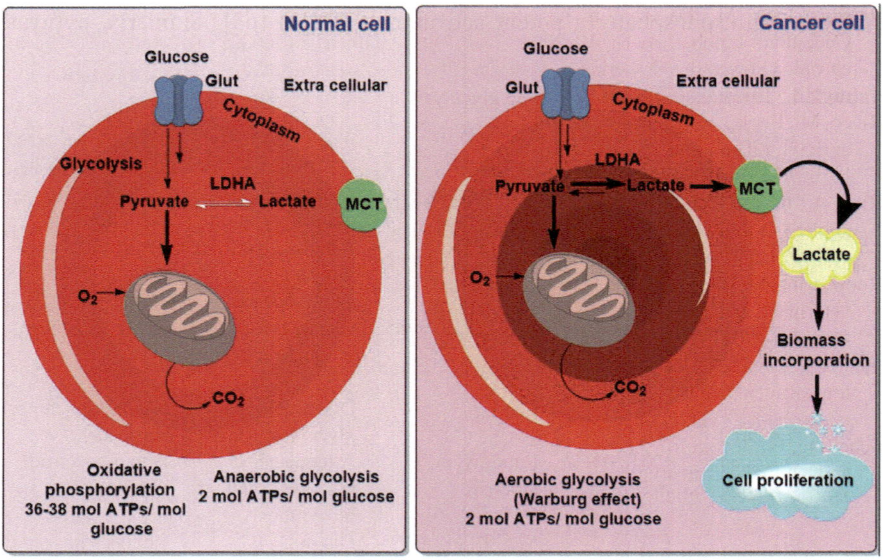

Fig. 2.3 Glycolytic mechanism in malignant versus normal cells

Exploiting redox homeostasis is another area of medicinal advancement. Through NADPH-dependent antioxidant mechanisms, cancer cells mitigate oxidative damage and generate ROS to drive signaling in a delicate equilibrium. NADPH production is decreased, and tumor cells become more susceptible to oxidative stress when the pentose phosphate pathway (mainly glucose-6-phosphate dehydrogenase) is inhibited. Similarly, cancer cells can be starved of C- and N-substrates necessary for biosynthesis by targeting glutaminolysis, i.e., a compensatory process to restore TCA cycle intermediates in conjunction with glycolytic blockage. Because of improved medication selectivity, bioavailability, and tumor accumulation, metabolic nanomedicine and delivery methods based on nanotechnology are transforming therapeutic delivery [68]. Targeting tumors selectively while reducing systemic toxicity is made possible by nanocarriers that include glycolytic inhibitors or siRNAs against metabolic enzymes. Furthermore, metabolic imaging sensors incorporated into these systems can offer real-time feedback on therapy efficacy through monitoring metabolic flow. Moreover, immunometabolism has recently emerged as a transformative dimension of metabolic therapy. The Warburg effect contributes to immunosuppression via depletion of glucose and production of lactic acid in high concentrations under the tumor microenvironment, which impairs cytotoxic T-cell and NK cell functions [69, 70]. Therefore, normalizing tumor metabolism can potentiate immune checkpoint blockade. Also, combining glycolysis inhibitors with PD-1/PD-L1 or CTLA-4 antibodies can reprogram the metabolic landscape of the tumor microenvironment to favor immune activation. Moreover, modulating metabolic enzymes in immune cells, such as increased oxidative metabolism in T cells or reduced glycolysis in regulatory T cells, can augment antitumor immunity [71]. Again, a particularly promising concept is metabolic synthetic lethality, in which dual inhibition of complementary metabolic pathways leads to selective tumor death. For example, co-targeting glycolysis and OXPHOS can trap cancer cells in an energetic crisis from which they cannot recover. Similarly, combining mitochondrial complex I blockers with LDH inhibition induces oxidative stress in cancer cells, which in turn triggers apoptosis. In order to maintain metabolic plasticity, these approaches avail use of metabolic rigidity that sets cancer cells apart from healthy tissues. Future developments will probably come from incorporating predictive models powered by artificial intelligence with metabolic profile which will enable physicians to create individualized metabolic intervention plans. Glycolytic inhibition combined with immunotherapy, redox regulation, and dietary restriction could result in an entirely new phase of cancer treatment in which tumor metabolic weaknesses are turned into therapeutic opportunities [72].

2.8 Clinical Perspectives of Metabolic Intervention

Over the past 10 years, the practical use of metabolic findings has increased significantly due to developments in systems biology, metabolomics, and molecular imaging. As tumor metabolism is so diverse, treatment must be dynamic and precisely targeted. Therefore, in order to ensure that treatments aimed against tumor metabolism are not only clinically feasible and safe but also biologically logical, translational research must connect mechanistic understanding with clinical applicability. Metabolic imaging that allows for real-time visualization of metabolic fluxes within tumors is a fundamental component of this translation. By taking advantage of the greater consumption of glucose in cancer, methods like PET employing ^{18}F-fluorodeoxyglucose have already transformed the detection of cancer [73]. To provide a more noticeable metabolic fingerprint of the tumor, the next generation of metabolic imaging aims to measure other metabolic intermediates such as lactate, glutamine, and acetate in addition to glucose. Hyperpolarized ^{13}C magnetic resonance spectroscopy is a highly effective technique that enables real-time evaluation of glycolytic activity and therapeutic responses by directly observing metabolic conversions like pyruvate to lactate. Targeting metabolic pathways in clinical trials has grown significantly and exhibits encouraging results in a variety of cancer types [74, 75]. LDH-A inhibitors, MCT blockers, and PKM2 activators have shown promising efficacy with manageable toxicity profiles in early-phase trials, particularly when used in conjunction with conventional chemotherapy or radiation therapy. For example, LDH-A inhibition decreases lactate deposits and increases oxygen consumption, which increases the vulnerability of tumors to radiation-induced DNA damage. The lactate-dependent synergy among glycolytic and oxidative tumor cell populations may also be disrupted by MCT1 inhibitors [76]. Another translational approach is to repurpose current medications that unintentionally interfere with metabolic processes. A common antidiabetic medication, metformin, inhibits mitochondrial complex I, which lowers ATP synthesis and activates AMPK. This is followed by suppression of mTOR signaling and glycolysis. Interest in the potential of metformin as an adjuvant metabolic therapy is sparked by epidemiological evidence that links its usage to better outcomes and a lower incidence of cancer [77, 78]. Another repurposed substance that reverses the Warburg phenotype is dichloroacetate, which activates pyruvate dehydrogenase and switches metabolism from glycolysis to OXPHOS. These known pharmacokinetics, safety, and toxicity characteristics of medicine provide useful translational benefits. One of the biggest obstacles in implementing metabolic treatments is the tumor microenvironment. The metabolic relationships between tumor cells, stromal fibroblasts, and immunological infiltrates are altered by hypoxia, acidosis, and nutritional scarcity. In order to target these interactions, such as lactate transport blockage or stromal glycolysis inhibition, medicines that can modify both malignant and noncancerous cells within the tumor ecosystem are needed. To restore the tumor microenvironment and get past treatment resistance, new combinatorial regimens that combine metabolic targeting with anti-angiogenic or immune checkpoint medicines are being investigated [79].

Finding metabolic dependence indicators is crucial from a clinical standpoint for therapy monitoring and patient classification. Certain metabolic abnormalities are significantly correlated with genomic signatures like MYC amplification, KRAS mutation, or PTEN loss, which can help to decide on a treatment. Additionally, levels of metabolic enzyme expression and circulating metabolites in blood or biopsy specimens may act as dynamic markers of treatment effectiveness. Clinical results can be improved by optimizing dose, timing, and combination strategies through the integration of metabolic biomarkers in adaptive clinical trial designs [80, 81]. Systemic toxicity, compensatory metabolic cascades, and tumor heterogeneity are some of the challenges that clinical translation must overcome. Because normally proliferating tissues such as intestinal epithelium and haematopoietic cells also depend on glycolysis, it is still a significant challenge to attain selectivity. To improve tumor selectivity, targeted delivery methods such as antibody-drug conjugates and drug carriers mediated by nanoparticles are being explored. In order to increase tolerance, metabolic cycle techniques or intermittent dosage may provide temporary inhibition of glycolysis while preserving healthy tissues. Personalized metabolic oncology, integration of multiomics data, patient-derived organoids, and AI-guided modeling to forecast tumor metabolic dependencies along with best drug combinations will all influence the clinical landscape of metabolic therapy in the future [82]. There may be synergistic effects from combined glycolytic inhibition with treatments that target lipid production, amino acid metabolism, and mitochondrial function. Through the use of circulating biomarkers and real-time imaging to track metabolic adaptations during therapy, physicians will be able to modify treatment plans in real time and thereby prevent the development of resistance. Metabolic therapies may potentially be used as preventive measures in high-risk groups in a more comprehensive translational framework. The potential of metabolic regulators, including NAD^+ precursors, along with dietary modification and caloric restriction mimetics to reverse early carcinogenic metabolic alterations is being studied [83].

2.9 Conclusions and Future Outlooks

The Warburg effect, which combines cellular energetics, biosynthesis, redox control, and immune evasion, has evolved beyond its original definition as an abnormality in energy generation to become a fundamental component of cancer biology. The deliberate metabolic reprogramming that gives cancer cells survival and proliferation advantages is reflected in the maintenance of aerobic glycolysis even in oxygen-rich settings. It becomes clear that addressing cancer metabolism necessitates a multimodal strategy that takes into consideration tumor heterogeneity, adaptability, and microenvironmental dynamics by coupling metabolic understanding with molecular precision. The next generation of anticancer therapies involves a combination of metabolic inhibitors with immune-based and conventional medicines. The Warburg effect may eventually change from being a sign of cancer persistence to therapeutically defeating it via dissecting and deliberately upsetting interdependent metabolic pathways that support tumor life. The development of an integrative awareness of the Warburg effect as a dynamic and context-dependent phenomenon rather than a static marker of malignancy is crucial for the future of research on cancer metabolism. Because of their exceptional metabolic adaptability, cancer cells can alternate between fatty acid metabolism, glutaminolysis, oxidative phosphorylation and glycolysis in response to oncogenic cues and environmental restrictions.

Future research must thus concentrate on adopting integrated multiomics techniques to trace intricate chemistry between signaling networks and metabolic flow and hence, gain insight into this metabolic plasticity at the systems level. Precision metabolic therapy will eventually be made possible by this comprehensive understanding, which will assist in detecting context-specific vulnerabilities, i.e., unique to each form of tumor. Exploiting these vulnerabilities with tailored therapies that target particular metabolic circuits within the tumor ecosystem is one of the main future objectives. Microenvironmental pressures and tissue origin that alter metabolic inhibitors based on the metabolic genotype and phenotype of the patient will improve treatment efficacy while reducing systemic toxicity, as tumors possess unique metabolic signatures based on oncogenic drivers. Since reprogramming tumor metabolism can restore immune surveillance through reversing the immunosuppressive microenvironment, combining metabolic targeting with immunotherapy offers another exciting prospect. Furthermore, a combination of glycolytic inhibitors with radiation or angiogenesis blockers may intensify treatment effects by interfering with both energy metabolism and nutrient transport. Overcoming tumor metabolic flexibility and adaptive resistance is still a major obstacle in this area. Many malignancies can compensate for reduced glycolysis through adjustment in amino acid metabolism, increasing mitochondrial respiration, or initiating autophagy. In order to address this adaptability, combination medicines that are logically planned and target numerous metabolic pathways at once in order to prevent compensatory survival strategies will be necessary. Co-targeting glycolytic and mitochondrial needs can kill cancer cells selectively while preserving healthy tissues. Alongside these initiatives, physicians will be able to track tumor metabolism in real time due to developments in metabolic imaging technologies like single-cell metabolic flux analysis and hyperpolarized ^{13}C MRI. Future treatments must consider metabolic interaction within the tumor microenvironment in addition to tumor cell-intrinsic metabolism. Tumor growth and treatment resistance are determined by metabolic relationships among cancer cells, stromal fibroblasts, endothelial cells, and immune cells. These cooperative networks can be disrupted and treatment effects improved by lactate mobility inhibition, reverse Warburg effect disruption, or acidosis normalization through carbonic anhydrase inhibition. Moreover, tumor-induced immunosuppression may be reversed and sensitivity to immunotherapeutic drugs enhanced by reprogramming stromal and immune cell metabolism to a greater oxidative phenotype.

References

1. Koppenol WH, Bounds PL, Dang CV. Otto Warburg's contributions to current concepts of cancer metabolism. Nat Rev Cancer. 2011;11(5):325–37.
2. Lu CL, Qin L, Liu HC, Candas D, Fan M, Li JJ. Tumor cells switch to mitochondrial oxidative phosphorylation under radiation via mTOR-mediated hexokinase II inhibition-a Warburg-reversing effect. PLoS One. 2015;10(3):e0121046.
3. Herst PM, Carson GM, Eccles DA, Berridge MV. Bioenergetic and metabolic adaptation in tumor progression and metastasis. Front Oncol. 2022;12:857686.

4. San-Millán I, Brooks GA. Reexamining cancer metabolism: lactate production for carcinogenesis could be the purpose and explanation of the Warburg effect. Carcinogenesis. 2017;38(2):119–33.
5. Courtnay R, Ngo DC, Malik N, Ververis K, Tortorella SM, Karagiannis TC. Cancer metabolism and the Warburg effect: the role of HIF-1 and PI3K. Mol Biol Rep. 2015;42(4):841–51.
6. Fuentes-Lemus E, Reyes JS, Figueroa JD, Davies MJ, López-Alarcón C. The enzymes of the oxidative phase of the pentose phosphate pathway as targets of reactive species: consequences for NADPH production. Biochem Soc Trans. 2023;51(6):2173–87.
7. Broecker-Preuss M, Becher-Boveleth N, Bockisch A, Dührsen U, Müller S. Regulation of glucose uptake in lymphoma cell lines by c-MYC-and PI3K-dependent signaling pathways and impact of glycolytic pathways on cell viability. J Transl Med. 2017;15(1):158.
8. Manley SJ, Liu W, Welch DR. The KISS1 metastasis suppressor appears to reverse the Warburg effect by shifting from glycolysis to mitochondrial beta-oxidation. J Mol Med. 2017;95(9):951–63.
9. Pérez-Tomás R, Pérez-Guillén I. Lactate in the tumor microenvironment: an essential molecule in cancer progression and treatment. Cancer. 2020;12(11):3244.
10. Zhou X, Chen R, Xie W, Ni Y, Liu J, Huang G. Relationship between 18F-FDG accumulation and lactate dehydrogenase A expression in lung adenocarcinomas. J Nucl Med. 2014;55(11):1766–71.
11. Apostolova I, Wedel F, Brenner W. Imaging of tumor metabolism using positron emission tomography (PET). Metab Cancer. 2016;207:177–205.
12. Mahundi P, Manwa L. Energy nutrient metabolism: the inter-conversions and the chain reaction leading to oxidative-phosphorilation and production of adenosine tri-phosphate (ATP). J Emerg Trends Educ Res Policy Stud. 2015;6(5):383–90.
13. Anderson R, Pladna KM, Schramm NJ, Wheeler FB, Kridel S, Pardee TS. Pyruvate dehydrogenase inhibition leads to decreased glycolysis, increased reliance on gluconeogenesis and alternative sources of acetyl-CoA in acute myeloid leukemia. Cancer. 2023;15(2):484.
14. Vaz CV, Marques R, Alves MG, Oliveira PF, Cavaco JE, Maia CJ, Socorro S. Androgens enhance the glycolytic metabolism and lactate export in prostate cancer cells by modulating the expression of GLUT1, GLUT3, PFK, LDH and MCT4 genes. J Cancer Res Clin Oncol. 2016;142(1):5–16.
15. Marin-Hernandez A, Gallardo-Perez JC, Ralph SJ, Rodriguez-Enriquez S, Moreno-Sanchez R. HIF-1α modulates energy metabolism in cancer cells by inducing over-expression of specific glycolytic isoforms. Mini Rev Med Chem. 2009;9(9):1084–101.
16. Hu L, Zeng Z, Xia Q, Liu Z, Feng X, Chen J, Huang M, Chen L, Fang Z, Liu Q, Zeng H. Metformin attenuates hepatoma cell proliferation by decreasing glycolytic flux through the HIF-1α/PFKFB3/PFK1 pathway. Life Sci. 2019;239:116966.
17. Pan S, Fan M, Liu Z, Li X, Wang H. Serine, glycine and one-carbon metabolism in cancer. Int J Oncol. 2021;58(2):158–70.
18. Sandforth L, Ammar N, Dinges LA, Roecken C, Arlt A, Sebens S, Schaefer H. Impact of the monocarboxylate transporter-1 (MCT1)-mediated cellular import of lactate on stemness properties of human pancreatic adenocarcinoma cells. Cancer. 2020;12(3):581.
19. Fan Q, Yang L, Zhang X, Ma Y, Li Y, Dong L, Zong Z, Hua X, Su D, Li H, Liu J. Autophagy promotes metastasis and glycolysis by upregulating MCT1 expression and Wnt/β-catenin signaling pathway activation in hepatocellular carcinoma cells. J Exp Clin Cancer Res. 2018;37(1):9.
20. Xiang S, Gu H, Jin L, Thorne RF, Zhang XD, Wu M. LncRNA IDH1-AS1 links the functions of c-Myc and HIF1α via IDH1 to regulate the Warburg effect. Proc Natl Acad Sci. 2018;115(7):E1465–74.
21. Tang HY, Guo JQ, Sang BT, Cheng JN, Wu XM. PDGFRβ modulates aerobic glycolysis in osteosarcoma HOS cells via the PI3K/AKT/mTOR/c-Myc pathway. Biochem Cell Biol. 2022;100(1):75–84.

22. Xiao Y, Peng H, Hong C, Chen Z, Deng X, Wang A, Yang F, Yang L, Chen C, Qin X. PDGF promotes the Warburg effect in pulmonary arterial smooth muscle cells via activation of the PI3K/AKT/mTOR/HIF-1α signaling pathway. Cell Physiol Biochem. 2017;42(4):1603–13.
23. Prigione A, Rohwer N, Hoffmann S, Mlody B, Drews K, Bukowiecki R, Blümlein K, Wanker EE, Ralser M, Cramer T, Adjaye J. HIF1 α modulates cell fate reprogramming through early glycolytic shift and upregulation of PDK1–3 and PKM2. Stem Cells. 2014;32(2):364–76.
24. Zeng L, Zhou HY, Tang NN, Zhang WF, He GJ, Hao B, Feng YD, Zhu H. Wortmannin influences hypoxia-inducible factor-1 alpha expression and glycolysis in esophageal carcinoma cells. World J Gastroenterol. 2016;22(20):4868.
25. Guo Y, Meng X, Ma J, Zheng Y, Wang Q, Wang Y, Shang H. Human papillomavirus 16 E6 contributes HIF-1α induced Warburg effect by attenuating the VHL-HIF-1α interaction. Int J Mol Sci. 2014;15(5):7974–86.
26. Woo YM, Shin Y, Lee EJ, Lee S, Jeong SH, Kong HK, Park EY, Kim HK, Han J, Chang M, Park JH. Inhibition of aerobic glycolysis represses Akt/mTOR/HIF-1α axis and restores tamoxifen sensitivity in antiestrogen-resistant breast cancer cells. PLoS One. 2015;10(7):e0132285.
27. Vazquez A, Liu J, Zhou Y, Oltvai ZN. Catabolic efficiency of aerobic glycolysis: the Warburg effect revisited. BMC Syst Biol. 2010;4(1):58.
28. Kukurugya MA, Rosset S, Titov DV. The Warburg effect is the result of faster ATP production by glycolysis than respiration. Proc Natl Acad Sci. 2024;121(46):e2409509121.
29. Vayakkattil AB, Pazhanchery AS, Andrews S, Vayakkattil U, Vayakkattil SU. The Warburg effect redefined: a kinetic and regulatory perspective. Cureus. 2025;17, 17(9)
30. Wu CA, Chao Y, Shiah SG, Lin WW. Nutrient deprivation induces the Warburg effect through ROS/AMPK-dependent activation of pyruvate dehydrogenase kinase. Biochimica et Biophysica Acta (BBA)-molecular Cell Res. 2013;1833(5):1147–56.
31. Nagdas S, Kashatus DF. The interplay between oncogenic signaling networks and mitochondrial dynamics. Antioxidants. 2017;6(2):33.
32. Liu Q, Sun Y, Fei Z, Yang Z, Duan K, Zi J, Cui Q, Yu M, Xiong W. Leptin promotes fatty acid oxidation and OXPHOS via the c-Myc/PGC-1 pathway in cancer cells. Acta Biochim Biophys Sin. 2019;51(7):707–14.
33. Lee WC, Ji X, Nissim I, Long F. Malic enzyme couples mitochondria with aerobic glycolysis in osteoblasts. Cell Rep. 2020;32(10):108108.
34. Wei R, Liu S, Zhang S, Min L, Zhu S. Cellular and extracellular components in tumor microenvironment and their application in early diagnosis of cancers. Anal Cell Pathol. 2020;2020(1):6283796.
35. Petersen C, Nielsen MD, Andersen ES, Basse AL, Isidor MS, Markussen LK, Viuff BM, Lambert IH, Hansen JB, Pedersen SF. MCT1 and MCT4 expression and lactate flux activity increase during white and brown adipogenesis and impact adipocyte metabolism. Sci Rep. 2017;7(1):13101.
36. Liu X, Qin H, Zhang L, Jia C, Chao Z, Qin X, Zhang H, Chen C. Hyperoxia induces glucose metabolism reprogramming and intracellular acidification by suppressing MYC/MCT1 axis in lung cancer. Redox Biol. 2023;61:102647.
37. Gómez V, Eykyn TR, Mustapha R, Flores-Borja F, Male V, Barber PR, Patsialou A, Green R, Panagaki F, Li CW, Fruhwirth GO. Breast cancer–associated macrophages promote tumorigenesis by suppressing succinate dehydrogenase in tumor cells. Sci Signal. 2020;13(652):eaax4585.
38. McDonald PC, Chafe SC, Dedhar S. Overcoming hypoxia-mediated tumor progression: combinatorial approaches targeting pH regulation, angiogenesis and immune dysfunction. Front Cell Dev Biol. 2016;4:27.
39. Chen G, Liu J, Guo Y, Sun P. Mechanisms for regulatory effects of exercise on metabolic diseases from the Lactate–Lactylation perspective. Int J Mol Sci. 2025;26(8):3469.
40. Chen J, Cao X, Li B, Zhao Z, Chen S, Lai SW, Muend SA, Nossa GK, Wang L, Guo W, Ye J. Warburg effect is a cancer immune evasion mechanism against macrophage immunosurveillance. Front Immunol. 2021;11:621757.

41. Guo S, Zhang C, Zeng H, Xia Y, Weng C, Deng Y, Wang L, Wang H. Glycolysis maintains AMPK activation in sorafenib-induced Warburg effect. Mol Metab. 2023;77:101796.
42. Granchi C, Fancelli D, Minutolo F. An update on therapeutic opportunities offered by cancer glycolytic metabolism. Bioorg Med Chem Lett. 2014;24(21):4915–25.
43. Dreute J, Stengel J, Becher J, van den Borre D, Pfisterer M, Bartkuhn M, Beutgen VM, Ndreshkjana B, Gärtner U, Graumann J, Huck M. Synergistic targeting of cancer cells through simultaneous inhibition of key metabolic enzymes. Cell Death Differ. 2025;32:1–8.
44. Yang H, Shu Z, Jiang Y, Mao W, Pang L, Redwood A, Jeter-Jones SL, Jennings NB, Ornelas A, Zhou J, Rodriguez-Aguayo C. 6-Phosphofructo-2-kinase/fructose-2, 6-biphosphatase-2 regulates TP53-dependent paclitaxel sensitivity in ovarian and breast cancers. Clin Cancer Res. 2019;25(18):5702–16.
45. Daneshmandi S, Wegiel B, Seth P. Blockade of lactate dehydrogenase-A (LDH-A) improves efficacy of anti-programmed cell death-1 (PD-1) therapy in melanoma. Cancer. 2019;11(4):450.
46. Ramos H, Calheiros J, Almeida J, Barcherini V, Santos S, Carvalho AT, Santos MM, Saraiva L. SLMP53-1 inhibits tumor cell growth through regulation of glucose metabolism and angiogenesis in a P53-dependent manner. Int J Mol Sci. 2020;21(2):596.
47. Duraj T, García-Romero N, Carrión-Navarro J, Madurga R, Ortiz de Mendivil A, Prat-Acin R, Garcia-Cañamaque L, Ayuso-Sacido A. Beyond the Warburg effect: oxidative and glycolytic phenotypes coexist within the metabolic heterogeneity of glioblastoma. Cells. 2021;10(2):202.
48. Shen K, Liu B, Zhou X, Ji Y, Chen L, Wang Q, Xue W. The evolving role of 18F-FDG PET/CT in diagnosis and prognosis prediction in progressive prostate cancer. Front Oncol. 2021;11:683793.
49. Zhang M, Ren Y, Li J, Yu J, Li Q, Zhao H, Wang Z, Chen X, Cheng J. Breaking glycolysis barriers to immunotherapy with nanomedicines. ACS Nano Med. 2025;1:149–92.
50. Lai H, Wu X, Tan J, Zhou X, Liao C, Zhang S. Regulation of tumor lactate metabolism by targeting glycolysis and mitochondrial OXPHOS for tumor metastasis inhibition. Ind Eng Chem Res. 2023;62(27):10290–300.
51. Ames S, Andring JT, McKenna R, Becker HM. CAIX forms a transport metabolon with monocarboxylate transporters in human breast cancer cells. Oncogene. 2020;39(8):1710–23.
52. Ma G, Li C, Zhang Z, Liang Y, Liang Z, Chen Y, Wang L, Li D, Zeng M, Shan W, Niu H. Targeted glucose or glutamine metabolic therapy combined with PD-1/PD-L1 checkpoint blockade immunotherapy for the treatment of tumors-mechanisms and strategies. Front Oncol. 2021;11:697894.
53. Fu XZ, Wang Y. Interferon-γ regulates immunosuppression in septic mice by promoting the Warburg effect through the PI3K/AKT/mTOR pathway. Mol Med. 2023;29(1):95.
54. Kawasaki Y, Sato K, Mashima K, Nakano H, Ikeda T, Umino K, Morita K, Izawa J, Takayama N, Hayakawa H, Tominaga K. Mesenchymal stromal cells inhibit aerobic glycolysis in activated T cells by negatively regulating hexokinase II activity through PD-1/PD-L1 interaction. Transplant Cell Ther. 2021;27(3):231–e1.
55. Zeng Y, Huang Y, Tan Q, Peng L, Wang J, Tong F, Dong X. Influence of lactate in resistance to anti-PD-1/PD-L1 therapy: mechanisms and clinical applications. Mol Med Rep. 2024;31(2):48.
56. Yuan L, Wang C, Du L, Chen W, Zhang X. Optimization of CAR-T therapy based on metabolic remodeling of the tumor immune microenvironment in diffuse large B-cell lymphoma. Am J Cancer Res. 2025;15(8):3338.
57. Eleftheriadis T, Pissas G, Antoniadi G, Spanoulis A, Liakopoulos V, Stefanidis I. Indoleamine 2, 3-dioxygenase increases p53 levels in alloreactive human T cells, and both indoleamine 2, 3-dioxygenase and p53 suppress glucose uptake, glycolysis and proliferation. Int Immunol. 2014;26(12):673–84.
58. Alwahsh M, Knitsch R, Marchan R, Lambert J, Hoerner C, Zhang X, Schalke B, Lee DH, Bulut E, Graeter T, Ott G. Metabolic profiling of thymic epithelial tumors hints to a strong Warburg effect, glutaminolysis and precarious redox homeostasis as potential therapeutic targets. Cancer. 2022;14(6):1564.

59. Wu W, Zhao S. Metabolic changes in cancer: beyond the Warburg effect. Acta Biochim Biophys Sin. 2013;45(1):18–26.
60. Lis P, Dyląg M, Niedźwiecka K, Ko YH, Pedersen PL, Goffeau A, Ułaszewski S. The HK2 dependent "Warburg effect" and mitochondrial oxidative phosphorylation in cancer: targets for effective therapy with 3-bromopyruvate. Molecules. 2016;21(12):1730.
61. Sun Z, Tan Z, Peng C, Yi W. HK2 is associated with the Warburg effect and proliferation in liver cancer: targets for effective therapy with glycyrrhizin. Mol Med Rep. 2021;23(5):343.
62. Wang L, Yang Q, Peng S, Liu X. The combination of the glycolysis inhibitor 2-DG and sorafenib can be effective against sorafenib-tolerant persister cancer cells. Onco Targets Ther. 2019:5359–73.
63. Fukushi A, Kim HD, Chang YC, Kim CH. Revisited metabolic control and reprogramming cancers by means of the Warburg effect in tumor cells. Int J Mol Sci. 2022;23(17):10037.
64. Huang X, He J, Sun H, Wu Y, Gu R, Li Z. PKM2-driven metabolic reprogramming in digestive system tumors: mechanisms, therapeutic advances, and clinical challenges. Front Immunol. 2025;16:1634786.
65. Elsisi A, Sokar S, El-Mahrouk S, Abu-Risha S. Potentiation of paclitaxel antitumor activity by galloflavin or oxamate as lactate dehydrogenase inhibitors. J Adv Med Pharm Res. 2021;2(2):64–76.
66. Hsu CY, Huang JW, Huang WR, Chen IC, Chen MS, Liao TL, Chang YK, Munir M, Liu HJ. Oncolytic avian reovirus σA-modulated upregulation of the HIF-1α/C-myc/glut1 pathway to produce more energy in different cancer cell lines benefiting virus replication. Viruses. 2023;15(2):523.
67. Pralea IE, Petrache AM, Tigu AB, Gulei D, Moldovan RC, Ilieş M, Nicoară R, Hegheş SC, Uifălean A, Iuga CA. Phytochemicals as regulators of tumor glycolysis and hypoxia signaling pathways: evidence from in vitro studies. Pharmaceuticals. 2022;15(7):808.
68. De Rosa V, Iommelli F, Monti M, Fonti R, Votta G, Stoppelli MP, Del Vecchio S. Reversal of Warburg effect and reactivation of oxidative phosphorylation by differential inhibition of EGFR signaling pathways in non–small cell lung cancer. Clin Cancer Res. 2015;21(22):5110–20.
69. Tian LR, Lin MZ, Zhong HH, Cai YJ, Li B, Xiao ZC, Shuai XT. Nanodrug regulates lactic acid metabolism to reprogram the immunosuppressive tumor microenvironment for enhanced cancer immunotherapy. Biomater Sci. 2022;10(14):3892–900.
70. Jadidi-Niaragh F, Atyabi F, Rastegari A, Kheshtchin N, Arab S, Hassannia H, Ajami M, Mirsanei Z, Habibi S, Masoumi F, Noorbakhsh F. CD73 specific siRNA loaded chitosan lactate nanoparticles potentiate the antitumor effect of a dendritic cell vaccine in 4T1 breast cancer bearing mice. J Control Release. 2017;246:46–59.
71. Patsoukis N, Bardhan K, Chatterjee P, Sari D, Liu B, Bell LN, Karoly ED, Freeman GJ, Petkova V, Seth P, Li L. PD-1 alters T-cell metabolic reprogramming by inhibiting glycolysis and promoting lipolysis and fatty acid oxidation. Nat Commun. 2015;6(1):6692.
72. Wu K, Han N, Mao Y, Li Y. Increased levels of PD1 and glycolysis in CD4+ T cells are positively associated with lymph node metastasis in OSCC. BMC Oral Health. 2023;23(1):356.
73. Choi BW, Jeong YJ, Park SH, Oh HK, Kang S. Reverse Warburg effect-related mitochondrial activity and 18F-FDG uptake in invasive ductal carcinoma. Nucl Med Mol Imaging. 2019;53(6):396–405.
74. Scroggins BT, Matsuo M, White AO, Saito K, Munasinghe JP, Sourbier C, Yamamoto K, Diaz V, Takakusagi Y, Ichikawa K, Mitchell JB. Hyperpolarized [1-13C]-pyruvate magnetic resonance spectroscopic imaging of prostate cancer in vivo predicts efficacy of targeting the Warburg effect. Clin Cancer Res. 2018;24(13):3137–48.
75. Macdonald EB, Begovatz P, Barton GP, Erickson-Bhatt S, Inman DR, Cox BL, Eliceiri KW, Strigel RM, Ponik SM, Fain SB. Hyperpolarized 13C magnetic resonance spectroscopic imaging of pyruvate metabolism in murine breast cancer models of different metastatic potential. Meta. 2021;11(5):274.
76. Vallée A, Lecarpentier Y, Guillevin R, Vallée JN. Aerobic glycolysis hypothesis through WNT/beta-catenin pathway in exudative age-related macular degeneration. J Mol Neurosci. 2017;62(3):368–79.

77. Tahtouh R, Wardi L, Sarkis R, Hachem R, Raad I, El Zein N, Hilal G. Glucose restriction reverses the Warburg effect and modulates PKM2 and mTOR expression in breast cancer cell lines. Cell Mol Biol. 2019;65(7):26–33.
78. Kozlov AM, Lone A, Betts DH, Cumming RC. Lactate preconditioning promotes a HIF-1α-mediated metabolic shift from OXPHOS to glycolysis in normal human diploid fibroblasts. Sci Rep. 2020;10(1):8388.
79. de Groof AJ, te Lindert MM, van Dommelen MM, Wu M, Willemse M, Smift AL, Winer M, Oerlemans F, Pluk H, Fransen JA, Wieringa B. Increased OXPHOS activity precedes rise in glycolytic rate in H-RasV12/E1A transformed fibroblasts that develop a Warburg phenotype. Mol Cancer. 2009;8(1):54.
80. Yoshida GJ. Beyond the Warburg effect: N-Myc contributes to metabolic reprogramming in cancer cells. Front Oncol. 2020;10:791.
81. Yeung SJ, Pan J, Lee MH. Roles of p53, MYC and HIF-1 in regulating glycolysis—the seventh hallmark of cancer. Cell Mol Life Sci. 2008;65(24):3981.
82. Chen Z, Kankala RK, Yang Z, Li W, Xie S, Li H, Chen AZ, Zou L. Antibody-based drug delivery systems for cancer therapy: mechanisms, challenges, and prospects. Theranostics. 2022;12(8):3719.
83. Wenger JB, Chun SY, Dang DT, Luesch H, Dang LH. Combination therapy targeting cancer metabolism. Med Hypotheses. 2011;76(2):169–72.

Glutamine Metabolism: Role in Cancer Cell Proliferation and Survival

3

Aganta Chakraborty, Sanket Pramanik, Shrabasti Mullick, Rajarshi Nath, Mohini Mondal, Radheshyam Pal, Sumel Ashique, and Mayukh Jana

Abbreviations

AKT	Protein Kinase B
AMPK	AMP-activated protein kinase
ASCT2	Alanine–Serine–Cysteine Transporter 2 (SLC1A5)
ATP	Adenosine Triphosphate
AZA	Azacytidine
Bcl-2	B-cell lymphoma 2
BPTES	Bis-2-(5-phenylacetamido-1,3,4-thiadiazol-2-yl)ethyl sulfide
CAF	Cancer-associated fibroblast
CAA	Cancer-associated adipocyte
CB-839	Telaglenastat (a GLS inhibitor)
CD	Cluster of Differentiation
CDK	Cyclin-dependent kinase
CRC	Colorectal Cancer
CSC	Cancer Stem Cell
DC	Dendritic Cell
DLBCL	Diffuse Large B-cell Lymphoma
DON	6-Diazo-5-oxo-L-norleucine
ECM	Extracellular Matrix
ENO1	Enolase 1
ETC	Electron Transport Chain
FA	Fatty Acids

A. Chakraborty · S. Pramanik · S. Mullick · R. Nath · M. Mondal · S. Ashique · M. Jana (✉)
Department of Pharmaceutical Technology, Bharat Technology, Uluberia, West Bengal, India

R. Pal
Department of Pharmacology, Bengal College of Pharmaceutical Technology, Dubrajpur, West Bengal, India

S. Ashique et al. (eds.), *Cancer Metabolism*, Cancer Treatment and Research 195, https://doi.org/10.1007/978-3-032-21861-2_3

FAO	Fatty Acid Oxidation
GFAT	Glutamine:fructose-6-phosphate amidotransferase
GCL	Glutamate cysteine ligase
GDH	Glutamate dehydrogenase
GLS	Glutaminase
Gln	Glutamine
Glu	Glutamate
GLUD	Glutamate dehydrogenase
GLUT	Glucose transporter
GSH	Reduced glutathione
GSSG	Oxidized glutathione
HBP	Hexosamine biosynthetic pathway
HCC	Hepatocellular carcinoma
HIF-1α	Hypoxia-inducible factor 1 alpha
HK2	Hexokinase 2
IDO	Indoleamine 2,3-dioxygenase
IFN-γ	Interferon gamma
IL	Interleukin
KEAP1	Kelch-like ECH-associated protein 1
KRAS	Kirsten rat sarcoma viral oncogene
LDHA	Lactate dehydrogenase A
LPS	Lipopolysaccharide
mTOR	Mammalian target of rapamycin
mTORC1	mTOR complex 1
MDSC	Myeloid-derived suppressor cell
ME1/ME2	Malic enzyme 1/2
MHC	Major histocompatibility complex
MSO	Methionine sulfoximine
NADPH	Nicotinamide adenine dinucleotide phosphate (reduced)
NK cell	Natural killer cell
OXPHOS	Oxidative phosphorylation
PDAC	Pancreatic ductal adenocarcinoma
PDH	Pyruvate dehydrogenase
PDK	Pyruvate dehydrogenase kinase
PD-L1	Programmed death ligand 1
PI3K	Phosphoinositide 3-kinase
PPP	Pentose phosphate pathway
ROS	Reactive oxygen species
SLC	Solute carrier family transporters
SIRT4	Sirtuin 4
SNAT	Sodium-coupled neutral amino acid transporter
TCA cycle	Tricarboxylic acid cycle
TAM	Tumor-associated macrophage
TCA	Tricarboxylic acid
TCR	T cell receptor
TGF-β	Transforming growth factor beta

Th1/Th2/Th17	T-helper cell subtypes
TILs	Tumor-infiltrating lymphocytes
TME	Tumor microenvironment
TNBC	Triple-negative breast cancer
TNF	Tumor necrosis factor
Treg	Regulatory T cell
Vps34	Vacuolar protein sorting 34
α-KG	Alpha-ketoglutarate

3.1 Introduction

3.1.1 Overview of Metabolic Reprogramming in Cancer

Metabolic reprogramming is one of the most common and essential hallmarks of cancer. However, unlike previously understood, this process can be dynamic or unstable based on the availability of substrates and the varying fertile metabolic demands for growth, invasion, proliferation, and survival of cells. Cancer cells alter their ability to break down proteins, lipids, and carbohydrates; however, not solely based on substrate availability. The adaptability of metabolic reprogramming of cancer cells, dependent on the tumor microenvironment (TME) and tumor environment, has been demonstrated to have a critical impact on the TME [1]. The term "metabolic reprogramming"commonly refers to a shared set of pathways observed in cancer cells or in highly proliferating tumors [2]. The Warburg effect explained that normal cells use oxidative phosphorylation (OXPHOS) to generate ATP, while cancer cells utilize aerobic glycolysis (converting glucose to lactate in the presence of oxygen). We have learned a significant amount about the purpose of aerobic glycolysis since Warburg investigated the phenomenon. More specifically, changes in oxidative metabolism, activation of oncogenes, and loss of tumor suppressor genes have all contributed to an increased ratio of glycolysis to oxygen consumption. Numerous vital molecular players engage in the complex molecular pathways that underlie the Warburg effect [3]. Recent studies indicate that multiple types of cancer demonstrate metabolic rewiring, such as aerobic glycolysis, glutamine dependence, accumulation of glycolytic intermediates, and increased lipid and amino acid synthesis to fulfill their high nutrient demands for building blocks and energy generation. In addition, metabolic reprogramming in cancer is known to be associated with oncogenic mutations, and these metabolic changes collectively affect tumor-microenvironment interactions and cancer progression [4]. Heterogeneity at a high level enables cancer cells to adapt to unfavorable tumor microenvironments (TMEs). TMEs are a challenge for cancer cells with limitations in nutrients, oxygen tension, and acidic pH that promote invasion and metastasis in conjunction with metabolic, genetic, and epigenetic alterations. It is possible that cancer cells metabolically adapted to a TME that is excessive were able to evade immune responses and cell death, in addition to contributing to drug resistance, recurrence, and poor prognosis in patients. Consequently, deciphering the mechanisms of adaptation in malignant cancer cells metabolically in TMEs is significant, and most are currently unknown. Recently, investigations have used single-cell interactions between cells to investigate how cancer cells are adapted into the TME [5].

3.1.2 Importance of Glutamine as a Metabolic Substrate

Glutamine is an amino acid that has unique and important metabolic functions. Glutamine is the most abundant free amino acid in plasma and intracellular sites, where it serves as a precursor for the biosynthesis of amino acids, proteins, nucleotides, and other important physiological molecules. Glutamine can also function as a substrate for gluconeogenesis, an oxidative fuel for rapidly proliferating cells and tissues, the primary end product of ammonia-trapping pathways in the liver, and the most significant precursor for ammonia genesis in the kidney. Glutamine may also have several important regulatory roles, such as promoting the synthesis of glycogen in the liver and stimulating protein synthesis and decreasing protein breakdown in skeletal muscle. It has been reconsidered the categorization of glutamine as a nonessential amino acid, and hence, the alternate theory has arisen to view glutamine as a conditionally essential nutrient since it has been corroborated that there are increases in tissue glutamine metabolism and decreases in glutamine concentrations within a number of catabolic-stressful disease processes [6]. As glutamine metabolism caters to ATP synthesis and the synthesis of protein, lipid, and nucleic acids, it enables cancer cells to maintain proliferation and survival. Glutamine metabolism could also modulate signal transduction and balance redox. In many instances, to support cell proliferation, significant amounts of glutamine are necessary to maintain your mitochondrial metabolism. Furthermore, glutamine acts in multiple roles that support healthy cell growth, function, and proliferation, as a nitrogen donor, redox regulator, and signal transducer [7]. The dependence of cancer cells on glutamine is due to the services glutamine provides as a carbon source to replenish the tricarboxylic acid (TCA) cycle and lipid biosynthesis pathways, and as a nitrogen source to facilitate biosynthesis of amino acids and nucleotides. The reliance of cancer cell viability on glutamine metabolism and supporting metabolic networks, e.g., aminotransferase, glutaminase, glutamine transporters, and homeostasis of redox state, has been well documented. Implementation of drug discovery targeting glutamine metabolism has produced promising approaches in cancer treatment, potential drug targets, and candidate drugs. There has also been considerable interest in the implications of glutamine blockade within the tumor microenvironment (TME) since immune checkpoint inhibitors have become part of routine cancer therapy [8]. The inhibition of glutaminase has shown powerful anticancer properties through pharmacological blockage, with CB-839, IACS-6274, and DRP-104 being examples of clinical trial compounds that suggest inhibition of glutaminase may play a considerable role in mediating tumor cell proliferation and apoptosis. Glutaminase inhibitor resistance may be treated through combination therapy of these inhibitors with other anticancer agents, which appear to have a synergistic effect. Investigating combination therapies and malignancies exhibiting increased glutaminolysis are overcoming resistance to glutaminase inhibitors and are interesting strategies to help treat certain cancers [9]. Researchers have shown that MYC promotes the circulation of TCA and glutathione synthesis fed with glutamine in the absence of oxygen by regulating glutamine transporters and inducing the expression of GLS at the mRNA and protein levels. In breast cancer, MYC can also drive the activation of downstream carcinogenic pathways such as mTOR, and interact with estrogen receptors (ER) and HER2 (also called ERBB2). Some studies indicate that triple-negative breast cancer cell lines are more glutamine-dependent than ER breast cancer cell lines [10].

3.2 Glutamine Metabolism: An Overview

The process whereby glutamine is metabolized into important intermediates is termed "glutaminolysis," and it is a crucial metabolic process for cellular energy, signaling, biosynthesis, and redox balance. The alterations to glutamine metabolism have big impacts on many different pathological states, including but not limited to cancers, metabolic, and neurological disorders. New research suggests that long noncoding RNA (lncRNA), circular RNA (circRNA), and oncogenic modifications to glutamine transporters and enzymes increase glutamine's availability as an alternative energy source, which supports cell survival and proliferation during times when nutrients and oxygen are limited. To counteract the pathogenic consequences of alterations in glutamine metabolism, scientists are designing inhibitors that specifically target enzymes and transporters implicated in glutaminolysis. These have the potential to decrease tumor growth and treat metabolic and neurological diseases by interfering with mechanisms supporting tumor cell growth [11].

3.2.1 Glutamine Transporters (SLC1A5, SLC7A5, SLC38A1, Etc.)

SLC1A5 (ASCT2) is a crucial sodium-dependent transporter that facilitates the transport of neutral amino acids by substituting for asparagine, serine, or threonine. Because of SLC1A5's high affinity for glutamine, particularly in acidic environments, the transporter is more effective at delivering glutamine to tumor cells that proliferate in acidic environments. It is strongly expressed in a number of solid tumors, including squamous lung carcinoma, where it accounts for 50% of glutamine uptake. A number of transcriptional regulators, including ATF4 and Myc, regulate SLC1A5 expression. Increased expression of both ATF4 and Myc is associated with poor survival outcomes in TNBC and has been linked to SLC1A5 overexpression. Additionally, in DLBCL cells, human colon adenocarcinoma cells, and mouse embryonic fibroblasts, Myc-dependent expression of ATF4 drives SLC1A5 expression when cells adapt to changes in metabolic stress. Significantly, a recent report demonstrated that HIF-2α, which induces overexpression of SLC1A5 isoforms in mitochondria, mediates chemotherapy resistance in pancreatic cancer cells as the cancer cells adapt to changes in regulating their glutamine metabolism [8]. SLC7A5 is an amino acid exchanger that behaves as a sodium-independent transporter by exchanging intracellular glutamine for large neutral amino acids such as leucine, phenylalanine, and tryptophan. In this way, it is able to maintain intracellular leucine, which is suspected of being a master regulator of the mTORC1 signaling, while providing amino acids to support cancer cells. In order to functionally express itself on the plasma membrane, SLC7A5 must heterodimerize with the heavy chain of SLC3A2. SLC7A5 has been reported to be highly expressed in multiple cancers, including lung adenocarcinoma, mouth cancers, and esophageal carcinoma. In several different cancers, SLC7A5 and the glutamine transporter SLC1A5 are co-expressed, suggesting that these transporters are functionally coupled to promote tumor growth [12]. Dysregulation of SLCs within neoplastic cells leads to alterations of metabolism, producing changes in levels of intracellular amino acids, which facilitates the progression of malignant cells into tumors. The neutral SLC7A5 and SLC1A5 appear to be associated with certain human cancers. SLC7A5 and SLC1A5, which have been shown to exist at the molecular level, have also been found in several neoplastic cells. Increased transcription of SLC1A5 promotes cloning and increases absorption of serine, which is important for the formation of purine nucleotides, which facilitate tumor formation [13]. SLC38A1 and SLC38A2 are sodium-coupled transporters for neutral amino acids, such as glutamine. Despite their neutrality, aromatic amino acid is not usable as substrates by the transporters. In mammalian tissues, both transporters are widely and consistently distributed. Because of their relatively narrow substrate specificity, transporters will be a major route for glutamine to enter cells under physiological conditions. Nearly all neurons in the central nervous system express SLC38A1 and SLC38A2, which are involved in the glutamate/GABA-glutamine cycle between neurons and astrocytes. Astrocytes internalize the neurotransmitter glutamate from both the synapse and extrasynaptic spaces, converting it into glutamine, which is then released into the extracellular space via system Ntransporters. The released glutamine is then taken up by neurons as a source of glutamate through SLC38A1 and SLC38A2, later released in the synaptic cleft upon neuronal activation. The glutamate/GABA-glutamine cycle is an integral component of glutamatergic neurotransmission. Analogously, a related metabolic cycle operates in GABAergic neurotransmission, due to the fact that glutamate is an intermediate and glutamine represents the precursor of GABA synthesis [14, 15]. Many distinct types of cancers are caused by the overexpression of SLC transporters. Overexpression of these genes initiates many pathways and mechanisms, including glutathione biosynthesis, glutaminolysis, MYC-mTOR, HIF-1 α-mTOR, P13K-AKT-mTOR, and PDK1-AKT-mTOR. These pathways regulate energy metabolism, cell migration, growth, and proliferation. Likewise, these mechanisms promote the survival and division of cancer cells by inhibiting apoptosis [13].

3.2.2 Connection to the TCA Cycle and Anaplerosis

Glutamine is metabolized to glutamate, aspartate, CO2, pyruvate, lactate, alanine, and citrate through the process of glutaminolysis. High-affinity membrane glutamine transporters (ASCT2 and SN2) facilitate intracellular glutamine transport.

Within cells, the majority of glutamine is either processed by glutaminases to glutamate (Glu) or used as a nitrogen donor to macromolecules. Glu has many fates. Glutathione cysteine ligase (GCL) is capable of directly converting it to glutathione (GSH), one of the most abundant mammalian cellular antioxidants and crucial for maintaining redox status in subcellular compartments. Glu can also be catabolized by either α-nitrogen removal via aminotransferases or by glutamate dehydrogenase (GDH), producing α-KG that can be incorporated into the TCA cycle for ATP production, or utilized as substrate for polyglutamated folic acid biosynthesis, or undergo further processing in mitochondria. Proline, which is an amino acid that is important for the creation of collagen and connective tissue, is formed upon cycling of glutamate. Other tissues can reductively carboxylate α-KG to form citrate, brown adipocyte cell lines and rat liver being two tissues that have been shown to do so. There is evidence that a fraction of carbon derived from glutamine can exit the TCA cycle as malate and become a substrate for malic enzymes 1, which produces NADPH [16]. With the involvement of several enzymes that are dysregulated in cancer, α-ketoglutarate enters the TCA cycle in the mitochondria and generates other organic molecules, including fumarate, malate, and citrate. For example, the malic isoenzymes (ME1 and ME2) have been identified as pro-tumorigenic and valid therapeutic targets as they are upregulated in several cancers. The pentose phosphate pathway (PPP) and ME1 have been demonstrated to be correlated. This suggests that ME1 is forming a hetero-oligomer with 6-phosphogluconate dehydrogenase (6PGD), which is the limiting enzyme in the PPP, and increases its affinity to the substrate 6-phosphogluconate, thus shunting glycolytic intermediates to PPP, and additionally, encourages the TCA cycle to become dependent on glutamine. Thus, glutamine serves as bioenergetics, as glucose is largely shunted to biosynthetic pathways [17]. The synthesis of reduced glutathione (GSH), which is the most abundant intracellular antioxidant molecule and the key component of the GSH–antioxidant system, comprised of GSH, oxidized glutathione (GSSG), glutathione reductase (GR), and glutathione peroxidases (GPXs), relies on glutamine (Gln). Glu can offer substrates for GSH production, but glutaminolysis restricts the oxidation of Gln and, therefore, oxidative phosphorylation (OXPHOS) and reactive oxygen species (ROS) that could otherwise disrupt normal cellular function. Potentially high levels of ROS produced in cancer cells could be harmful; however, they act as an essential signaling mechanism to support the homeostasis of the tumor. For this reason, the levels of ROS in the cell are finely tuned by a variety of antioxidant enzymes, including the isoenzymes of glutaminase (GA) [18]. Changes in glutamine metabolism have recently been shown to be implicated in the pathologic consequences of mitochondrial dysfunction. Glutamine is a pleiotropic molecule in that it provides an alternative carbon source to glucose under some conditions and has unique roles in cellular communication in neurons and astrocytes. Glutamine utilization and net catabolic flux may be altered heavily both under genetic mitochondrial defects and exposures to mitochondrial toxins. Further, alteration in glutamine metabolism is implicated, especially in neurodegenerative diseases. These include primary mitochondrial diseases such as Leigh syndrome (subacute necrotizing encephalopathy) and MELAS (mitochondrial myopathy with encephalopathy, lactic acidosis, and stroke-like episodes), and age-related neurodegenerative diseases including Alzheimer's disease and Parkinson's disease. Pharmacological interventions targeting glutamine metabolizing and catabolizing pathways have been shown to provide some benefit in the care of cell and animal models of these diseases, suggesting that glutamine metabolism may be a clinically relevant target [19].

3.3 Regulation of Glutamine Metabolism in Cancer

3.3.1 Oncogenic Regulation (Myc, KRAS, p53, HIF-1α, mTORC1)

It has been demonstrated that MYC, one of the most significant oncogenic drivers, is active in a number of cancer types and subtypes, including the most prevalent and aggressive tumors [20]. The Myc family, including MycL and MycN, is important for controlling the reprogramming of metabolism in a variety of human tumors. Apoptosis results from Myc overexpression by switching prosurvival signals (e.g., bcl-2) to prodeath signals [11]. The c-Myc transcription factor can transcriptionally induce Gln transporters (SLC1A5, SLC7A5, and SLC7A11), as well as the rate-limiting enzymes GLS1 and GS. It was found that c-Myc attaches to the GLS1 promoter near the transcriptional start site at the beginning of the 5′ UTR and reduces the post-transcriptional inhibition of GLS by miR-23a/b. In addition, c-Myc can impact deamination/transamination processes in tumor metabolism in several ways, specifically: (1) by increasing GDH and GOT1 in renal carcinoma; and (2) by orchestrating the overexpression of GOT1 and GPT2 in breast cancer malignancies. Interestingly, Gln shows reciprocal c-Myc expression regulation: Gln deprivation reduced c-Myc protein levels in HCT116 CRC cells due to 3′ UTR indirect translational inhibitions; however, Gln supplementation can restore c-Myc protein levels [21]. KRAS, a member of the RAS protein family, regulates several downstream effectors that are key regulators of autophagy and apoptosis. KRAS mutations constitutively activate this oncogene in tumor cells, resulting in stimulation of cell division, promotion of autophagy, inhibition of apoptosis, modulation of cell metabolism, alteration of motility and invasion properties, and alterations to the tumor microenvironment. Specifically, KRAS mutations have been reported to downregulate pro-apoptotic proteins (e.g., thymine-DNA glycosylase (TDG) and tumor necrosis factor (TNF)-related apoptosis-inducing ligand (TRAIL)) and upregulate anti-apoptotic proteins (e.g., survivin and Bel-xL). In addition, KRAS mutations also induce autophagy to enhance cell survival and promote tumor progression through modulation of PI3K and MAPK signaling. As a result, these mutations provide resistance to anticancer medication therapy, which leads to a bad prognosis [22]. The tumor suppressor p53 regulates Gln metabolic reprogramming to facilitate context-dependent survival of cancer cells. Mechanistically, p53 binds to the GLS2 promoter and increases GLS2 expression. p53 also promotes p53-mediated genome protection by facilitating Gln input into glutathione (GSH), which reduces reactive oxygen species (ROS) levels in cancer cells and regulates apoptosis. When Gln is unavailable, p53 triggers compensatory pathways by transcriptionally directing the arginine transporter SLC7A3 and the aspartate/Glu transporter SLC1A3. SLC7A3 supports mTORC1 activation by enhancing arginine intake, and SLC1A3 sustains the electron transport chain (ETC) and tricarboxylic acid (TCA) cycle by bringing in aspartate as an energy source. These mechanisms combine to control Gln metabolism and promote therapeutic resistance [21]. HIF-1α might inhibit the propagation of tumor cells through the regulation of glutamine catabolism. For instance, HIF1α interacts with GOT1 and GOT2 by blocking aspartate production from glutamine oxidation (GOT1) or glutamine reduction (GOT2) pathways specifically and directly in clear cell renal cell carcinoma. After HIF1α activation, this dual inhibition may lead to a significant decrease in the intracellular aspartate pool. Furthermore, because GOT1 can convert both aspartates generated by GOT2 and exogenous aspartate to glutamate, the dual inhibition of GOT2 and GOT1 may also prevent oxidative transport of malate-aspartate. The impact of HIF-1α on glutamine-dependent aspartate synthesis will effectively limit tumor growth because tumor cells will utilize aspartate at a lower rate than without HIF-1α.HIF1-α modulates glutamine metabolism through the inhibition of α-ketoglutarate dehydrogenase (α-KGDH), a significant mitochondrial enzyme, along with an increase in α-KG levels that push the reverse reaction of isocitrate dehydrogenase forward. Moreover, by competing with c-myc for sp1 binding, HIF1-α inhibits the transcriptional ability of c-myc, which allows for some cell-cycle arrest and inhibition of tumor-cell proliferation. Even with HIF-1 being generally characterized as having the potential to stimulate the proliferation of cancer cells, there may exist several compensatory mechanisms in tumors that suppress the inhibitory effects of HIF-1 [23]. To provide sufficient energy and metabolites to facilitate tumor dedifferentiation into cancer stem cells (CSCs), at both the material and mechanistic level, HIF-1α induces accelerated aerobic glycolysis in the cancer cells. Inhibition or silencing of HIF-1α, therefore, will improve patient prognosis and treatment, as it will reduce tumor food supply, discernibly preventing or reducing tumor dedifferentiation or even reducing cancer stem cell proportion [24]. mTORC1 promotes GS stability through post-translational downregulation of ubiquitination, linking energy balance and amino acid utilization during nutritional stress. mTORC1 enhances proliferative capacity via the transcriptional inhibition of mitochondrial sirtuin4 (SIRT4), which then activates GDH and promotes Glu-to-α-KG flux [21]. A multitude of amino acid-activated mTORC1 pathways have been detected to promote unregulated cell growth and proliferation in tumor cells during recent studies. Rag-dependent pathways comprise one of these. In tumor cells, SLC7A5 transports glutamine in exchange for essential amino acids, and one such amino acid is leucine. This interaction between glutamine and leucine affects several cellular functions, including growth and autophagy, by promoting glutaminolysis (especially the production of α-KG) and Rag-mediated mTORC1 recruitment to the lysosomal surface where mTORC1 is ultimately activated [23]. A recent study has reported that glutamine stimulates proliferation of intestinal epithelial cells through activation of mTORC1 signaling, which requires a functional lysosome and phospholipase D. Novel insight are provided for homeostasis of the intestinal epithelium, including potential implications for pig production [25].

3.3.2 Signaling Pathways Influencing Glutamine Utilization

There are many signaling pathways that are important for homeostasis in cells and disease, which can also regulate glutamine metabolism. The regulation of glutamine metabolism is centrally linked to a number of important signaling pathways, for example, c-Myc, mTOR, and KRAS. One potential for therapeutic targeting is the mTOR pathway, as it increases the flow and metabolism of glutamate in cancer cells. The mTOR pathway is an important regulator of growth and metabolism in cells. Other signaling pathways that have been shown to be involved in the regulation of glutamine metabolism include AMPK, AKT, and Wnt/β-catenin, and these may represent additional opportunities for therapeutic strategies. The development of novel therapies for diseases such as cancer, neurological disease, and metabolic syndromes (MetS) associated with dysregulation of glutamine metabolism may be formed upon a better understanding of how the complex networks of signaling regulate glutamine metabolism [11]. The prospective predictive MRGs in HCC uncovered that SLC38A1 regulated HCC growth and dissemination by regulating the PI3K/AKT/mTOR pathway via glutamine-dependent energy metabolism [26]. mTORC1 activation represses SIRT4 transcription, which promotes glutamine anaplerosis through activation of glutamate dehydrogenase. In RCCs, HIF supports and promotes reductive glutamine metabolism. HIF-1 increases the levels of ketoglutarate in malignancies by inducing GLS1 (glutaminase 1) expression, allowing for increased citrate production and fatty acids/lipids. Therefore, HIFs alter glutamine signaling and promote tumor growth by influencing amino acid metabolism [27]. Some of the target genes of c-Myc that are important in glutamine metabolism include GLS1, GLUD, and the amino acid transferases. Myc upregulates the expression of GLUL, an enzyme that is responsible for the de novo synthesis of glutamine from glutamate and ammonia. Within the active demethylation process that is activated by Thymine DNA glycosylase, another Myc transcriptional target, the expression of the glutamine synthetase (GS) promoter is increased. These demonstrate a unique biological link between glutamine metabolism and DNA demethylation in Myc-driven cancers [11]. C-Myc modulates the uptake and metabolism of glutamine through transporters like SLC3A2, SLC7A1, SLC5A1, GLS-1, and GLS-2 [28]. Mutant KRAS restructures glutamine metabolism to enhance the production of succinate from a-KG in a SLC25A22-dependent manner. Accumulation of succinate activates WNT/b-catenin signaling specifically, WNT targets associated with CRC stemness, such as LGR5, by blocking a-KG dependent epigenetic regulators. This observation employed various in vitro and in vivo models of KRAS-mutant CRC [29].

3.3.3 Epigenetic and Transcriptional Control Mechanisms

The dysregulation of amino acid metabolism can be altered with epigenetic changes such as methylation and acetylation that produce reducing potential to diminish the extreme redox state caused by abnormal energy metabolism. The corresponding high bioenergetic state and redox balance facilitate metabolic capacity for synthesizing key intermediates such as SAM and acetyl-CoA, as well as energy production in the form of ATP. This allows for further epigenetic regulation that can be exploited to reduce the expression of tumor suppressor genes while increasing the expression of important metabolic enzymes in cancer cells [30]. There are four major types of epigenetic modifications reported, including DNA methylation, chromatin remodeling, histone modification, and noncoding RNA-induced alteration [31]. Metabolites and epigenetic alterations in DNA facilitate metabolic reprogramming of cancer cells, influencing physiological processes, such as dysfunctional cell growth, immune evasion, and immune surveillance. Disruption of pathways influenced by metabolites, aberrant proliferation cues, and epigenetic changes can be detrimental, hastening cancer progression [32].

3.4 Glutamine in Cancer Cell Proliferation

The most abundant amino acid in the body, glutamine, is important for the biological synthesis of nucleotides and other nonessential amino acids during cell metabolism. Recent studies show that glutamine metabolic reprogramming is a key signal in cancer initiation and progression. This metabolic reprogramming in tumorigenic cells can facilitate cancer growth through various oncogenic and signal pathway activation. Furthermore, it may also regulate the tumor immune microenvironment and promote tumor treatment resistance [33].

3.4.1 Role in Nucleotide, Amino Acid, and Lipid Biosynthesis

The γ-nitrogen amide group of glutamines is a crucial nitrogen contributor in the de novo synthesis of hexosamines, such as glucosamine and galactosamine, as well as nucleobases purine and pyrimidine. Glutamate, which is generated from glutamine in mitochondria via the enzyme glutaminase, is the substrate for the processes in the second group. Glutamate is converted to α-ketoglutarate (α-KG) by anaplerosis to fuel the tricarboxylic acid (TCA) cycle. The α-nitrogen from glutamate is transferred to another amino acid and α-ketoglutarate by either glutamate dehydrogenase (GLUD1 and GLUD2 in humans) or a variety of aminotransferases. So, in glutamine-dependent cancer cells, α-ketoglutarate has been proposed as an essential metabolite for cell survival [34]. The uptake of Gln/Glu into lipids and fatty acids (FAs) was measured in primary neurons and a neuronal cell line, and the results were compared with those from primary cell cultures and non-neuronal cell lines under hypoxic conditions. In all the nonneuronal cells studied, the total uptake of

Gln/Glu into total lipids was lower or stable compared to constant and specific increases in neurons. Depending on substrate and cell type, uptake into total (esterified and free) FA ranged from 90% to 97% of substrate uptake into neuronal lipids. Collectively, these suggest a unique mechanism of adaptation for neural cells under hypoxia may involve FA production from Gln/Glu [35]. In a state of low oxygen (hypoxia), proliferating cells utilize more glutamine, which preferentially provides carbon for carbon fatty acid production via reductive carboxylation. The reductive carboxylation process occurs by isocitrate dehydrogenases through the conversion of glutamine-derived α-ketoglutarate to citric acid and the oxidation of NADPH to NADP+ [36]. Hypoxia regulates mitochondrial glutamine metabolism via HIF1α-GDH signaling, and the hypoxia-mediated GDH has been shown to promote drug resistance in human lung cancer cells. In lung cancer cells, hypoxia promotes the uptake and catabolism of glutamine, resulting in ATP production [37]. Glutamine supports the proliferation and survival of cancerous cells. First, glutamine acts as a nitrogen substrate that is a requirement for producing nonessential amino acids and nucleotides. Second, the TCA cycle continues to use glutamine as a carbon substrate for manufacturing α-ketoglutarate (α-KG), which is required to manufacture fatty acids and citrate. Third, glutamine maintains redox balance and aids in the manufacture of glutathione. Finally, glutamine increases the supply of amino acids, mainly leucine, which activates the mTOR pathway. Moreover, the process of glutaminolysis, specifically loading the downstream molecule Rag with guanosine triphosphate (GTP), is a potential activation pathway for mTORC1. Glutaminase (GLS1) converts intracellular glutamine to glutamate, which is a precursor of alpha-ketoglutarate (α-KG). The majority of nonessential amino acids are precursors of glutamate, which include aspartate (Asp), alanine (Ala), arginine (Arg), and proline (Pro). In ER-negative breast cancer, overexpression of glutaminase (GLS1) in cancer cells is known to increase amino acid production and is thought to correlate with poorer prognosis. Glutamine addiction is another drug target that occurs in some subsets of breast cancer and, in particular, tumors overexpressing MYC, the major subtype being triple negative breast cancer (TNBC) [38].

3.4.2 Maintenance of Redox Homeostasis (NADPH Production, Glutathione Synthesis)

Glutamine is essential in maintaining the redox homeostasis of tumor cells. It is one of the key amino acids involved in glutathione synthesis. Specifically, glutamate can polymerize with cysteine to form gamma-glutamylcysteine, which can then undergo condensation with glycine to become GSH. Besides, malate generated in the TCA cycle can be catalyzed by malic enzyme to NADPH. NADPH has a role in reducing oxidized glutathione to GSH and cystine to cysteine for participation in the de novo synthesis of GSH. GSH is an important endogenous antioxidant eliminating the oxidative damage caused by excessive ROS. As a result, targeting glutamine metabolism in cancer cells could be a potential treatment approach by disrupting their redox balance. By targeting cell autophagy through the mTOR pathway activation and ROS removal, glutamine may also inhibit tumor growth. Conversely, ammonia produced from glutamine metabolism could promote cell autophagy and tumor growth. The exact role of glutamine in the modulation of cell autophagy is still unclear [39]. The oxidation of glutathione can regenerate itself when NADPH is converted to NADP+. The mitochondrial glutamine transporter is linked with floatation-based NADPH production, and glutamine generates NADPH in pancreatic cancer cells via a noncanonical metabolism of glutamine. Furthermore, NADPH is produced through IDH1-dependent reductive metabolism of glutamine to reduce mitochondrial ROS during the growth of anchorage independent. All in all, glutamine provides reducing power as NADPH for tumor growth and drives glutathione production to maintain cellular redox equilibrium [40].

3.4.3 Contribution to Bioenergetics and Mitochondrial Function

A hallmark of cancer is altered cellular energy metabolism. Cancer cells can repurpose their metabolic pathways to meet their needs for energy and building blocks to grow and survive. Mitochondrial carbon pool replenishment is essential for maintaining mitochondrial integrity, as proliferating cells consume precursors deriving from the tricarboxylic acid (TCA) cycle intermediates. Cancer cells utilize glutamine (Gln), an essential source of both nitrogen and carbon, to provide for this mitochondrial anaplerosis. Glutaminase (GLS) metabolizes glutamate and ammonia (NH4+) in mitochondria, and glutamate dehydrogenase (GDH) or transaminases convert Gln into α-ketoglutarate (αKG), a TCA cycle intermediate, to replenish the carbon pool in mitochondria. The main anaplerotic pathway in cells that are growing or dividing is the incorporation of αKG derived from Gln into the TCA cycle. This is particularly relevant because oncogene-induced carcinogenesis depends on mitochondrial Gln metabolism, and several cancer cells show increased TCA cycle intermediates and enhanced mitochondrial Gln anaplerosis [41]. In the first place, the main source of the TCA cycle anaplerosis is glutamine. Glutamine can be readily converted to α-ketoglutarate, which enters the TCA cycle to generate NADH and FADH2. The electron transport and OXPHOS use NADH and FADH2 to produce ATP. This generates TCA cycle intermediates that support multiple biosynthetic pathways, including gluconeogenesis. In addition, α-ketoglutarate from glutamine can be reductively carboxylated to citrate in hypoxic or mitochondrial-deficient conditions, thereby supporting the maintenance of anabolic pathways [42]. Alterations in signal transduction pathways can affect mitochondrial proteins that are important elements in regulating the membrane potential, for example, UCP2 (uncoupling protein 2), components of MPTP (mitochondrial permeability transition pore), and components of oxPhos (oxidative phosphorylation) complexes, or regulating cell life and death, for example, the Bcl-2 (B-cell lymphoma 2) protein family. Additionally, effective regulation of these mitochondrial functions is important for the growth of tumors since mitochondrial bioenergetics and dynamics influence cell life and death as well [43].

3.4.4 Cross Talk with Glycolysis and Fatty Acid Metabolism

Hexosamine biosynthesis connects glucose and glutamine metabolism since the enzyme glutamine fructose-6-phosphate amidotransferase (GFAT) puts the γ-amino group of glutamine onto a hexose sugar which is the limiting step. GlcNAc and N-linked glycosylation of the IL-3 receptor α-chain were necessary for IL-3 to stimulate glutamine uptake and proliferation of cells in hematopoietic cells [44]. In terms of cell production, both glutamine and glucose are essential nutrients. Otto Warburg proposed almost a century ago that cancer cells generate the necessary biosynthetic precursors through glycolysis even in the presence of oxygen, resulting in lactate production and diminished availability of acetyl-CoA. Immune surveillance largely modulates cancer development. They rely on both innate and adaptive immune system elements. Natural killer T (NKT) cells consume glutamine at a higher rate than $CD4^+$ T cells when activated, and in terms of NKT cells, glutamine plays a vital role in glycosylation, mitochondrial function, and REDOX homeostasis [45]. In most tumor cells, glucose is the main lipogenic substrate. The TCA cycle cannot be viewed as a carbon sink, as the production of fatty acids depends solely on the outflow of citrate from the mitochondria. Glucose-derived pyruvate will be converted into acetyl-CoA by PDH, which then enters the TCA cycle, where it is converted into citrate. Citrate will then leave the mitochondria and return to the cytosol, where it is utilized for de novo fatty acid production. Glutamine, in addition to glucose, can also assist in producing citrate through forward flow through the TCA cycle and can replenish TCA cycle intermediates through a-ketoglutarate production [46]. In cancer, lipid metabolism is also reprogrammed. The membrane of cancer cells consists of active cholesterol and fatty acid synthesis, which produces signaling molecules. Fatty acid oxidation is one important energy source for swiftly growing cancers [47]. One method by which hypoxia increases glycolytic flux is through the activation of hypoxia-inducible factor (HIF) and its downstream target genes, which contain many glycolytic enzymes. Hypoxia and Ras decrease the flux of glucose into the TCA cycle by activating pyruvate dehydrogenase kinase (PDK), which inhibits pyruvate dehydrogenase (PDH). In this setting, other substrates, such as glutamine, may support the TCA cycle. This is possibly because Ras activity and hypoxia are more important for cell growth and survival, leading to a greater dependence on glutamine as either a bioenergetic substrate or as an anabolic precursor for lipids, acetyl-CoA, or amino acids [48]. MYC overexpression stimulates glutamine metabolism through the transcriptional activation of genes involved in glutaminolysis, and the high rate of glutaminolysis enhances cellular survival and proliferation [49]. As per a recent study, a common cellular response to impaired mitochondrial metabolism is glutamine-dependent reductive carboxylation [50].

3.5 Glutamine in Cancer Cell Survival and Stress Adaptation

3.5.1 Role of Autophagy and Stress Response

Micro-autophagy, also known as autophagy, is a homeostatic process that degrades cellular organelles and proteins, which maintain cellular biosynthesis during metabolic stress [51]. It is also a proteolytic process by which the cell mediates the lysosomal-dependent breakdown of long-lived, damaged organelles and misfolded proteins, which provides stability to cells. It contributes to immunity, infection, cancer, irritation, and suspension [52]. Glutamine is an essential amino acid and has the highest concentration in human blood among other amino acids [53]. The Warburg effect of Glutamine explains the excessive demand for Glutamine as it is highly required to sustain proper oxidative phosphorylation to supply the tri-carboxylic acid (TCA) intermediates [40]. Autophagy plays a major role in tumor suspension and also reduces stress tolerance that enables tumor cells to survive under critical condition, stress in tumor cells is compounded by the high metabolic demand associated with rapid cell proliferation, which also induces tumors in hypoxic regions [54]. Autophagy fundamentally forms a bi-layer membrane around random cytosolic compounds. This develops vesicles, which are called autophagosm which bind with lysosomes to mediate cargo degradation. More than 30 enzymes associated with autophagy have been discovered, most of which regulate autophagosome development [55]. The initiation of autophagy is controlled by the ULK1 (human homolog of ATG1) kinase complex, which consists of ULK1, Atg13, and Atg17, and integrates stress signals from mTOR complex 1 (mTORC1) [56, 57]. When mTORC1 kinase activity is inhibited, autophagosome formation can occur. This involves vacuolar sorting protein 34 (Vps34), a class III phosphoinositide 3-kinase (PI3K) that forms a complex with Beclin 1. The production of PtIns3P by the Beclin 1/Vps34 complex is essential for the recruitment of other autophagy-related gene (Atg) products that are critical for autophagosome formation [58]. During the initiation phase, formation of the Atg5-Atg12-Atg16 complex promotes the recruitment and conversion of cytosolic-associated protein light chain 3 (LC3-I) to the membrane-bound, lipidated form, LC3-II [59]. LC3 is conjugated to phosphatidyl ethanolamine and incorporated into the membrane by an Atg7- and Atg3-dependent activation and transfer cascade that follows cleavage of LC3 by the cysteine protease Atg4 [60]. Beclin 1 is a protein required for autophagy induction, and Beclin 1þ/ mice were shown to be tumor-prone, indicating that Beclin 1 is a haploinsufficient tumor suppressor gene [61]. In contrast, excessive stimulation of autophagy due to Beclin 1 overexpression can inhibit tumor development [62]. A potential molecular link between defective autophagy and tumorigenesis involves the accumulation of p62/SQSTM1 protein aggregates, damaged mitochondria, and misfolded proteins that lead to the production of ROS. This causes DNA damage that can lead to genomic instability [63]. Knockdown of p62/SQSTM1 in autophagy-defective cells prevented ROS and the DNA damage response. The relationship between defective autophagy and p62/SQSTM1 accumulation with tumorigenesis was also shown in a study in which p62/SQSTM1/mice were protected from Ras-induced lung carcinomas compared with wild-type animals [64]. Autophagy may also protect against tumorigenesis by limiting necrosis and chronic inflammation, which are associated with the release of proinflammatory HMGB1 [65]. Cancer cells have high metabolic demands due to increased cellular proliferation, and in in vivo models, exposure to metabolic stress was shown to impair survival in autophagy-deficient cells compared with autophagy-proficient cells [63]. Cytotoxic and metabolic stresses, including hypoxia and nutrient deprivation, can activate autophagy for recycling of ATP and to maintain cellular biosynthesis and survival. Autophagy is induced in hypoxic tumor cells from regions that are distal to blood vessels, and HIF-1a-dependent and -independent activation have been described. HIF-1a can also increase the expression of angiogenic factors, such as vascular endothelial growth factor, platelet-derived growth factor, and nitric oxide synthase [66]. Recent data indicate that human cancer cell lines bearing activating mutations in H-ras or K-ras have high basal levels of autophagy even in the presence of abundant nutrients [67]. In these cells, suppression of essential autophagy proteins was shown to inhibit cell growth, indicating that autophagy maintains tumor cell survival and suggesting that blocking autophagy in tumors that are addicted to autophagy, such as Ras-driven cancers, may be an effective treatment approach.

3.5.2 Interaction with Tumor Microenvironment (TME)

TME is a complex and dynamic cellular environment that is composed of tumor cells and immune cells, such as macrophages and lymphocytes; it is also composed of nonimmune cells, such as cancer-associated fibroblasts (CAFs) and tumor endothelial cells, and extracellular matrix [68]. Glutamine is involved in a variety of metabolic processes in the TME, which helps for growth, metabolism, and biosynthesis of tumor cells, immune and nonimmune cells in the TME. Glutamine is not only vital for tumor cells but is also an essential nutrient for the immune system. It supports several key lymphocyte functions, including the release of signaling molecules, cell growth, and overall survival of these immune cells [69]. The immune system uses a highly coordinated network of biological processes involving both innate and adaptive immunity, which together influence how tumors begin and progress. The innate immune system includes many types of immune and nonimmune cells—such as monocytes, macrophages, neutrophils, eosinophils, basophils, natural killer (NK) cells, dendritic cells (DCs), platelets, epithelial cells, and fibroblasts. These cells act as the body's first line of defense, helping block infections and maintain internal balance [70]. The adaptive immune system relies on controlled interactions between T cells, B cells, and antigen-presenting cells. These interactions trigger pathogen-specific immune responses, help form immune memory, and maintain the stability of the immune environment [71]. Immune cells can detect changes in the TME and adjust their activity accordingly. Altered levels of nutrients and metabolites—such as lactic acid, glucose, and glutamine—can directly influence how immune cells function. Moreover, tumor cells and immune cells often compete for these nutrients within the TME, which may weaken immune cell effectiveness [72]. A growing body of research shows that glutamine can regulate immune-cell behavior within the TME through several molecular pathways. This suggests that targeting glutamine metabolism could potentially enhance the success of anticancer immunotherapies. In the TME, cancer cells are highly dependent on glutamine for proliferation, and their unique metabolic pattern, known as glutamine addition, which increases the transport of glutamine in the plasma membrane [73]. Tumor cells transport glutamine into cells through specific transporters which is (such as solute carrier family 1 neutral amino acid transporter member 5, SLC1A5; also known as alanine, serine, cysteine-preferring transporter 2, ASCT2), and then convert it into glutamate under the action of glutaminase (GLS), and further convert it into α-ketoglutarate (α-KG), which enters the tricarboxylic acid (TCA) cycle and participates in the onset, development and dissemination of tumors [74]. For example, glutamine metabolites in tumor cells provide energy for tumor progression after entering the TCA cycle [75]. After a large amount of glutamine enters tumor cells, it is catabolized into glutamate and ammonia by GLS, which provides a carbon source for the TCA cycle [76]. In addition, approximately half of the nonessential amino acids are required for Protein Synthesis in tumor cells [77].

3.6 Glutamine Metabolism and Tumor Microenvironment

3.6.1 Role in Immune Evasion and Suppression (T Cells, Macrophages)

T cell plays an important role in the antitumor immune response. It helps to regulate T-cell proliferation [78]. Different types of T cells have different requirements for glutamine, which control T-cell function. In the resting state, the metabolic rate of native T cells is low, so the demand for glutamine is low. This low level of glutamine metabolism maintains its survival [79]. Effector T cells (Teff) require rapid proliferation and require a higher rate of glutamine metabolism. Different types of T cells have different ways of immune response against cancer [80]. When activated, CD^{4+} helper T cell 1 (Th1) cells fight cancer by secreting interferon-γ (IFN-γ) to activate macrophages and natural killer (NK) T cells, activated $CD8^{+}$T cells have direct cytotoxic effects against tumors [81]. Regulatory T cells (Treg) and activated CD^{4+} helper T cells to promote the amino suppressive environment that cancer creates [82]. CD^{4+} helper T cell 17 (Th 17 cells) can either support or inhibit the tumor. Progression depends on the specific condition. When cytokine levels shift, such as under limited glutamine availability, that balance may move from a Th1 dominant response to a Th2 dominant one. Glutamine metabolism is essential for controlling the activity of Y and T cells, which generate interleukin 17 (IL 17) in the skin tissue of patients with psoriasis [82]. The glutamine transporter plays a critical role in T cells. The differentiation and functional activity of $CD4^{+}$ Th1 and $CD8^{+}$ T cells are influenced by glutamine, which enhances the transcription factor T-bet while suppressing the mTORC1 and IL-2 signaling cascades. This suppression ultimately limits Th17 cell development [83]. Moreover, the absence of GLS1 results in reduced α-KG levels, disrupting normal Th17 cell differentiation [84]. Glutamine transporters—such as ASCT2, SLC7A5 (Solute Carrier Family 7 Member 5), and the Sodium-coupled Neutral Amino Acid Transporters (SNAT)—are essential for $CD4^+$ Th1 and Th17 lineage commitment; blocking these transport systems hinders their differentiation. Among them, SLC7A5-driven glutamine uptake is crucial for activating c-MYC-dependent effector T cells. Under glutamine-limited conditions, effector T cells exhibit decreased c-MYC protein levels, restricted proliferation, and weakened immune capacity [85]. Additionally, glutamine scarcity enhances the development of regulatory T cells (Tregs) through the AMPK–mTORC1 axis, further shifting immune balance. According to Suzuki et al., through restricting cell metabolism, the cancer suppressor menin stops activated CD8 + T lymphocytes from developing functional abnormalities [86]. Vallion et al. found that the stability of Treg lacking mTOR decreases [87].

Macrophages are innate immune cells. Macrophages are used to control host inflammation and preserve tissue homeostasis [88]. Macrophages are of two types: M1 and M2 macrophages. M1 macrophages present in the positive immune responses and play the role in immune surveillance by secreting inflammatory cytokines and chemokines [89]. M2 macrophages have weak antigen-presenting ability and secrete anti-inflammatory cytokines such as IL10, TGF-β, and downregulate the immune response [90]. A distinct or unique group of macrophages is called tumor-associated macrophages (TAMs). It is often categorized as M2-like, but evidence shows that M1 like. During the early phases of tumor formation, it shows an inflammatory reaction, and in later stages, they shift toward the immunosuppressive phenotype that facilitates tumor progression [91]. According to Du et al., l-methionine sulfoximine (MSO) controls TAMs' glutamine metabolism and causes them to polarize toward the M1 phenotype [92]. The consumption of glutamine by the cancer cells in clear cell renal cell carcinoma (ccRCC) results in the local deprivation of extracellular glutamine. This, in turn, triggers the release of IL-23 by cancer-infiltrating macrophages via the activation of hypoxia-inducible factor 1α (HIF1α) [93]. The polarization of macrophages toward M1 or M2 states is closely connected to glutamine metabolism. It remains unclear whether inhibiting M2 polarization results in stronger antitumor immunity than enhancing M1-driven responses, especially since M2 macrophages utilize more glutamine than M1 cells. Liu et al. demonstrated that dimethyl α-KG supports M1 polarization by preventing IKKβ activation, which subsequently blocks NF-κB signaling. This regulation appears to depend on PHD-mediated hydroxylation of specific serine residues on IKKβ [94]. Glutamine metabolism plays an important regulatory role in determining macrophage phenotypes. Early in vivo studies showed that glutamine availability is necessary for cytokine production (e.g., IL-1, IL-6, TNFα), antigen presentation, and phagocytic activity in macrophages [95]. Glutaminolysis drives M1 polarization, and the uptake and metabolism of glutamine in LPS-activated M1 cells help sustain α-KG levels. This supports succinate production, enhances HIF-1α activity, and boosts pro-inflammatory cytokines such as IL-1 [96]. M2 macrophages, however, require more glutamine than M1 cells. Glutamine tends to accumulate in M2 macrophages and supports pathways associated with M2 polarization [97]. One explanation is that α-KG, produced from glutamine, activates gene expression programs consistent with an anti-inflammatory M2-like state. Additionally, M1 macrophages express low levels of glutamine synthase (GS), while M2 macrophages express high levels [98]. Recent studies further show that in IL-4–induced M2 cells, glutamine fuels both the tricarboxylic acid (TCA) cycle and the hexosamine biosynthetic pathway (HBP). The HBP produces UDP-GlcNAc, which serves as a substrate for N-glycosylation of M2-associated proteins such as CD206 and supports transcription factors like KLF4, IRF4, and CCL22, which promote M2 polarization. Some tumor-derived macrophages (e.g., TAMs from Lewis lung carcinoma) have been observed to express high levels of glutamine-metabolizing enzymes, including glutaminase, transaminases, and glutamine synthetase [99]. Furthermore, Nelson Liu et al. discovered that glutamine-mediated alternate activation of macrophages requires the nuclear receptor peroxisome proliferator-activated receptor γ (PPARγ) [100].

3.6.2 Metabolic Competition in the TME

The TME is highly intricate and diverse, containing cancer cells along with immune cells, endothelial cells, fibroblasts, and others, all interacting within a shared but specialized space [101]. Tumor cells possess elevated metabolic activity, and the surrounding cells may either compete with them—creating metabolic conflict—or assist them, leading to metabolic cooperation. Because multiple cell types within the TME depend on limited nutrients, metabolic competition is common. To overcome this, tumors often modify their metabolic pathways to either directly enhance their own proliferation or reshape the surrounding microenvironment in ways that support tumor survival. For instance, tumor cells secrete various cytokines, lactate, and the enzyme indoleamine 2,3-dioxygenase (IDO), all of which suppress T-cell growth and activity. Activation of oncogenes and increased HIF signaling also strengthen metabolic fitness in cancer cells, depriving stromal cells of essential nutrients such as glucose and glutamine [102]. This metabolic struggle contributes to immune suppression, largely through the exhaustion of immune cells [103]. In response, antitumor immune cells—including effector T cells and cytotoxic T lymphocytes (CTLs)—shift their metabolism toward increased glycolysis and glutaminolysis, placing them in direct metabolic conflict with tumor cells. Meanwhile, tumor-promoting immune populations such as Tregs, myeloid-derived suppressor cells (MDSCs), and M2 tumor-associated macrophages (TAMs) exploit metabolites generated by tumor cells, forming metabolically cooperative relationships within the TME. Research over the past twenty years has identified CAFs as major drivers of tumor progression and cell proliferation. CAFs often influence tumor growth via paracrine signaling. For example, conditioned medium from CAF cultures derived from oral carcinoma has been shown to enhance the proliferation of tongue cancer cells, indicating that a paracrine system contributes to tumor progression [104]. Additionally, CAFs isolated from prostate cancer tissue can increase proliferation rates even in normal prostate epithelial cells [105], underscoring their growth-promoting role. In a similar manner, adipocytes near the tumor site can undergo phenotypic changes in the TME and become cancer-associated adipocytes (CAA), which further support tumor development [106].

3.7 Targeting Glutamine Metabolism for Cancer Therapy

3.7.1 Pharmacological Inhibitors

GLS (Glutaminase) is an important inhibitor used in the metabolism of cancer and plays a crucial role in tumor cell survival [107]. To verify the role of GLS in cancer, there are various GLS inhibitors, common examples are CB 839, DON (6–diazido 5-oxolucine), JHU 083, BPTES, 968, and Ebselen. Among these, 968 and BPTES show antitumor potential [104]. CB 839 are orally bioavailable allosteric inhibitor derived from BPTES with greater potency and is currently under evaluation in clinical trials [108]. Previous research has shown that BPTES treatment promoted pro-inflammatory M1-like activation of macrophages, which enhances the body's antitumor immune response [94]. BPTES was also found to elevate PD-L1 expression, which can suppress the tumor-killing function of immune cells when PD-L1 binds to PD-1 on their surface [109].

CB 839 is a GLS 1 inhibitor, which influences several T cells response which, causing diverse effects on immune regulation. In vitro studies show that CB 839 treatment promoted the differentiation of CD^{4+}Th1 cells and CD^{8+} cytotoxic T lymphocytes and induced both cell types to secrete more cytokines [110]. It is found that CB 839 could bind with other anticancer drugs to enhance the therapeutic effects, and KRAS mutation increases the glucose and glutamine metabolism in ovarian cancer cells, which is inhibited by the combination of metformin and CB 839 [111]. Research has shown that pairing CB 839 with azacytidine (AZA) produces a synergistic response. This is demonstrated in a single-arm, open-label phase 1b/2 clinical trial involve patient with MDS syndrome. This trial was conducted with six participants in the dose escalation stage and twenty-four participants in the dose expansion stage. The combination therapy was generally well tolerated, achieving 70% objective remission and 53% complete remission in patients [112]. There are currently numerous studies investigating the combination of CB-839 with other drugs. For instance, in ovarian clear cell carcinoma xenograft mice, it was discovered that immune checkpoint blockage using anti-PD-L1 antibody and glutaminase inhibitor CB-839 works in concert when ARID1A inactivation is present [113]. And it is worth noting that many KRas-dependent tumors develop resistance to mTORC1 inhibition by upregulating glutamine metabolism, but the combination of mTORC1 inhibition with CB-839 can overcome this resistance [114].

Several antibiotics secreted by streptomyces bacteria, such as 6-nitro-5-oxo L norlucine (L-DON), nitroacetylserine, and glutamine analogs [115]. L-DON is an irreversible competitive inhibitor of glutamine transferase and glutaminase [116]. L-DON is a first-generation antimetabolite that inhibits glutamine enzymes and promotes a strong antitumor effect and systemic toxicity limits and provides clinical applications [117]. To address this problem, researchers developed JHU 083, which is a prodrug from L-DON, whose function is to activate the L-DON after entering the TME, which reduces its systemic toxicity and improves the antitumor immune response [118]. L-DON prevents the induction of PPAT and PAICS by glutamine and reduces Pyruvate kinase activity [119]. Another prodrug form of L-DON, which is known as sirpiglenastat (DRP 104), attempts to avoid the toxic side effects which is produced by L-DON [120]. In lung cancer with KEAP1/NRF2 mutations, DRP 104 combined with L-DON can enhance antitumor immunity [121]. Studies found that PDAC, in the absence of Glutamine, it can inhibit the synthesis of ASn to exert the tumor-suppressive effect [122].

3.7.2 Combination Strategies with Chemotherapy, Radiotherapy, and Immunotherapy

Combining therapeutic agents that target distinct metabolic routes is increasingly viewed as a more promising strategy to inhibit tumor progression. This approach is particularly valuable in situations involving synthetic lethality, where two agents jointly trigger cancer cell death, although each one alone is insufficient. Because glutamine plays a central part in numerous cellular pathways, blocking GLS activity emerges as a strong candidate for multidrug regimens. Elgogary et al. demonstrated that using BPTES together with metformin produced superior antitumor responses in pancreatic cancer compared with administering either drug independently. Metformin, an FDA-approved therapy for type 2 diabetes, disrupts glycolysis and glycogen formation. In this paired approach, BPTES interferes with glutamine utilization, while metformin limits glucose-dependent pathways, collectively generating a more effective suppression of tumor growth [123]. Additional agents that display synthetic lethality when combined with GLS inhibition include inhibitors of GLUT2q1, mTOR, and activators of ATF4 [75]. More recently, researchers have increasingly adopted combination-based strategies across diverse cancer models [124]. For example, Parlati et al. evaluated the co-administration of CB-839 and pomalidomide in myeloma models [125]. Momcilovic et al. applied a CB-839 and erlotinib regimen in lung cancer, reporting marked decreases in both glucose and glutamine uptake [126]. Emberley et al. further assessed the use of CB-839 with CDK4/6 inhibitors and PARP inhibitors across colorectal cancer (CRC), triple-negative breast cancer (TNBC), ovarian cancer, and non-small cell lung cancer [127]. Chemoradiotherapy and immunotherapy have significantly improved cancer treatment outcomes, but a considerable proportion of patients still fail to respond adequately. One major reason is the ability of tumor cells to reprogram Gln metabolism, allowing them to evade immune surveillance and develop resistance to radiation. Consequently, inhibiting Gln utilization may enhance the therapeutic efficacy of diverse anticancer modalities that act through distinct biological mechanisms. In head and neck squamous cell carcinoma, radiation exposure elevates intracellular Gln levels and upregulates the Gln transporter SLC1A5. When Gln inhibition is combined with radiotherapy, the resulting metabolic stress promotes antitumor immunity. Mechanistically, radiation increases interferon regulatory factor 1 (IRF1) through stimulation of the interferon-signaling cascade. IRF1 induction enhances transferrin receptor expression, boosts intracellular Fe^{2+} accumulation, disrupts iron homeostasis, and triggers ferroptosis in cancer cells. Blocking Gln metabolism amplifies this ferroptotic response [128]. Animal studies further demonstrate that mice lacking the Gln-synthetase gene (Gls1) show markedly improved survival following radiation treatment. These Gls1-deficient mice also present elevated natural killer cell activity and higher levels of interferon-α/γ relative to mice with normal Gls1 expression, supporting the idea that defective Gln metabolism can modulate innate immune pathways that determine radiosensitivity [129]. Mukha et al. reported that radiation-resistant prostate cancer (PCa) cells and PCa CSCs have an increased dependence on Gln [130]. Enhanced Gln metabolism not only preserves tumor cell redox balance and decreases radiation responsiveness but also maintains CSC populations by influencing α-ketoglutarate-dependent chromatin-modifying dioxygenases. Suppression of key metabolic regulators such as GLS and MYC—or restricting Gln availability—enhances radiosensitivity, reduces CSC populations in vivo, and limits tumor progression in xenograft studies. Importantly, combining Gln-targeting inhibitors with radiotherapy does not induce toxicity in nonmalignant prostate tissue. PCa cells resistant to Gln inhibition may survive radiation by activating ATG-dependent autophagy [131]. Thus, dual targeting of Gln metabolism and autophagy pathways may offer a promising strategy for treating advanced PCa. Gln inhibition may also counteract chemotherapy resistance. For example, Kim et al. demonstrated that suppressing Gln uptake increases ovarian cancer cell sensitivity to paclitaxel by inhibiting mTORC1/S6K signaling, lowering Mcl-1 expression, and enhancing Bcl-2 phosphorylation [132]. Gln metabolism can interfere with SERCA activity by lowering intracellular GSH, a process that may subsequently elevate PD-L1 expression. Combining Gln-metabolism inhibition with PD-L1 blockade has been shown to strengthen T-cell–mediated antitumor immunity [133]. Research by Tang et al. demonstrated that molybdenum disulfide (MoS2), a biocompatible and durable nanomaterial, can effectively deliver anti-PD-L1 antibodies (αPDL1) and V9302, reduce Gln uptake in cancer cells, and enhance the infiltration and activation of $CD8^+$ T cells within tumors. This combination also facilitates the movement of $CD8^+$ T cells from the tumor margins toward the central tumor region, leading to improved immunotherapy outcomes [134]. In gastric cancer models, GPNA suppresses Gln uptake by targeting the SLC1A5 transporter, thereby intensifying the antitumor effect of cetuximab in both in vivo and in vitro studies [135]. DON, a Gln structural analog, enhances $CD8^+$ T-cell cytotoxicity while inhibiting Gln metabolism in cancer cells. It has shown encouraging anticancer potential in preclinical and clinical settings; however, its clinical advancement has been hindered by gastrointestinal toxicity observed during late-phase trials. To overcome these limitations, efforts are underway to develop DON prodrugs that improve therapeutic outcomes. Among these, JHU395—a DON prodrug—exhibits superior tumor penetration and greater efficacy than DON itself. JHU395 reduces tumor growth and promotes apoptosis in high-MYC medulloblastoma models, ultimately prolonging survival [136]. DRP-104, another prodrug currently under clinical evaluation

(NCT04471415), is selectively activated within tumors, limiting systemic toxicity [137]. Metabolomic data indicate that DRP-104 strongly inhibits Gln metabolism, reduces immunosuppressive metabolites, enhances immune-cell infiltration, and drives TAMs toward an M1-like phenotype. Consequently, DRP-104 alone or in combination with immune checkpoint inhibitors may improve clinical outcomes in cancer therapy [138].

3.8 Emerging Insights and Future Directions

3.8.1 Metabolic Plasticity and Adaptive Resistance

Metabolic plasticity is now widely recognized as a key feature that enables tumor cells to grow and survive. A major example of this flexibility is the Warburg effect, where cancer cells preferentially use glycolysis instead of OXPHOS for ATP production even when oxygen is present, a process known as aerobic glycolysis [139]. Glycolysis are less ATP than OXPHOS, which is helpful in cancer because it supports rapid glucose breakdown and supplies metabolic intermediates to help synthesize nucleic acids, proteins, and lipids [140]. This metabolic reprogramming not only accelerates cell proliferation but also acidifies the tumor microenvironmentTME through lactate accumulation, which enhances invasion and weakens immune defenses [141]. Cancer therapies mainly target rapidly dividing tumor cells that depend heavily on glycolysis [142]. Some studies show that glycolytic cancer cells possess higher metabolic flexibility. They can switch between glycolysis and oxidative phosphorylation depending on the surrounding nutrient and oxygen levels [143]. Cancer metabolism is far more complex than the Warburg effect alone. Tumors display heterogeneous and adaptable metabolic behaviors, shifting between glycolysis and OXPHOS depending on intrinsic factors such as oncogenic mutations and extrinsic influences like oxygen levels, nutrient supply, or treatment stress [144]. This flexibility enables tumor cells to adapt to diverse and hostile conditions and supports survival, progression, and relapse. Cancer stem cells (CSCs) and therapy-resistant cells frequently rely on mitochondrial metabolism (e.g., increased OXPHOS or fatty acid oxidation) when stressed or in quiescent states [145]. Their metabolic profile varies not only across tumor types and patients but even within different regions of the same tumor [146]. Such variability results from a complex interaction of genetic, epigenetic, and microenvironmental cues that together regulate metabolic pathways and enzyme activity [2]. While the Warburg effect remains a foundational idea in tumor biology, recent insights show that it represents only a fragment of a broader, adaptive metabolic reprogramming characteristic of cancer. The capacity of tumor cells to dynamically switch between glycolysis and OXPHOS in response to microenvironmental changes is a major driver of tumor development and therapeutic resistance. Oncogenes such as MYC and KRAS are well-known for promoting cell proliferation, but they also exert strong control over metabolic processes. For instance, MYC enhances several metabolic pathways, including glycolysis, the TCA cycle, glutaminolysis, the pentose phosphate pathway (PPP), and fatty acid oxidation (FAO) [147]. It also stimulates glycolytic genes and transporters such as GLUT1, HK2, PFK, PDK1, and ENO1, while promoting lactate formation (via LDHA) and glutaminolysis (through MCT1, GLS, and ASCT2) [148]. These coordinated metabolic shifts increase glucose and glutamine flux into biosynthetic routes, providing precursors necessary for tumor growth. KRAS activation similarly boosts MYC expression through the MEK/ERK pathway, enhancing glucose metabolism [149]. It also promotes glycolysis (via glucose transporters and glycolytic enzymes) and alters mitochondrial function, further reinforcing cancer cell reprogramming. Cancer displays significant diversity at genetic, metabolic, and phenotypic levels, which creates major obstacles for effective treatment, as tumor cells can alter their behavior to survive in varied and often challenging microenvironments. Among the defining features of cancer metabolism, glycolysis continues to be a central therapeutic target because it is essential for sustaining cancer cell growth, survival, and tumor development. Current glycolysis-focused therapeutic strategies use small-molecule inhibitors against enzymes such as HK2, LDHA, and PKM2, as well as agents that influence lactate transport and tumor microenvironment acidification [150]. Dichloroacetate (DCA), an inhibitor of PDK1, serves as a key example of this therapeutic approach. By suppressing PDK1 activity, DCA reactivates PDH, increasing the conversion of pyruvate into acetyl-CoA and encouraging its utilization within the TCA cycle. In hepatocellular carcinoma models, DCA reduced glycolytic markers such as p-PDH/PDH, LDHA, and HK2, while simultaneously restoring mitochondrial OXPHOS function [151]. This metabolic reprogramming resulted in increased mitochondrial ROS, membrane damage, and ultimately cell-cycle arrest and apoptosis both in vitro and in vivo. Comparable effects were observed in ovarian cancer, where DCA enhanced oxidative activity and apoptosis in cisplatin-sensitive A2780 cells, which rely on glycolysis and OXPHOS [152]. However, these benefits were diminished in cisplatin-resistant A2780/DDP cells, which are predominantly glycolytic and express elevated levels of UCP2 and PDK1proteins that play a central role in regulating the glycolysis–OXPHOS metabolic switch.

3.8.2 Personalized Metabolic Therapy Approaches

The inhibition of mitochondrial complex I by this drug leads to reduced NADH oxidation and ATP synthesis, activates AMPK, and pushes metabolism toward catabolic pathways [153]. This metabolic disruption is especially harmful to OXPHOS-dependent tumor cells, including CSCs. However, despite promising preclinical observations and some epidemiological support, clinical outcomes have been inconsistent, creating uncertainty about its usefulness as an anticancer agent [154]. These mixed results highlight the need for more rigorous and carefully structured trials to accurately determine its therapeutic benefit. Because mitochondrial metabolism includes several enzyme targets within the ETC, additional OXPHOS inhibitors—such as phenformin, IACS-010759, IM156, BAY87–2243, ME-344, and VLX600—are being explored [155]. Studies show that metformin is used as a dual metabolic pathway inhibitor. Primarily, it is used as an antidiabetic medication. Recently, its anticancer properties have been identified; it inhibits cancer cell survival by suppressing glycolysis and oxidative phosphorylation [156]. Metformin also reduces glycolysis in liver cancer cells and removes prostate and colon cancer cells by radiotherapy. Studies show that metformin reduces OXPHOS activity by inhibiting complex I in the ETC [157]. For a patient with both diabetes and cancer, metformin was able to improve the overall prognosis. A similar diabetic drug, Phenformin also able to remove trigger cell death in lung cancer cells [158]. Metabolic plasticity is essential for CSC survival; exploiting these metabolic shifts is crucial for improving therapeutic responses. Research should prioritize understanding metabolic regulators such as transcription factors (MYC, KRAS, HIF-1α), epigenetic programs, and post-translational modifications that influence CSC behavior [144]. Mitochondrial processes, including fusion, fission, and mitophagy, have emerged as central drivers of CSC metabolism, particularly in governing the glycolysis-to-OXPHOS switch, and thus may serve as promising therapeutic points [159]. Because metabolic pathways are regulated differently depending on the signaling environment, targeting upstream regulators may enhance treatment precision and efficacy. Preclinical findings show that simultaneously blocking glycolysis and OXPHOS can restrain CSC metabolic adaptation and reduce treatment resistance [160]. Using metabolic inhibitors alongside agents that disrupt CSC-specific pathways—such as Wnt or Notch—may further improve therapeutic outcomes. CSCs that remain largely quiescent yet strongly depend on mitochondrial activity appear especially vulnerable to OXPHOS inhibitors [161]. For example, ClpP agonists interrupt mitochondrial homeostasis, induce redox imbalance, and impair one-carbon and proline metabolism, collectively reducing CSC function [162]. Leveraging nutrient dependencies, such as glutamine metabolism, may also offer effective strategies for suppressing CSC-specific metabolic programs linked to stemness and survival [163]. Differences in CSC metabolic phenotypes often arise from tumor heterogeneity, genetic variation, and methodological inconsistencies. Emerging tools such as spatial transcriptomics and single-cell metabolomics provide high-resolution insights into CSC metabolism and its interaction with the tumor microenvironment. These technologies make it possible to study how metabolic states vary across individual CSCs and how these changes relate to spatial and functional differences within the tumor. For instance, Liu et al. (2024) applied spatial transcriptomics to squamous cell carcinoma and identified spatially distinct metabolic programs linked to immune suppression [164]. Compared to bulk or dissociated single-cell approaches, spatial transcriptomics preserves tissue architecture, allowing researchers to observe metabolic interactions in situ. Single-cell metabolomics can further identify heterogeneous metabolic signatures, reveal regulatory mechanisms, and clarify the drivers of metabolic shifts. These tools also help uncover how treatment-induced stress reshapes CSC metabolism. As a result, metabolic profiling can significantly improve the identification of biomarkers with diagnostic, prognostic, and therapeutic relevance. Moreover, these technologies can detect tumor-specific metabolic vulnerabilities suitable for precision treatments.

3.9 Conclusion

Glutamine is a critical nexus in cancer metabolism, simultaneously fueling the TCA cycle, biosynthetic processes (amino acids, nucleotides, lipids), and redox homeostasis (glutathione) to support proliferation and survival. Oncogenic programs (MYC, KRAS, p53, HIF-1α) rewire glutamine uptake and catabolism, integrating with mTORC1 and growth signals to drive tumor expansion. Within the tumor microenvironment, malignant cells' "glutamine addiction" (e.g., via ASCT2) competes with immune cells for this nutrient, skewing T cells and macrophages toward an immunosuppressive phenotype. Because of its centrality, glutamine metabolism is a prime therapeutic target; blocking glutaminase (e.g., with CB-839) impairs tumor growth, and combining glutamine blockade with chemotherapy, radiotherapy, or immunotherapy can overcome adaptive resistance. Finally, the metabolic plasticity of tumors—their ability to switch pathways under stress—underscores the need for dual-targeted and personalized strategies. Advanced metabolic profiling and single-cell techniques promise to identify glutamine-dependent vulnerabilities and guide precision therapies.

References

1. Navarro C, Ortega Á, Santeliz R, Garrido B, Chacín M, Galban N, Vera I, De Sanctis JB, Bermúdez V. Metabolic reprogramming in cancer cells: emerging molecular mechanisms and novel therapeutic approaches. Pharmaceutics. 2022;14(6):1303.
2. Faubert B, Solmonson A, DeBerardinis RJ. Metabolic reprogramming and cancer progression. Science. 2020;368(6487):eaaw5473.
3. Schiliro C, Firestein BL. Mechanisms of metabolic reprogramming in cancer cells supporting enhanced growth and proliferation. Cells. 2021;10(5):1056.
4. Min HY, Lee HY. Oncogene-driven metabolic alterations in cancer. Biomol Ther. 2017;26(1):45.
5. Nakahara R, Maeda K, Aki S, Osawa T. Metabolic adaptations of cancer in extreme tumor microenvironments. Cancer Sci. 2023;114(4):1200–7.
6. Smith RJ. Glutamine metabolism and its physiologic importance. J Parenter Enter Nutr. 1990;14:40S–4S.
7. Daye D, Wellen KE. Metabolic reprogramming in cancer: unraveling the role of glutamine in tumorigenesis. InSeminars in cell & developmental biology 2012 (Vol. 23, no. 4, pp. 362–369). Academic Press.
8. Jin J, Byun JK, Choi YK, Park KG. Targeting glutamine metabolism as a therapeutic strategy for cancer. Exp Mol Med. 2023;55(4):706–15.
9. Cyriac R, Lee K. Glutaminase inhibition as potential cancer therapeutics: current status and future applications. J Enzyme Inhib Med Chem. 2024;39(1):2290911.
10. Li S, Zeng H, Fan J, Wang F, Xu C, Li Y, Tu J, Nephew KP, Long X. Glutamine metabolism in breast cancer and possible therapeutic targets. Biochem Pharmacol. 2023;210:115464.
11. Kumar MA, Baba SK, Khan IR, Khan MS, Husain FM, Ahmad S, Haris M, Singh M, Akil AS, Macha MA, Bhat AA. Glutamine metabolism: molecular regulation, biological functions, and diseases. MedComm. 2025;6(7):e70120.
12. El Ansari R, Craze ML, Miligy I, Diez-Rodriguez M, Nolan CC, Ellis IO, Rakha EA, Green AR. The amino acid transporter SLC7A5 confers a poor prognosis in the highly proliferative

breast cancer subtypes and is a key therapeutic target in luminal B tumours. Breast Cancer Res. 2018;20(1):21.
13. Hossen MS, Islam MS, Yasin M, Ibrahim M, Das A. A review on the role of human solute carriers transporters in cancer. Health Science Reports. 2025;8(1):e70343.
14. Bhutia YD, Ganapathy V. Glutamine transporters in mammalian cells and their functions in physiology and cancer. Biochimica et Biophysica Acta (BBA)-Mol Cell Res. 2016;1863(10):2531–9.
15. Bak LK, Schousboe A, Waagepetersen HS. The glutamate/GABA-glutamine cycle: aspects of transport, neurotransmitter homeostasis and ammonia transfer. J Neurochem. 2006;98(3):641–53.
16. Chen JQ, Russo J. Dysregulation of glucose transport, glycolysis, TCA cycle and glutaminolysis by oncogenes and tumor suppressors in cancer cells. Biochimica et Biophysica Acta (BBA)-Rev Cancer. 2012;1826(2):370–384.
17. Martins F, Gonçalves LG, Pojo M, Serpa J. Take advantage of glutamine anaplerosis, the kernel of the metabolic rewiring in malignant gliomas. Biomolecules. 2020;10(10):1370.
18. De los Santos-Jiménez J, Campos-Sandoval JA, Alonso FJ, Márquez J, Matés JM. GLS and GLS2 glutaminase isoenzymes in the antioxidant system of cancer cells. Antioxidants. 2024;13(6):745.
19. Bornstein R, Mulholland MT, Sedensky M, Morgan P, Johnson SC. Glutamine metabolism in diseases associated with mitochondrial dysfunction. Mol Cell Neurosci. 2023;126:103887.
20. Tambay V, Raymond VA, Bilodeau M. MYC rules: leading glutamine metabolism toward a distinct cancer cell phenotype. Cancer. 2021;13(17):4484.
21. Chen T, Xu Y, Yang F, Pan Y, Ji N, Li J, Zeng X, Chen Q, Jiang L, Shen YQ. Crosstalk of glutamine metabolism between cancer-associated fibroblasts and cancer cells. Cell Signal. 2025;133:111874.
22. Ferreira A, Pereira F, Reis C, Oliveira MJ, Sousa MJ, Preto A. Crucial role of oncogenic KRAS mutations in apoptosis and autophagy regulation: therapeutic implications. Cells. 2022;11(14):2183.
23. Li X, Peng X, Li Y, Wei S, He G, Liu J, Li X, Yang S, Li D, Lin W, Fang J. Glutamine addiction in tumor cell: oncogene regulation and clinical treatment. Cell Commun Signal. 2024;22(1):12.
24. Zeng Y, Tao Y, Du G, Huang T, Chen S, Fan L, Zhang N. Advances in the mechanisms of HIF-1α-enhanced tumor glycolysis and its relation to dedifferentiation. Prog Biophys Mol Biol. 2025;197:1.
25. Zhu M, Lu EQ, Yan L, Liu G, Huang K, Xu E, Zhang YY, Li XG. Phospholipase D mediates glutamine-induced mTORC1 activation to promote porcine intestinal epithelial cell proliferation. J Nutr. 2024;154(4):1119–29.
26. Feng HG, Wu CX, Zhong GC, Gong JP, Miao CM, Xiong B. Integrative analysis reveals that SLC38A1 promotes hepatocellular carcinoma development via PI3K/AKT/mTOR signaling via glutamine mediated energy metabolism. J Cancer Res Clin Oncol. 2023;149(17):15879–98.
27. Badoiu SC, Greabu M, Miricescu D, Stanescu-Spinu II, Ilinca R, Balan DG, Balcangiu-Stroescu AE, Mihai DA, Vacaroiu IA, Stefani C, Jinga V. PI3K/AKT/mTOR dysregulation and reprogramming metabolic pathways in renal cancer: crosstalk with the VHL/HIF axis. Int J Mol Sci. 2023;24(9):8391.
28. Wise DR, DeBerardinis RJ, Mancuso A, Sayed N, Zhang XY, Pfeiffer HK, Nissim I, Daikhin E, Yudkoff M, McMahon SB, Thompson CB. Myc regulates a transcriptional program that stimulates mitochondrial glutaminolysis and leads to glutamine addiction. Proc Natl Acad Sci. 2008;105(48):18782–7.
29. Wong CC, Xu J, Bian X, Wu JL, Kang W, Qian Y, Li W, Chen H, Gou H, Liu D, Luk ST. In colorectal cancer cells with mutant KRAS, SLC25A22-mediated glutaminolysis reduces DNA demethylation to increase WNT signaling, stemness, and drug resistance. Gastroenterology. 2020;159(6):2163–80.
30. Li X, Zhang HS. Amino acid metabolism, redox balance and epigenetic regulation in cancer. FEBS J. 2024;291(3):412–29.

31. Xu X, Peng Q, Jiang X, Tan S, Yang Y, Yang W, Han Y, Chen Y, Oyang L, Lin J, Xia L. Metabolic reprogramming and epigenetic modifications in cancer: from the impacts and mechanisms to the treatment potential. Exp Mol Med. 2023;55(7):1357–70.
32. Gao Y, Zhang X, Du Y, Ni T, Hao S. Crosstalk between metabolic and epigenetic modifications during cell carcinogenesis. Iscience. 2024;27(12)
33. Xiao-Yan W, Xiao-Xia Y, Peng-Fei S, Zong-Xue Z, Xiu-Li G. Metabolic reprogramming of glutamine involved in tumorigenesis, multidrug resistance and tumor immunity. Eur J Pharmacol. 2023;940:175323.
34. Zhu Y, Li T, Ramos da Silva S, Lee JJ, Lu C, Eoh H, Jung JU, Gao SJ. A critical role of glutamine and asparagine γ-nitrogen in nucleotide biosynthesis in cancer cells hijacked by an oncogenic virus. MBio. 2017;8(4):10–128.
35. Brose SA, Marquardt AL, Golovko MY. Fatty acid biosynthesis from glutamate and glutamine is specifically induced in neuronal cells under hypoxia. J Neurochem. 2014;129(3):400–12.
36. Wang Y, Bai C, Ruan Y, Liu M, Chu Q, Qiu L, Yang C, Li B. Coordinative metabolism of glutamine carbon and nitrogen in proliferating cancer cells under hypoxia. Nat Commun. 2019;10(1):201.
37. Jiang ZF, Wang M, Xu JL, Ning YJ. Hypoxia promotes mitochondrial glutamine metabolism through HIF1α-GDH pathway in human lung cancer cells. Biochem Biophys Res Commun. 2017;483(1):32–8.
38. Cha YJ, Kim ES, Koo JS. Amino acid transporters and glutamine metabolism in breast cancer. Int J Mol Sci. 2018;19(3):907.
39. Fan Y, Xue H, Li Z, Huo M, Gao H, Guan X. Exploiting the Achilles' heel of cancer: disrupting glutamine metabolism for effective cancer treatment. Front Pharmacol. 2024;15:1345522.
40. Yoo HC, Yu YC, Sung Y, Han JM. Glutamine reliance in cell metabolism. Exp Mol Med. 2020;52(9):1496–516.
41. Jeong SM, Hwang S, Park K, Yang S, Seong RH. Enhanced mitochondrial glutamine anaplerosis suppresses pancreatic cancer growth through autophagy inhibition. Sci Rep. 2016;6(1):30767.
42. Alam MM, Lal S, FitzGerald KE, Zhang L. A holistic view of cancer bioenergetics: mitochondrial function and respiration play fundamental roles in the development and progression of diverse tumors. Clin Transl Med. 2016;5(1):3.
43. Solaini G, Sgarbi G, Baracca A. Oxidative phosphorylation in cancer cells. Biochimica et Biophysica Acta (BBA)-Bioenergetics. 2011;1807(6):534–42.
44. Rajagopalan KN, DeBerardinis RJ. Role of glutamine in cancer: therapeutic and imaging implications. J Nucl Med. 2011;52(7):1005–8.
45. Li J, Xiang L, Wang S, Zhang Y, Zhao S, Zhang D, Meng X, Zhang Y, Lin JM. Targeting the crosstalk between glutamine metabolism and tumor immune microenvironment for lung cancer immunotherapy. Interdisciplinary Medicine. 2025;3(2):e20240069.
46. Li Z, Zhang H. Reprogramming of glucose, fatty acid and amino acid metabolism for cancer progression. Cell Mol Life Sci. 2016;73(2):377–92.
47. Ge T, Gu X, Jia R, Ge S, Chai P, Zhuang A, Fan X. Crosstalk between metabolic reprogramming and epigenetics in cancer: updates on mechanisms and therapeutic opportunities. Cancer Commun. 2022;42(11):1049–82.
48. Fan J, Kamphorst JJ, Mathew R, Chung MK, White E, Shlomi T, Rabinowitz JD. Glutamine-driven oxidative phosphorylation is a major ATP source in transformed mammalian cells in both normoxia and hypoxia. Mol Syst Biol. 2013;9(1):712.
49. Thorén MM, Vaapil M, Staaf J, Planck M, Johansson ME, Mohlin S, Påhlman S. Myc-induced glutaminolysis bypasses HIF-driven glycolysis in hypoxic small cell lung carcinoma cells. Oncotarget. 2017;8(30):48983.
50. Mullen AR, Wheaton WW, Jin ES, Chen PH, Sullivan LB, Cheng T, Yang Y, Linehan WM, Chandel NS, DeBerardinis RJ. Reductive carboxylation supports growth in tumour cells with defective mitochondria. Nature. 2012;481(7381):385–8.

51. Degenhardt K, Mathew R, Beaudoin B, Bray K, Anderson D, Chen G, Mukherjee C, Shi Y, Gélinas C, Fan Y, Nelson DA. Autophagy promotes tumor cell survival and restricts necrosis, inflammation, and tumorigenesis. Cancer Cell. 2006;10(1):51–64.
52. Dikic I, Elazar Z. Mechanism and medical implications of mammalian autophagy. Nat Rev Mol Cell Biol. 2018;19(6):349–64.
53. Cruzat V, Macedo Rogero M, Noel Keane K, Curi R, Newsholme P. Glutamine: metabolism and immune function, supplementation and clinical translation. Nutrients. 2018;10(11):1564.
54. Amaravadi RK, Yu D, Lum JJ, Bui T, Christophorou MA, Evan GI, Thomas-Tikhonenko A, Thompson CB. Autophagy inhibition enhances therapy-induced apoptosis in a Myc-induced model of lymphoma. J Clin Invest. 2007;117(2):326–36.
55. Mizushima N, Yoshimori T, Ohsumi Y. The role of Atg proteins in autophagosome formation. Annu Rev Cell Dev Biol. 2011;27(1):107–32.
56. Jung CH, Jun CB, Ro SH, Kim YM, Otto NM, Cao J, Kundu M, Kim DH. ULK-Atg13-FIP200 complexes mediate mTOR signaling to the autophagy machinery. Mol Biol Cell. 2009;20(7):1992–2003.
57. Mizushima N. The role of the Atg1/ULK1 complex in autophagy regulation. Curr Opin Cell Biol. 2010;22(2):132–9.
58. Pattingre S, Espert L, Biard-Piechaczyk M, Codogno P. Regulation of macroautophagy by mTOR and Beclin 1 complexes. Biochimie. 2008;90(2):313–23.
59. Matsushita M, Suzuki NN, Obara K, Fujioka Y, Ohsumi Y, Inagaki F. Structure of Atg5·Atg16, a complex essential for autophagy. J Biol Chem. 2007;282(9):6763–72.
60. Satoo K, Noda NN, Kumeta H, Fujioka Y, Mizushima N, Ohsumi Y, Inagaki F. The structure of Atg4B–LC3 complex reveals the mechanism of LC3 processing and delipidation during autophagy. EMBO J. 2009;28(9):1341–50.
61. Qu X, Yu J, Bhagat G, Furuya N, Hibshoosh H, Troxel A, Rosen J, Eskelinen EL, Mizushima N, Ohsumi Y, Cattoretti G. Promotion of tumorigenesis by heterozygous disruption of the beclin 1 autophagy gene. J Clin Invest. 2003;112(12):1809–20.
62. Liang XH, Jackson S, Seaman M, Brown K, Kempkes B, Hibshoosh H, Levine B. Induction of autophagy and inhibition of tumorigenesis by beclin 1. Nature. 1999;402(6762):672–6.
63. Mathew R, Karp CM, Beaudoin B, Vuong N, Chen G, Chen HY, Bray K, Reddy A, Bhanot G, Gelinas C, DiPaola RS. Autophagy suppresses tumorigenesis through elimination of p62. Cell. 2009;137(6):1062–75.
64. Duran A, Linares JF, Galvez AS, Wikenheiser K, Flores JM, Diaz-Meco MT, Moscat J. The signaling adaptor p62 is an important NF-κB mediator in tumorigenesis. Cancer Cell. 2008;13(4):343–54.
65. Tang D, Kang R, Livesey KM, Cheh CW, Farkas A, Loughran P, Hoppe G, Bianchi ME, Tracey KJ, Zeh HJ III, Lotze MT. Endogenous HMGB1 regulates autophagy. J Cell Biol. 2010;190(5):881–92.
66. Semenza GL. HIF-1: upstream and downstream of cancer metabolism. Curr Opin Genet Dev. 2010;20(1):51–6.
67. Guo JY, Chen HY, Mathew R, Fan J, Strohecker AM, Karsli-Uzunbas G, Kamphorst JJ, Chen G, Lemons JM, Karantza V, Coller HA. Activated Ras requires autophagy to maintain oxidative metabolism and tumorigenesis. Genes Dev. 2011;25(5):460–70.
68. Quail DF, Joyce JA. Microenvironmental regulation of tumor progression and metastasis. Nat Med. 2013;19(11):1423–37.
69. Huang R, Wang H, Hong J, Wu J, Huang O, He J, Chen W, Li Y, Chen X, Shen K, Wang Z. Targeting glutamine metabolic reprogramming of SLC7A5 enhances the efficacy of anti-PD-1 in triple-negative breast cancer. Front Immunol. 2023;14:1251643.
70. Edwards DN, Ngwa VM, Raybuck AL, Wang S, Hwang Y, Kim LC, Cho SH, Paik Y, Wang Q, Zhang S, Manning HC. Selective glutamine metabolism inhibition in tumor cells improves antitumor T lymphocyte activity in triple-negative breast cancer. J Clin Invest. 2021;131(4)
71. Spada M, Piras C, Diana G, Leoni VP, Frau DV, Serreli G, Simbula G, Loi R, Noto A, Murgia F, Caria P. Glutamine starvation affects cell cycle, oxidative homeostasis and metabolism in colorectal cancer cells. Antioxidants. 2023;12(3):683.

72. Newsholme P, Curi R, Curi TP, Murphy CJ, Garcia C, De Melo MP. Glutamine metabolism by lymphocytes, macrophages, and neutrophils: its importance in health and disease. J Nutr Biochem. 1999;10(6):316–24.
73. Abou Ziki R, Colnot S. Glutamine metabolism, a double agent combating or fuelling hepatocellular carcinoma. JHEP Reports. 2024;6(5):101077.
74. Zhang J, Pavlova NN, Thompson CB. Cancer cell metabolism: the essential role of the nonessential amino acid, glutamine. EMBO J. 2017;36(10):1302–15.
75. Altman BJ, Stine ZE, Dang CV. From Krebs to clinic: glutamine metabolism to cancer therapy. Nat Rev Cancer. 2016;16(10):619–34.
76. Yang L, Venneti S, Nagrath D. Glutaminolysis: a hallmark of cancer metabolism. Annu Rev Biomed Eng. 2017;19:163–94.
77. Wang B, Pei J, Xu S, Liu J, Yu J. A glutamine tug-of-war between cancer and immune cells: recent advances in unraveling the ongoing battle. J Exp Clin Cancer Res. 2024;43(1):74.
78. Jayarajan S, Daly JM. The relationships of nutrients, routes of delivery, and immunocompetence. Surgical Clinics. 2011;91(4):737–53.
79. Buck MD, O'sullivan D, Pearce EL. T cell metabolism drives immunity. J Exp Med. 2015;212(9):1345.
80. Ma G, Zhang Z, Li P, Zhang Z, Zeng M, Liang Z, Li D, Wang L, Chen Y, Liang Y, Niu H. Reprogramming of glutamine metabolism and its impact on immune response in the tumor microenvironment. Cell Communication and Signaling. 2022;20(1):114.
81. Bailey SR, Nelson MH, Himes RA, Li Z, Mehrotra S, Paulos CM. Th17 cells in cancer: the ultimate identity crisis. Front Immunol. 2014;5:276.
82. Li G, Liu L, Yin Z, Ye Z, Shen N. Glutamine metabolism is essential for the production of IL-17A in γδ T cells and skin inflammation. Tissue Cell. 2021;71:101569.
83. Johnson MO, Wolf MM, Madden MZ, Andrejeva G, Sugiura A, Contreras DC, Maseda D, Liberti MV, Paz K, Kishton RJ, Johnson ME. Distinct regulation of Th17 and Th1 cell differentiation by glutaminase-dependent metabolism. Cell. 2018;175(7):1780–95.
84. Xiao M, Yang H, Xu W, Ma S, Lin H, Zhu H, Liu L, Liu Y, Yang C, Xu Y, Zhao S. Inhibition of α-KG-dependent histone and DNA demethylases by fumarate and succinate that are accumulated in mutations of FH and SDH tumor suppressors. Genes Dev. 2012;26(12):1326–38.
85. Loftus RM, Assmann N, Kedia-Mehta N, O'Brien KL, Garcia A, Gillespie C, Hukelmann JL, Oefner PJ, Lamond AI, Gardiner CM, Dettmer K. Amino acid-dependent cMyc expression is essential for NK cell metabolic and functional responses in mice. Nat Commun. 2018;9(1):2341.
86. Suzuki J, Yamada T, Inoue K, Nabe S, Kuwahara M, Takemori N, Takemori A, Matsuda S, Kanoh M, Imai Y, Yasukawa M. The tumor suppressor menin prevents effector CD8 T-cell dysfunction by targeting mTORC1-dependent metabolic activation. Nat Commun. 2018;9(1):3296.
87. Vallion R, Divoux J, Glauzy S, Ronin E, Lombardi Y, Lubrano di Ricco M, Grégoire S, Nemazanyy I, Durand A, Fradin D, Lucas B. Regulatory T cell stability and migration are dependent on mTOR. J Immunol. 2020;205(7):1799–809.
88. Kieler M, Hofmann M, Schabbauer G. More than just protein building blocks: how amino acids and related metabolic pathways fuel macrophage polarization. FEBS J. 2021;288(12):3694–714.
89. Biswas SK, Mantovani A. Macrophage plasticity and interaction with lymphocyte subsets: cancer as a paradigm. Nat Immunol. 2010;11(10):889–96.
90. Xue J, Schmidt SV, Sander J, Draffehn A, Krebs W, Quester I, De Nardo D, Gohel TD, Emde M, Schmidleithner L, Ganesan H. Transcriptome-based network analysis reveals a spectrum model of human macrophage activation. Immunity. 2014;40(2):274–88.
91. Biswas SK, Allavena P, Mantovani A. Tumor-associated macrophages: functional diversity, clinical significance, and open questions. InSeminars in immunopathology 2013 (Vol. 35, no. 5, pp. 585–600). Berlin/Heidelberg: Springer Berlin Heidelberg.

92. Du B, Jiao Q, Bai Y, Yu M, Pang M, Zhao M, Ma H, Yao H. Glutamine metabolism-regulated nanoparticles to enhance chemoimmunotherapy by increasing antigen presentation efficiency. ACS Appl Mater Interfaces. 2022;14(7):8753–65.
93. Fu Q, Xu L, Wang Y, Jiang Q, Liu Z, Zhang J, Zhou Q, Zeng H, Tong S, Wang T, Qi Y. Tumor-associated macrophage-derived interleukin-23 interlinks kidney cancer glutamine addiction with immune evasion. Eur Urol. 2019;75(5):752–63.
94. Liu PS, Wang H, Li X, Chao T, Teav T, Christen S, Di Conza G, Cheng WC, Chou CH, Vavakova M, Muret C. α-Ketoglutarate orchestrates macrophage activation through metabolic and epigenetic reprogramming. Nat Immunol. 2017;18(9):985–94.
95. Tannahill GÁ, Curtis AM, Adamik J, Palsson-McDermott EM, McGettrick AF, Goel G, Frezza C, Bernard NJ, Kelly B, Foley NH, Zheng L. Succinate is an inflammatory signal that induces IL-1β through HIF-1α. Nature. 2013;496(7444):238–42.
96. Jha AK, Huang SC, Sergushichev A, Lampropoulou V, Ivanova Y, Loginicheva E, Chmielewski K, Stewart KM, Ashall J, Everts B, Pearce EJ. Network integration of parallel metabolic and transcriptional data reveals metabolic modules that regulate macrophage polarization. Immunity. 2015;42(3):419–30.
97. Ren W, Xia Y, Chen S, Wu G, Bazer FW, Zhou B, Tan B, Zhu G, Deng J, Yin Y. Glutamine metabolism in macrophages: a novel target for obesity/type 2 diabetes. Adv Nutr. 2019;10(2):321–30.
98. Palmieri EM, Menga A, Martín-Pérez R, Quinto A, Riera-Domingo C, De Tullio G, Hooper DC, Lamers WH, Ghesquière B, McVicar DW, Guarini A. Pharmacologic or genetic targeting of glutamine synthetase skews macrophages toward an M1-like phenotype and inhibits tumor metastasis. Cell Rep. 2017;20(7):1654–66.
99. Colegio OR, Chu NQ, Szabo AL, Chu T, Rhebergen AM, Jairam V, Cyrus N, Brokowski CE, Eisenbarth SC, Phillips GM, Cline GW. Functional polarization of tumour-associated macrophages by tumour-derived lactic acid. Nature. 2014;513(7519):559–63.
100. Nelson VL, Nguyen HC, Garcìa-Cañaveras JC, Briggs ER, Ho WY, DiSpirito JR, Marinis JM, Hill DA, Lazar MA. PPARγ is a nexus controlling alternative activation of macrophages via glutamine metabolism. Genes Dev. 2018;32(15–16):1035–44.
101. Hanahan D, Coussens LM. Accessories to the crime: functions of cells recruited to the tumor microenvironment. Cancer Cell. 2012;21(3):309–22.
102. Wang T, Liu G, Wang R. The intercellular metabolic interplay between tumor and immune cells. Front Immunol. 2014;5:358.
103. Ho PC, Bihuniak JD, Macintyre AN, Staron M, Liu X, Amezquita R, Tsui YC, Cui G, Micevic G, Perales JC, Kleinstein SH. Phosphoenolpyruvate is a metabolic checkpoint of anti-tumor T cell responses. Cell. 2015;162(6):1217–28.
104. Usart M, Hansen N, Stetka J, Almeida Fonseca T, Guy A, Kimmerlin Q, Rai S, Hao-Shen H, Roux J, Dirnhofer S, Skoda RC. The glutaminase inhibitor CB-839 targets metabolic dependencies of JAK2-mutant hematopoiesis in MPN. Blood Adv. 2024;8(9):2312–25.
105. Izar B, Joyce CE, Goff S, Cho NL, Shah PM, Sharma G, Li J, Ibrahim N, Gold J, Hodi FS, Garraway LA. Bidirectional cross talk between patient-derived melanoma and cancer-associated fibroblasts promotes invasion and proliferation. Pigment Cell Melanoma Res. 2016;29(6):656–68.
106. Romero IL, Mukherjee A, Kenny HA, Litchfield LM, Lengyel E. Molecular pathways: trafficking of metabolic resources in the tumor microenvironment. Clin Cancer Res. 2015;21(4):680–6.
107. Wang JB, Erickson JW, Fuji R, Ramachandran S, Gao P, Dinavahi R, Wilson KF, Ambrosio AL, Dias SM, Dang CV, Cerione RA. Targeting mitochondrial glutaminase activity inhibits oncogenic transformation. Cancer Cell. 2010;18(3):207–19.
108. Gross MI, Demo SD, Dennison JB, Chen L, Chernov-Rogan T, Goyal B, Janes JR, Laidig GJ, Lewis ER, Li J, MacKinnon AL. Antitumor activity of the glutaminase inhibitor CB-839 in triple-negative breast cancer. Mol Cancer Ther. 2014;13(4):890–901.

109. Byun JK, Park M, Lee S, Yun JW, Lee J, Kim JS, Cho SJ, Jeon HJ, Lee IK, Choi YK, Park KG. Inhibition of glutamine utilization synergizes with immune checkpoint inhibitor to promote antitumor immunity. Mol Cell. 2020;80(4):592–606.
110. Yang WH, Qiu Y, Stamatatos O, Janowitz T, Lukey MJ. Enhancing the efficacy of glutamine metabolism inhibitors in cancer therapy. Trends in cancer. 2021;7(8):790–804.
111. Wu H, Zhang J, Wang Q, Li Z, Li L, Xie Y. Metformin combined with CB-839 specifically inhibits KRAS-mutant ovarian cancer. Sci Rep. 2025;15(1):6072.
112. DiNardo CD, Verma D, Baran N, Bhagat TD, Skwarska A, Lodi A, Saxena K, Cai T, Su X, Guerra VA, Poigaialwar G. Glutaminase inhibition in combination with azacytidine in myelodysplastic syndromes: a phase 1b/2 clinical trial and correlative analyses. Nature Cancer. 2024;5(10):1515–33.
113. Wu S, Fukumoto T, Lin J, Nacarelli T, Wang Y, Ong D, Liu H, Fatkhutdinov N, Zundell JA, Karakashev S, Zhou W. Targeting glutamine dependence through GLS1 inhibition suppresses ARID1A-inactivated clear cell ovarian carcinoma. Nature cancer. 2021;2(2):189–200.
114. Matés JM, Campos-Sandoval JA, de Los S-JJ, Márquez J. Glutaminases regulate glutathione and oxidative stress in cancer. Arch Toxicol. 2020;94(8):2603–23.
115. Nitenberg G, Dechelotte P. Is immune nutrition the Holy Grail for cancer patients. In Nestle Nutr Workshop Ser Clin Perform Programme 2000 (Vol. 4, pp. 255–72).
116. Villalba M, Lopez-Royuela N, Krzywinska E, G Rathore M, A Hipskind R, Haouas H, Allende-Vega N. Chemical metabolic inhibitors for the treatment of blood-borne cancers. Anti-Cancer Agents in Medicinal Chemistry (Formerly Current Medicinal Chemistry-Anti-Cancer Agents). 2014;14(2):223–32.
117. Magill GB, Myers WP, Reilly HC, Putnam RC, Magill JW, Sykes MP, Escher GC, Karnofsky DA, Burchenal JH. Pharmacological and initial therapeutic observations on 6-Diazo-5-Oxo-L-Norleucine (Don) in human neoplastic disease. Cancer. 1957;10(6):1138–50.
118. Rais R, Jancarik A, Tenora L, Nedelcovych M, Alt J, Englert J, Rojas C, Le A, Elgogary A, Tan J, Monincova L. Discovery of 6-diazo-5-oxo-l-norleucine (DON) prodrugs with enhanced CSF delivery in monkeys: a potential treatment for glioblastoma. J Med Chem. 2016;59(18):8621–33.
119. Yang WH, Qiu Y, Stamatatos O, Janowitz T, Lukey MJ. Enhancing the efficacy of glutamine metabolism inhibitors in cancer therapy. Trend Cancer. 2021;7(8):790–804.
120. Encarnacion-Rosado J, Sohn AS, Biancur DE, Lin EY, Osorio-Vasquez V, Rodrick T, González-Baerga D, Zhao E, Yokoyama Y, Simeone DM, Jones DR. Targeting pancreatic cancer metabolic dependencies through glutamine antagonism. Nat Cancer. 2024;5(1):85–99.
121. Blatt EB, DeBerardinis RJ. Glutamine antagonists may KEAP lung cancer in check. Science Advances. 2024;10(13):eado7808.
122. Recouvreux MV, Grenier SF, Zhang Y, Esparza E, Lambies G, Galapate CM, Maganti S, Duong-Polk K, Bhullar D, Naeem R, Scott DA. Glutamine mimicry suppresses tumor progression through asparagine metabolism in pancreatic ductal adenocarcinoma. Nature cancer. 2024;5(1):100–13.
123. Elgogary A, Xu Q, Poore B, Alt J, Zimmermann SC, Zhao L, Fu J, Chen B, Xia S, Liu Y, Neisser M. Combination therapy with BPTES nanoparticles and metformin targets the metabolic heterogeneity of pancreatic cancer. Proc Natl Acad Sci. 2016;113(36):E5328–36.
124. Meng Y, Xu XI, Luan H, Li L, Dai W, Li Z, Bian J. The progress and development of GLUT1 inhibitors targeting cancer energy metabolism. Future Med Chem. 2019;11(17):2333–52.
125. Parlati F, Gross M, Janes J, Lewis E, MacKinnon A, Rodriguez M, Shwonek P, Bennett M. Glutaminase inhibitor CB-839 synergizes with pomalidomide in preclinical multiple myeloma models. Blood. 2014;124(21):4720.
126. Momcilovic M, Bailey ST, Lee JT, Fishbein MC, Magyar C, Braas D, Graeber T, Jackson NJ, Czernin J, Emberley E, Gross M. Targeted inhibition of EGFR and glutaminase induces metabolic crisis in EGFR mutant lung cancer. Cell Rep. 2017;18(3):601–10.

127. Emberley ED, Bennett M, Chen J, Gross M, Huang T, Makkouk A, Marguier G, Pan A, Spurlock SM, Steggerda S, Parlati F. The glutaminase inhibitor CB-839 synergizes with CDK4/6 and PARP inhibitors in pre-clinical tumor models. Cancer Res. 2018;78(13_Supplement):3509.
128. Song A, Wu L, Zhang BX, Yang QC, Liu YT, Li H, Mao L, Xiong D, Yu HJ, Sun ZJ. Glutamine inhibition combined with CD47 blockade enhances radiotherapy-induced ferroptosis in head and neck squamous cell carcinoma. Cancer Lett. 2024;588:216727.
129. Patel R, Cooper DE, Kadakia KT, Allen A, Duan L, Luo L, Williams NT, Liu X, Locasale JW, Kirsch DG. Targeting glutamine metabolism improves sarcoma response to radiation therapy in vivo. Commun Biol. 2024;7(1):608.
130. Mukha A, Kahya U, Linge A, Chen O, Löck S, Lukiyanchuk V, Richter S, Alves TC, Peitzsch M, Telychko V, Skvortsov S. GLS-driven glutamine catabolism contributes to prostate cancer radiosensitivity by regulating the redox state, stemness and ATG5-mediated autophagy. Theranostics. 2021;11(16):7844.
131. Mukha A, Kahya U, Dubrovska A. Targeting glutamine metabolism and autophagy: the combination for prostate cancer radiosensitization. Autophagy. 2021;17(11):3879–81.
132. Kim G, Jang SK, Kim YJ, Jin HO, Bae S, Hong J, Park IC, Lee JH. Inhibition of glutamine uptake resensitizes paclitaxel resistance in SKOV3-TR ovarian cancer cell via mTORC1/S6K signaling pathway. Int J Mol Sci. 2022;23(15):8761.
133. Wang JJ, Siu MK, Jiang YX, Leung TH, Chan DW, Wang HG, Ngan HY, Chan KK. A combination of glutaminase inhibitor 968 and PD-L1 blockade boosts the immune response against ovarian cancer. Biomolecules. 2021;11(12):1749.
134. Tang Y, Wang S, Li Y, Yuan C, Zhang J, Xu Z, Hu Y, Shi H, Wang S. Simultaneous glutamine metabolism and PD-L1 inhibition to enhance suppression of triple-negative breast cancer. J Nanobiotechnol. 2022;20(1):216.
135. Ma H, Wu J, Zhou M, Wu J, Wu Z, Lin L, Huang N, Liao W, Sun L. Inhibition of glutamine uptake improves the efficacy of cetuximab on gastric cancer. Integr Cancer Ther. 2021;20:15347354211045349.
136. Pham K, Maxwell MJ, Sweeney H, Alt J, Rais R, Eberhart CG, Slusher BS, Raabe EH. Novel glutamine antagonist JHU395 suppresses MYC-driven medulloblastoma growth and induces apoptosis. J Neuropathol Exp Neurol. 2021;80(4):336–44.
137. Rais R, Lemberg KM, Tenora L, Arwood ML, Pal A, Alt J, Wu Y, Lam J, Aguilar JM, Zhao L, Peters DE. Discovery of DRP-104, a tumor-targeted metabolic inhibitor prodrug. Sci Adv. 2022;8(46):eabq5925.
138. Yokoyama Y, Estok TM, Wild R. Sirpiglenastat (DRP-104) induces antitumor efficacy through direct, broad antagonism of glutamine metabolism and stimulation of the innate and adaptive immune systems. Mol Cancer Ther. 2022;21(10):1561–72.
139. DeBerardinis RJ, Chandel NS. We need to talk about the Warburg effect. Nat Metab. 2020;2(2):127–9.
140. Liberti MV, Locasale JW. The Warburg effect: how does it benefit cancer cells? Trends Biochem Sci. 2016;41(3):211–8.
141. Wang ZH, Peng WB, Zhang P, Yang XP, Zhou Q. Lactate in the tumour microenvironment: from immune modulation to therapy. EBioMedicine. 2021;73
142. Sancho P, Barneda D, Heeschen C. Hallmarks of cancer stem cell metabolism. Br J Cancer. 2016;114(12):1305–12.
143. Kogure A, Kosaka N, Ochiya T. Cross-talk between cancer cells and their neighbors via miRNA in extracellular vesicles: an emerging player in cancer metastasis. J Biomed Sci. 2019;26(1):7.
144. Phan LM, Yeung SC, Lee MH. Cancer metabolic reprogramming: importance, main features, and potentials for precise targeted anti-cancer therapies. Cancer Biol Med. 2014;11(1):1–9.
145. Pastò A, Bellio C, Pilotto G, Ciminale V, Silic-Benussi M, Guzzo G, Rasola A, Frasson C, Nardo G, Zulato E, Nicoletto MO. Cancer stem cells from epithelial ovarian cancer patients privilege oxidative phosphorylation, and resist glucose deprivation. Oncotarget. 2014;5(12):4305.

146. Lu CL, Qin L, Liu HC, Candas D, Fan M, Li JJ. Tumor cells switch to mitochondrial oxidative phosphorylation under radiation via mTOR-mediated hexokinase II inhibition-a Warburg-reversing effect. PLoS One. 2015;10(3):e0121046.
147. Dong Y, Tu R, Liu H, Qing G. Regulation of cancer cell metabolism: oncogenic MYC in the driver's seat. Signal Transduct Target Ther. 2020;5(1):124.
148. Nong S, Han X, Xiang Y, Qian Y, Wei Y, Zhang T, Tian K, Shen K, Yang J, Ma X. Metabolic reprogramming in cancer: mechanisms and therapeutics. MedComm. 2023;4(2):e218.
149. Mukhopadhyay S, Vander Heiden MG, McCormick F. The metabolic landscape of RAS-driven cancers from biology to therapy. Nat Cancer. 2021;2(3):271–83.
150. Chelakkot C, Chelakkot VS, Shin Y, Song K. Modulating glycolysis to improve cancer therapy. Int J Mol Sci. 2023;24(3):2606.
151. Deng X, Wang Q, Cheng M, Chen Y, Yan X, Guo R, Sun L, Li Y, Liu Y. Pyruvate dehydrogenase kinase 1 interferes with glucose metabolism reprogramming and mitochondrial quality control to aggravate stress damage in cancer. J Cancer. 2020;11(4):962.
152. Zhou L, Liu L, Chai W, Zhao T, Jin X, Guo X, Han L, Yuan C. Dichloroacetic acid upregulates apoptosis of ovarian cancer cells by regulating mitochondrial function. Onco Targets Ther. 2019;Volume 12:1729–39.
153. Amengual-Cladera E, Morla-Barcelo PM, Morán-Costoya A, Sastre-Serra J, Pons DG, Valle A, Roca P, Nadal-Serrano M. Metformin: from diabetes to cancer—unveiling molecular mechanisms and therapeutic strategies. Biology. 2024;13(5):302.
154. Lord SR, Harris AL. Is it still worth pursuing the repurposing of metformin as a cancer therapeutic? Br J Cancer. 2023;128(6):958–66.
155. Xiao Y, Yu TJ, Xu Y, Ding R, Wang YP, Jiang YZ, Shao ZM. Emerging therapies in cancer metabolism. Cell Metab. 2023;35(8):1283–303.
156. Mastropasqua F, Girolimetti G, Shoshan M. PGC1α: friend or foe in cancer? Genes. 2018;9(1):48.
157. Chesney J. 6-phosphofructo-2-kinase/fructose-2, 6-bisphosphatase and tumor cell glycolysis. Curr Opin Clin Nutr Metab Care. 2006;9(5):535–9.
158. García Rubiño ME, Carrillo E, Ruiz Alcalá G, Domínguez-Martín AA, Marchal J, Boulaiz H. Phenformin as an anticancer agent: challenges and prospects. Int J Mol Sci. 2019;20(13):3316.
159. Trotta AP, Chipuk JE. Mitochondrial dynamics as regulators of cancer biology. Cell Mol Life Sci. 2017;74(11):1999–2017.
160. Bacci M, Giannoni E, Fearns A, Ribas R, Gao Q, Taddei ML, Pintus G, Dowsett M, Isacke CM, Martin LA, Chiarugi P. miR-155 drives metabolic reprogramming of ER+ breast cancer cells following long-term estrogen deprivation and predicts clinical response to aromatase inhibitors. Cancer Res. 2016;76(6):1615–26.
161. Sriramkumar S, Sood R, Huntington TD, Ghobashi AH, Vuong TT, Metcalfe TX, Wang W, Nephew KP, O'Hagan HM. Platinum-induced mitochondrial OXPHOS contributes to cancer stem cell enrichment in ovarian cancer. J Transl Med. 2022;20(1):246.
162. De Luca A, Fiorillo M, Peiris-Pagès M, Ozsvari B, Smith DL, Sanchez-Alvarez R, Martinez-Outschoorn UE, Cappello AR, Pezzi V, Lisanti MP, Sotgia F. Mitochondrial biogenesis is required for the anchorage-independent survival and propagation of stem-like cancer cells. Oncotarget. 2015;6(17):14777.
163. Zhong Y, Li X, Ji Y, Li X, Li Y, Yu D, Yuan Y, Liu J, Li H, Zhang M, Ji Z. Pyruvate dehydrogenase expression is negatively associated with cell stemness and worse clinical outcome in prostate cancers. Oncotarget. 2017;8(8):13344.
164. Liu Z, Zhang Z, Zhang Y, Zhou W, Zhang X, Peng C, Ji T, Zou X, Zhang Z, Ren Z. Spatial transcriptomics reveals that metabolic characteristics define the tumor immunosuppression microenvironment via iCAF transformation in oral squamous cell carcinoma. Int J Oral Sci. 2024;16(1):9.

Lipid Metabolism and Oncogenesis

4

Mirunalini Gobinath, Pratik Phalke,
Parikshit Roychowdhury, Alberto Ouro Villasante,
and Naina Mohamed Pakkir Maideen

4.1 Introduction

The changes in lipid metabolism have been considered as an important cancer hallmark, which allows tumor cells to acquire plenty of nutrients from the external environment or under stressful events, which helps tumor cells to maintain activities such as membrane biosynthesis, energy production, and bioactive lipid signaling, that are necessary for rapid development, proliferation, and survival. Lipid metabolic pathways consist of anabolic activities such as de novo lipogenesis, fatty acid (FA) synthesis, desaturation, and triglyceride synthesis, as well as catabolic processes like lipolysis and mitochondrial β-oxidation, which are essential in sustaining cellular lipid homeostasis [1].

M. Gobinath
Department of Pharmacognosy & Phytopharmacy, JSS College of Pharmacy, JSS Academy of Higher Education & Research, Ooty, Tamil Nadu, India

P. Phalke · P. Roychowdhury
Department of Pharmaceutics, JSS College of Pharmacy, JSS Academy of Higher Education & Research, Ooty, Tamil Nadu, India

A. O. Villasante
NeuroAging Laboratory (NEURAL) Group, Clinical Neurosciences Research Laboratory (LINC), Health Research Institute of Santiago de Compostela (IDIS), Hospital Clínico Universitario, Santiago de Compostela, Spain

Centro de Investigación Biomédica en Red en Enfermedades Neurodegenerativas (CIBERNED), Instituto de Salud Carlos III, Madrid, Spain
e-mail: alberto.ouro.villasante@sergas.es

N. M. P. Maideen (✉)
Clinical Associate Professor of Pharmacology, College of Medicine, Mohammed Bin Rashid, University of Medicine and Health Sciences, Dubai, UAE

Dubai Health, Dubai, UAE
e-mail: nmmaideen@dubaihealth.ae

S. Ashique et al. (eds.), *Cancer Metabolism*, Cancer Treatment and Research 195, https://doi.org/10.1007/978-3-032-21861-2_4

Lipid metabolism modifications could lead to the buildup of lipid components, also known as deposited lipid droplets, in the tumor microenvironment (TME). This also impairs antitumor immunity via reducing antigen presentation of dendritic cells, depleting T cells, and engaging lipid mediators secreted by cancer-associated fibroblasts, which further induce angiogenesis and remodeling of the extracellular matrix and promote tumor progression [2]. Lipidomics is the study of lipid profiles and their molecular structure and physiology. With the help of analytical tools like Mass spectroscopy, researchers have discovered more about lipids, their structural, functional, and metabolic networks, which were previously considered as simple fat deposits [3]. This helps in knowing the molecular links between cancer-associated signaling and changes in lipid metabolism offers novel strategies for precision oncology, such that metabolic profiling may influence the selection of targeted lipid metabolism therapies and estimate therapeutic response [4].

Metabolic modifications in lipid metabolism commonly contributed by oncogenic drivers such as Myc, PI3K/Akt/mTOR, decreased tumor suppressors like p53 and PTEN, and HIF-1α, together cause altered biosynthesis of lipids, which leads to the formation of aggressive tumors that are resistant to therapies [5]. Moreover, biomolecules like sphingolipids (SPh), phospholipids (PLs), eicosanoids, phosphoinositide, etc., modulate the TME and promote immune evasion, angiogenesis, and inflammation. The flexibility and plasticity nature of tumors assist them to adapt frequently to stressful events, hypoxia, nutrient fluctuations, and gather biomolecules from the surroundings [6]. Thus, in this chapter, we will discuss in depth the role of lipid metabolism in cancer oncogenesis and therapeutic strategies.

4.2 Understanding Lipid Metabolism

At the cellular level, biomolecules such as lipids, proteins, and carbohydrates play a crucial role in biogenesis and molecular metabolism of cells. Lipids, which are categorized as hydrophobic molecules that are made up of fatty acids, phospholipids, tri-acyl-glycerides, cholesterol, and sphingolipids, are eventually distributed to cell organelles and perform their respective functions in energy metabolism, cellular signaling, structural and barrier integrity, and secondary messengers [7]. Lipids are often portrayed as a primary factor that leads to the global epidemic obesity crisis. It is believed that the fast-food and sedentary culture has contributed to the rise in body mass index (BMI), which correlates with adverse health effects. Recent research has demonstrated that the site at which fat accumulation occurs, for instance, the abdomen and facial fat, is important in diagnosing further health hazards. These individuals have elevated risks of cancer and other metabolic diseases, such as cardiovascular disease and diabetes [8].

Lipids have an indispensable role in cellular functions that preserve homeostasis. They produce ATP and take part in producing vitamins, hormones, bile salts, eicosanoids, and cellular membranes, as well as in cellular signaling. Cholesterol and phospholipids are key constituents of cellular membranes. The anabolic and catabolic processes of lipids could be differentiated. Anabolism predominantly happens in the cytosol and endoplasmic reticulum, while catabolism largely takes place in the mitochondria [9].

Lipid biology is essential to understand the production of lipid molecules, the catabolism of lipids, which helps in generating ATP, and the signaling of lipid molecules. Fatty acids (FA), triglycerides (TG), sphingolipids (SPh), Phospholipids (PL), and cholesterol undergo various steps for their synthesis and degradation in lipid metabolism [10]. In perspectives of oncology, altered lipid metabolism is directly related to uncontrolled proliferation and survival of tumor cells. Metabolic pathways such as lipogenesis, β- oxidation of FA, desaturation, elongation, lipolysis, esterification, de novo synthesis, and Kennedy pathways happen in order to maintain homeostasis and molecular lipid metabolism. Metabolic changes often lead to tumorigenesis, as seen in the Warburg effect, which is due to altered glycolysis [11].

FA synthesis is generally considered as de novo synthesis of lipids, which occurs primarily in the cytosol of the liver, adipose tissue, and newly proliferating cells such as cancer cells. Citrates that are released from the citric acid cycle or TCA cycle in the mitochondria. FAs are crucial building blocks of various lipids such as PL, SPh, and TG, and consist of a carboxylic acid group with a hydrocarbon chain of different lengths with degrees of desaturation [12]. These together form complex lipid molecules, including tri-acyl-glycerides, phosphatidylethanolamine, phosphatidic acid, diacylglycerides, and phosphatidylserine, that plays significant role in membrane fluidity, biological barriers, such as cell membranes, and secondary messengers in cellular signaling pathways, to preserve homeostasis. In cancer biology, when tumor cells undergo metabolic stress, FA assists in rapid proliferation and provides essential energy for tumorigenesis. This makes the tumor more resistant to apoptosis and other chemicals like chemotherapeutic drugs and radiation [13].

How do tumor cells make fatty acids?

At the cellular level in mammals, FAs could either be acquired through exogenous direct uptake, which is from the TME surroundings, or could be fabricated de novo with the help of nutrients such as glucose and glutamine. In this process of remodeling, cancer cells could influence changes in their metabolic processes and alter the transport of FAs, storage of lipids, de novo lipogenesis, and β-oxidation for producing more ATP for energy [14]. Figure 4.1 represents lipid metabolism in nutrient-replete and nutrient-depleted conditions of the tumor.

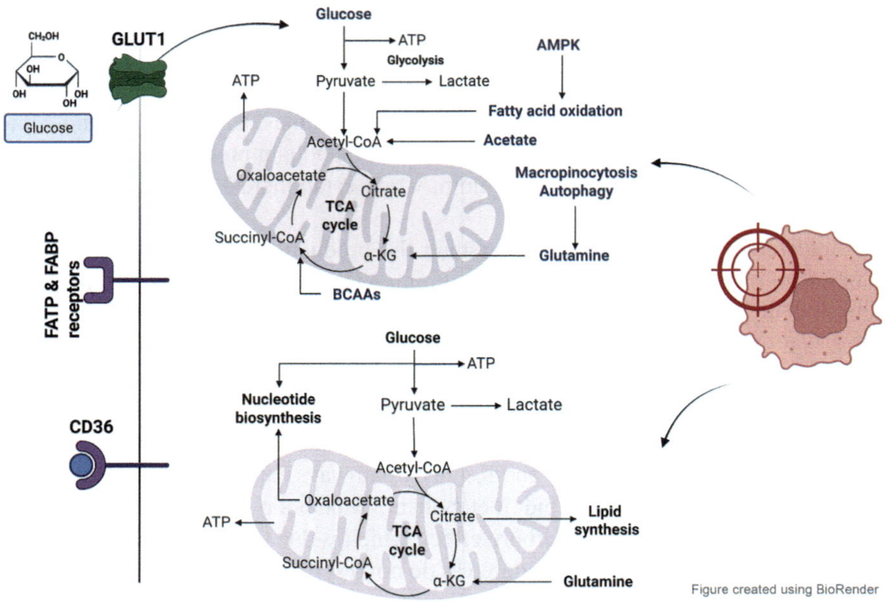

Fig. 4.1 Lipid metabolism in tumor cells. (Figure created using BioRender)

4.3 Alterations in Lipid Metabolism in Cancer

4.3.1 Causes of Dysfunction in Lipid Metabolism

Lipid programming, such as sterol regulatory element-binding protein (SERBP) driven FA and cholesterol gene networks, is activated by oncogenic signaling and transcriptional regulation, which also increases the production of enzymes like fatty acid synthase (FASN), Acetyl-CoA carboxylase (ACC), and 3-hydroxy-3-methylglutaryl-CoA reductase (HMGCR), hypoxia, nutritional stress, and storage of lipids often through transporters like Fatty acid binding proteins (FABPs) and CD36 [15]. Lipids and cytokines in the TME alter metabolism: IFN-γ-driven alteration can make people more sensitive to lipid peroxidation and ferroptosis, leptin encourages β-oxidation, and adiponectin decreases LDLR (low-density lipoprotein receptor)-mediated uptake. Cross talk between metabolic pathways facilitates reprogramming: under hypoxia, glutamine or acetate backfill acetyl-CoA, while glycolysis provides citrate for lipogenesis; these changes sustain membrane synthesis and signaling lipids [16].

4.3.2 Imbalance in Cellular Homeostasis & Composition of Lipids

Cancer cells raise membrane phospholipid synthesis and adjust saturation: SCD activity adds monounsaturated fatty acids (MUFAs), enhancing membrane fluidity and resisting ferroptosis when MUFAs replace oxidation prone poly-unsaturated FAs (PUFAs). Lipid droplet accumulation causes increased levels of excessive lipids in the TME, which acts as a fuel for tumor cell growth. But, sometimes, excessive lipid droplets are also related to the chemotherapy resistance or apoptotic mechanism resistance in tumors [17].

When a huge amount of lipids is deposited, cells usually undergo abrupt stressful changes and modify their metabolic pathways. FAs give rise to acetyl-CoA, which is a key for histone acetylation and can interfere with the palmitoylation of transporter proteins that act as temporary nutrition. These steep changes enable cells to manage NAD+ and NADH levels, which in turn causes either carbohydrate metabolism or glycolysis [18]. In hypoxic conditions, FA desaturation makes the condition difficult due to the absence of oxygen, like in normoxic situations. Hence, cells start depending more on external unsaturated FAs. At the same time, they produce more triglycerides [19]. All these changes alter the homeostasis, leading to high lipid production, different rates of elimination and lipid biosynthesis, and excess storage deposits. Altogether, gets accumulated near the cell membrane, leading to disrupted cell signaling [20].

4.3.3 Dysregulation in Cholesterol Metabolism

It is well known that cancer increases the production and absorption of cholesterol, and then makes it difficult to eliminate. Why? For the purpose of creating new membranes, maintaining the activity of those lipid rafts, and keeping the division machinery running, cells require additional cholesterol. Many malignancies have elevated levels of certain well-known enzymes and players, such as SREBP2, HMGCR, *SQLE*, and squalene synthase. In many patient groups, such reasons correspond to a worse prognosis and greater spreading [21].

Cell migration and invasion are increased in laboratory models of lung, breast, melanoma, and oral malignancies when cholesterol is changed or simply eliminated. The action of cholesterol in cells also affects immunity. Adjusting cholesterol in conjunction with immunotherapy may be a wise move because it can either slow down or accelerate the body's defenses against malignancies. The mevalonate pathway being switched on is interpreted by researchers examining pancreatic, colorectal, breast, and glioma malignancies as an indication that the disease is progressing or that the patient is avoiding therapy. Sometimes, such enzyme blockers work well with chemotherapy. At least in lab models, they impede tumor growth and reduce the growth of new blood vessels [22].

4.4 Lipid Metabolism and Cancer: Linking Mechanisms

4.4.1 Factors That Influence Tumor Microenvironment

The progression and growth of cancer are greatly affected by the TME. It consists of, apart from cancer cells, blood vessels, extracellular matrix, immune cells, stromal cells, and a host of signaling molecules. Lipid metabolism shapes the TME by a set of interconnected processes. The altered metabolism of cancer cells is also a significant contributing factor [23]. Cancer cells alter their metabolism pathways to allow for the growth of larger tumors by increased production and uptake of fatty acids. With their metabolism shift, cancer cells also produce and release increased numbers of metabolites into the TME, including lipid products and lactate, which are released and act on other adjacent noncancer cells. High lipid contents of the TME have immunosuppressive activities, which repress immune responses against tumors and promote the survival of tumors. As a case in point, we are aware that some tumors are supplied by adipocytes located near them with fatty acids, thereby giving a boost to their growth and their resistance to therapy [24].

In addition, lipid metabolism occurs in hypoxic conditions, which leads to lower levels of oxygen, and this condition is so frequent in solid tumors. Tumor cells, with hypoxic TME, depend upon anaerobic pathways and tend to switch their energy sources from aerobic respiration to other sources, thus increasing dependence on lipid oxidation. Subsequently, switching between metabolisms helps tumors, as well as stromal cells, and outer layers to increase lipid droplet production, enabling tumors to withstand difficult conditions better [25].

Another essential element of the microenvironment is cholesterol and its metabolites. They modify cell membrane structure, regulate platforms of signaling (e.g., lipid rafts), and are involved in the synthesis of bioactive metabolites, which manipulate cell communication between immune cells, stromal cells, and cancer cells [26]. High cholesterol consumption might also contribute to immune evasion by activating inhibitory immunological cell subsets, regulatory T cells, or myeloid-derived suppressor cells (MDSCs). In parallel to metabolic alterations, products of lipid peroxidation, growth factors, cytokines, and reactive oxygen species (ROS) also modify the microenvironment to favor tumor invasion, metastasis, and cell survival [27].

4.4.2 Role of Lipid Mediators in Cell Signaling

Lipid-derived compounds, which are also known as lipid mediators, are critical for cell coordination of signaling pathways in cancer conditions. The lipid mediators comprise several compounds, such as prostaglandins, leukotrienes, sphingosine-1-phosphate (S1P), lysophosphatidic acid (LPA), and a few oxylipins, which are synthesized by fatty acid- and cholesterol-derived sources [28]. Prostaglandin E2 (PGE_2), synthesized by arachidonic acid, has the ability to promote tumor development by inducing cell division, angiogenesis, and immunosuppression. Similarly, leukotrienes, which are also synthesized by arachidonic acid, are involved in promoting tumor cell motility, inflammation, and metastatic procedures [29]. Sphingolipids, of which S1P is a prominent type that influences several biological processes, including cell migration, growth, and survival, by interacting at specific cell membrane surface receptors. In addition, active compounds in sphingolipid metabolism like S1P and ceramides cause apoptosis, which is also called programmed cell death, and depends upon their own concentration and its coexisting environment, which has both pros and cons based upon the situation of tumor cells [30].

LPA, being yet another lipid mediator, induces cell motility, proliferation, invasion, and survival of various malignancies through activation of G protein-coupled receptors. Activities of these mediators are stringently controlled by individual enzymes, and perturbation of their synthesis or degradation by their own enzymes does have a considerable impact on tumor behavior [31]. Furthermore, lipid mediators usually also involve metabolic process pathways and gene regulation by acting on protein-based signaling. With such action, it is possible for cancer cells to alter their communication with stromal and immune cells, react rapidly to stresses of the environment, and modulate growth signals [32].

4.4.3 Inflammatory Mechanisms and Immune Modulation

Lipid metabolism is involved primarily in the integration of immune response and inflammation, both of which are central to cancer initiation. Several lipid mediators of immune cell recruitment and activation act as inflammatory signals. Acute inflammation can aid in clearing damaged cells during the early stages of tumor growth [33]. However, when tumors grow, lipid-derived signals such as prostaglandins and some oxylipins tend to contribute to the development of chronic inflammation. Chronic inflammatory condition aids cancer development by inducing cell survival, division, angiogenesis, and remodeling of tissues [34]. Also impacted are the immune cells of the TME. For instance, tumor-associated macrophages (TAMs) become lipid-storing and end their promotion of antitumor activity, instead choosing the release of anti-inflammatory cytokines for promotion of tumor growth. FA metabolism may be critical for regulatory T cells within their microenvironment, to allow for suppression of immune responses and a promotion of immunologic tolerance to cancer [35]. The emergence of immunosuppressive cell populations, such as myeloid-derived suppressor cells (MDSCs), in conjunction with lipid metabolism stress-caused direct suppression of cytotoxic T lymphocytes and natural killer cells exemplifies lipid-linked immune evasion [36].

The cell division can become deregulated and bypass a programmed cell death, termed apoptosis, due to lipid metabolism disturbances. For example, increased levels of cholesterol, as well as FA synthesis and absorption, enhance some signaling pathways, suppressing apoptosis and boosting cell membrane integrity. Otherwise, lipid peroxidation products, if not controlled, will induce oxidative stress and activate cell death pathways, including a novel type of iron- and lipid peroxide-dependent regulated cell death called ferroptosis. Ferroptosis is also being explored as a novel target for cancer treatment based on targeting tumors' lipid metabolism vulnerabilities [37, 38].

4.5 Sphingolipids and Their Mechanisms in Oncology

Sphingolipid biology is important in regulating cellular signaling networks, structural integrity of cells and organelle membranes, and cell metabolic functions such as apoptosis, proliferation, and angiogenesis. These are extensive classes of lipid rafts and mostly phospholipids, which are often involved in tumorigenesis. In the cancer cell cycle, lipid regulation plays a key role in oncogenesis, which could even modify genes that are involved in oncogenesis [39]. A diverse class of biomolecules, such as ceramides, cerebrosides, globosides, sphingosine, sphingomyelins, sulfatides, gangliosides, glycosphingolipids, and sphingosine-1-phosphate (S1P), are categorized under sphingolipid pathways. These processes, through rate-limiting steps, along with enzymes such as sphingosine kinase and ceramidase, are involved in de novo synthesis and salvage pathways [40].

Firstly, in the de novo synthesis of sphingolipids, serine amino acids fuse together with palmitoyl-CoA with the enzyme palmitoyl transferase (SPT), which reduces 3-keto-dihydroxysphingosine, which is further reduced into dihydroxy-sphingosine, dihydroxy-ceramide, and ceramides with the help of 3-keto-sphinganine reductase (KDHR), ceramide synthase (CerS), and dihydroxy-ceramide desaturase (DES) [41]. When the key component ceramide is formed, they undergo different steps to form sphingomyelin by the enzyme sphingomyelin synthase, ceramide-1-phosphate by the enzyme ceramide kinase, sphingosine by the enzyme ceramidase, and further it is reduced into S1P by the enzyme sphingosine kinase, and it further gets cleaved into hexadecenal and ethanolamine-1-phosphate by S1P lyase. In addition, enzymes like glucosylceramide synthase or galactosyl ceramide synthase give rise to cerebrosides, glucosylceramide, galactosylceramide, and further into glycosphingolipids, globosides, gangliosides, and sulfatide [42].

In this sphingolipid biogenesis, protumor effect is demonstrated by sphingomyelin causing proliferation and apoptosis, ceramide-1-phosphate causing inflammation and proliferation, S1P causes angiogenesis, inflammation, proliferation, and apoptosis, cerebrosides initiate apoptosis and proliferation. Whereas in antitumor effect, sphingosine leads to apoptosis, and ceramide causes autophagy and apoptosis. The central molecule of sphingolipid biology is ceramide, which could either be generated by de novo synthesis or catabolic pathways, i.e., reverse pathways through the enzymes like ceramide synthase and others [43]. Figure 4.2 describes pathways involved in sphingolipid metabolism.

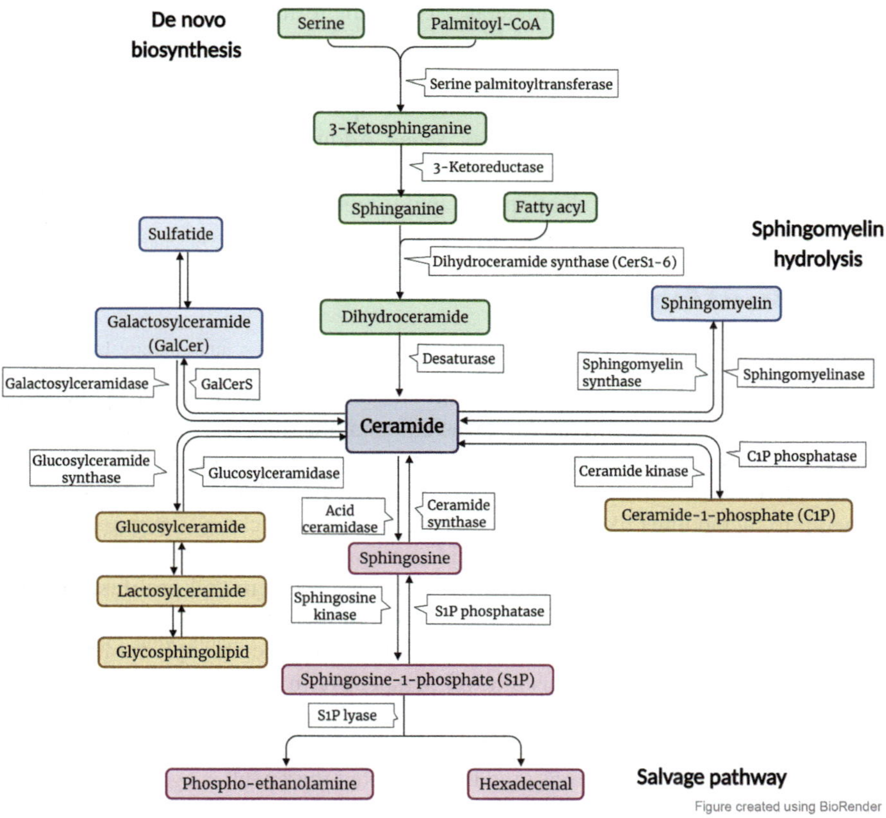

Fig. 4.2 Metabolic pathways involved in sphingolipid biosynthesis. (Figure created using BioRender)

4.6 Role of Lipid Metabolism in Specific Cancer Types

4.6.1 Colorectal Cancer

Colorectal cancer (CRC) shows drastic changes in lipid metabolism, which allow for tumor growth, invasion, and treatment resistance. Two major characteristics are increased uptake of extracellular lipids and increased de novo FA synthesis. Cancer cells display an upregulation of enzymes like FASN, which, besides being involved in new FA synthesis, aids antiapoptosis and metastasis. Moreover, certain tumor milieus cause increased expression of fatty acid transporter CD36, increasing FA uptake from extracellular sources [44]. It is critical to target synthesis pathways, as cancer cells compensate by boosting their lipid intake from dietary sources or local tissues to meet their membrane synthesis and energy demands. High CD36 expression is related to increased metastasis and the formation of epithelial-mesenchymal transition (EMT). Consequently, cells usually employ FAs for their β-oxidation, which drives additional cell division and migration. Dietary deficiency or circadian disturbances may serve to increase lipid-based oncogenic processes or oncogenes and reduce tumor suppressor genes. Additionally, lipid metabolism disruptions and SREBP activity led to the progression of colorectal cancer by supporting lipid and cholesterol production for rapid tumor growth [45].

4.6.2 Breast Cancer

Breast cancer exhibits drastic changes in lipid metabolism as cancer cell causes increase in both FA uptake through CD36 and other transporters and lipogenesis, which helps sustain proliferation, invasion, and therapy resistance of cancers. Elevated FASN and sterol-CoA desaturase sources, fatty acids oxidation (FAO) is upregulated to meet energy needs under metabolic stress [46]. Cholesterol is converted into metabolites like 27-hydroxycholesterol, which can also promote cancer progression. The synthesis of glycolipids and sphingolipids is also involved in triple-negative breast cancer (TNBC). This encourages stem cell proliferation and metastasis, which is abnormal. In addition, each of these targets is suppressed, and tumor progression is slowed, by the accumulation of specific sphingolipids like ceramides [47]. This approach is a novel perspective in targeted intervention, as a TME provides additional lipid and paracrine signaling, predominantly when breast tissue contains more fat in its TME. Moreover, lipid networks could pose complicated challenges on a daily basis, and thus, targeted therapeutics against the important and active lipid enzymes are crucial [48].

4.6.3 Skin Cancer

In melanoma, lipid metabolism supports the aggressive growth of the tumor and immune evasion. Increased uptake of lipids, especially via CD36 and FABP5, could increase lipid accumulation within melanoma cells and the TME. This acts as a fuel for tumor proliferation and contributes to treatment resistance and metastasis. Fatty acids oxidation (FAO) is a key metabolic adaptation, where melanoma cells increase FAO (carnitine palmitoyl transferase, CPT1) to survive metabolic stress, promoting metastasis [49]. Another crucial feature is that excessive lipid accumulation in the tumor can suppress antitumor immunity, particularly by driving T-cell exhaustion. Upregulated cholesterol metabolism, often via acyl-CoA: cholesterol acyltransferase (ACAT1), sustains tumor growth and modulates the immune checkpoint environment. On the other hand, enhanced de novo lipogenesis (FASN/SCD1) promotes cell survival and immune evasion, reducing the effectiveness of immunotherapies in melanoma. Thus, both lipid metabolic rewiring and its immunological impact are central in melanoma pathophysiology [50].

4.6.4 Lung Cancer

Lung cancer cells shift their lipid metabolism to promote growth, drug resistance, and adaptation to hypoxic conditions. Non-small cell lung cancers (NSCLC), the most common type, often upregulate both lipid uptake and FA synthesis. This is sometimes driven by Epidermal Growth Factor Receptor (EGFR) signaling mechanisms, which affect SREBP1 activity and increase lipogenesis and cholesterol synthesis. Tumor cells use these lipids to build new membranes and signaling molecules, helping them proliferate rapidly [51]. The function of FAO is associated with chemoresistance and helps lung cancer cells tolerate metabolic stress. Potential therapeutic approaches include blocking SREBP activation by employing EGFR inhibitors or targeting key metabolic enzymes, for example, FASN or SCD1. The need for their comprehension and interference for lung cancer's lipid metabolic dependences is further fortified by information supporting changed cholesterol homeostasis affecting tumor progression and sensitivity to targeted treatments [52].

4.6.5 Miscellaneous

Notable alterations in lipid metabolism are also seen across several malignancies, including pancreatic, ovarian, and prostate cancer. Prostate cancer, for example, shows a change in phospholipid composition, a rise in de novo lipogenesis, and a dependence on fatty acid uptake from expanse adipose tissue. Such factors affect responsiveness to treatment as well as the spread of the tumor to other areas. Ovarian and pancreatic cancer rely on increased fatty acid oxidation, increased CD36-dependent uptake, and altered cholesterol homeostasis, by which invasion is favored and resistance to therapy ensues, and in which ovarian cancer is highly sensitive to alterations of the lipid-dense microenvironment of the tumor [53]. A trend toward increased fatty acid synthesis and uptake, protective mechanisms against lipotoxicity by altered lipid droplet management, and redistributed cholesterol metabolism supporting proliferative potential and immune avoidance become common traits across those and other kinds of cancer. Lipid metabolic reprogramming is thus a major hallmark in solid tumors, influencing both cancer progression and response to existing experimental therapies [54].

4.7 Targeting Lipid Metabolism in Cancer Therapy and Existing Research Updates

Targeting lipid metabolism in cancer therapy is a rapidly expanding research area, motivated by the observation that many tumors depend on altered lipid pathways for growth, survival, and metastasis. Instead of relying only on traditional treatments, researchers are now investigating how disrupting lipid metabolism can weaken cancer cells or make them more sensitive to chemotherapy, immunotherapy, or radiation therapy. Several promising discoveries and clinical trial results have increased hope for this approach, though challenges remain in finding patient subgroups that benefit most from these therapies and in overcoming resistance mechanisms adopted by tumors [55].

4.7.1 Fatty Acid Synthesis and Uptake Inhibition

Inhibition of FASN, which generates fatty acids for new membrane and other cell structure synthesis, is a principal therapeutic approach. Preclinical and early clinical activity have been described for agents such as TVB-2640 and TVB-3664, particularly for glioblastomas and lung adenocarcinomas with KRAS mutations. FASN inhibitors can induce a "lipid crisis" for cancer cells, resulting in a surplus of toxic saturated fats, eventually leading to cell death via apoptosis [56]. However, dependency of FASN is not a universal phenomenon for all types of cancer, for there are certain subtypes against which it is ineffective, and thus limitation of their potency is felt for their respective drugs of pharmacopoeia. Another key target is stearoyl-CoA desaturase 1 (SCD1), an enzyme playing a role in the regulation of membrane fluidity and the mitigation of cell death (ferroptosis) by bringing about a conversion of saturated fatty acids to their respective unsaturated species [57]. SCD1 inhibition has advanced to the clinical stage in other diseases and might enhance antitumor immunity or sensitize tumors to immune checkpoint inhibitors. Those targets, through which fatty acid uptake is possible from the microenvironment of tumors, e.g., transporters of CD36, are of immense potential. CD36 blocking may restrict energy sources for metastases, thereby boosting the efficiency of immunotherapy along with chemotherapy. Other research focuses on determining an optimum combination of inhibitors of fatty acid synthesis and absorption for specific types of cancer [1].

4.7.2 Cholesterol Pathway Modulation

Steps in the mevalonate pathway of cholesterol synthesis are often discovered to be overexpressed in neoplasms, thereby fueling membranes and signaling processes necessary for tumor growth. Even though preclinical studies and epidemiologic research have suggested potential advantages of statin therapies (HMG-CoA reductase inhibitors) and other agents affecting the cholesterol metabolism pathway, debate regarding their value for cancer patients persists. Researchers are busily investigating inhibitors of transporters of cholesterol as well as downstream enzymes, including squalene synthase and SQLE [58]. Interestingly, closure of the cholesterol biosynthesis process, at times, might operate to enhance levels of immunity to tumors or reverse resistance to chemical agents, thereby unveiling potential avenues for combination therapeutic agents. Clinical investigations of dietary intervention (e.g., low-lipid or ketogenic diets) as complementary metabolic therapy are also on the rise. However, dietary manipulation as cancer therapy remains controversial and needs more robust clinical trials and evidence before routine use [59].

4.7.3 Biomarkers and Precision Approach

Not all cancer patients benefit equally from targeting lipid metabolites. One of the major research focuses on identifying the biomarkers—such as high FASN or CD36 expression—that predict response to lipid pathway inhibitors. The "selective lipid metabolism therapy benefit hypothesis" suggests that with better biomarker-driven selection, more patients will see significant benefits while minimizing unnecessary side effects [60].

4.7.4 Ongoing Clinical Trials and Future Directions

Currently, many clinical studies are being conducted, including those focusing on FASN inhibitors for a variety of solid tumors, including liver, brain, and lung cancer, as well as lipid pathway inhibitors being reevaluated for application across the landscape of cancer treatments. Initial findings indicate it should be possible to obtain tumor control, at least for groups of patients who have a particular genetic predisposition or a particular metabolic vulnerability. Even so, many questions are unanswered: Which transporter or enzyme is best for each type of cancer? What is the best way to combine metabolic inhibitors with immunotherapy or diet therapy? What are the mechanisms of resistance to therapy? [61]. To find out answers to these questions, future research should wholly focus on integrating multiomics strategies like lipidomics, transcriptomics, genomics, metabolomics, and proteomics, which could revolutionize the treatment of cancer targeting biosynthetic pathways. Development of selective blockers of lipid metabolism, such as FASN, ACLY, ACC, and SCD1, offers precision oncology therapies [19].

4.8 Conclusion

In conclusion, lipid metabolism plays an indispensable role in oncogenesis, assisting as a structural membranous support for rapidly proliferating cancer cells. They also modulate metabolic signaling networks, redox homeostasis, and survival of tumors in harsh environments and metabolic stress. Future research of lipid metabolic pathways in cancer progression mainly depends on the integration of various emerging advancements such as CRISPR-Cas gene editing techniques, precision medicine, precision oncology, nanotechnology, artificial intelligence, and machine learning. This deepens the understanding of lipid metabolic role in the pathophysiology of cancer and assists in designing and developing novel therapeutic agents that halt these pathways, which could enhance patient outcomes and treatment modalities in the future.

References

1. Gupta A, Das D, Taneja R. Targeting dysregulated lipid metabolism in cancer with pharmacological inhibitors. Cancer. 2024;16(7):1313.
2. Wang D, Ye Q, Gu H, Chen Z. The role of lipid metabolism in tumor immune microenvironment and potential therapeutic strategies. Front Oncol. 2022;12:984560.
3. Weng X, Gonzalez M, Angelia J, Piroozmand S, Jamehdor S, Behrooz AB, et al. Lipidomics-driven drug discovery and delivery strategies in glioblastoma. Biochim Biophys Acta (BBA) - Mol Basis Dis. 2025;1871(3):167637.
4. Delmas D, Mialhe A, Cotte AK, Connat JL, Bouyer F, Hermetet F, et al. Lipid metabolism in cancer: exploring phospholipids as potential biomarkers. Biomed Pharmacother. 2025;187:118095.
5. Jiang M, Zhang K, Zhang Z, Zeng X, Huang Z, Qin P, et al. PI3K/AKT/mTOR Axis in cancer: from pathogenesis to treatment. MedComm. 2025;6(8):e70295.
6. Sebestyén A, Dankó T, Sztankovics D, Moldvai D, Raffay R, Cervi C, et al. The role of metabolic ecosystem in cancer progression—metabolic plasticity and mTOR hyperactivity in tumor tissues. Cancer Metastasis Rev. 2021;40(4):989–1033.
7. Gu Q, Wang Y, Yi P, Cheng C. Theoretical framework and emerging challenges of lipid metabolism in cancer. Semin Cancer Biol. 2025;108:48–70.
8. Broadfield LA, Pane AA, Talebi A, Swinnen JV, Fendt SM. Lipid metabolism in cancer: new perspectives and emerging mechanisms. Dev Cell. 2021;56(10):1363–93.
9. Jones PJH, Lichtenstein AH. Chapter 4 - Lipids. In: Marriott BP, Birt DF, Stallings VA, Yates AA, editors. Present knowledge in nutrition (11th ed.) [Internet]. Academic Press; 2020 [cited 2025 Oct 8]. p. 51–69. Available from: https://www.sciencedirect.com/science/article/pii/B9780323661621000044
10. Vasseur S, Guillaumond F. Lipids in cancer: a global view of the contribution of lipid pathways to metastatic formation and treatment resistance. Oncogene. 2022;11(1):46.
11. Vogel FCE, Chaves-Filho AB, Schulze A. Lipids as mediators of cancer progression and metastasis. Nat Cancer. 2024;5(1):16–29.
12. Röhrig F, Schulze A. The multifaceted roles of fatty acid synthesis in cancer. Nat Rev Cancer. 2016;16(11):732–49.
13. Koundouros N, Poulogiannis G. Reprogramming of fatty acid metabolism in cancer. Br J Cancer. 2020;122(1):4–22.
14. Corn KC, Windham MA, Rafat M. Lipids in the tumor microenvironment: from cancer progression to treatment. Prog Lipid Res. 2020;80:101055.
15. Jin HR, Wang J, Wang ZJ, Xi MJ, Xia BH, Deng K, et al. Lipid metabolic reprogramming in tumor microenvironment: from mechanisms to therapeutics. J Hematol Oncol. 2023;16(1):103.
16. Luo X, Cheng C, Tan Z, Li N, Tang M, Yang L, et al. Emerging roles of lipid metabolism in cancer metastasis. Mol Cancer. 2017;16(1):76.
17. Fu Y, Zou T, Shen X, Nelson PJ, Li J, Wu C, et al. Lipid metabolism in cancer progression and therapeutic strategies. MedComm. 2021;2(1):27–59.
18. Mylonis I, Simos G, Paraskeva E. Hypoxia-inducible factors and the regulation of lipid metabolism. Cells. 2019;8(3):214.
19. Munir R, Lisec J, Swinnen JV, Zaidi N. Lipid metabolism in cancer cells under metabolic stress. Br J Cancer. 2019;120(12):1090–8.
20. Liu Q, Luo Q, Halim A, Song G. Targeting lipid metabolism of cancer cells: a promising therapeutic strategy for cancer. Cancer Lett. 2017;401:39–45.
21. Snaebjornsson MT, Janaki-Raman S, Schulze A. Greasing the wheels of the cancer machine: the role of lipid metabolism in cancer. Cell Metab. 2020;31(1):62–76.
22. Huang B, Song B, liang, Xu C. Cholesterol metabolism in cancer: mechanisms and therapeutic opportunities. Nat Metab. 2020;2(2):132–41.
23. Liu X, Zhang P, Xu J, Lv G, Li Y. Lipid metabolism in tumor microenvironment: novel therapeutic targets. Cancer Cell Int. 2022;22(1):224.

24. Mallick R, Bhowmik P, Duttaroy AK. Targeting fatty acid uptake and metabolism in cancer cells: a promising strategy for cancer treatment. Biomed Pharmacother. 2023;167:115591.
25. Du A, Wang Z, Huang T, Xue S, Jiang C, Qiu G, et al. Fatty acids in cancer: metabolic functions and potential treatment. MedComm—Oncologia. 2023;2(1):e25.
26. Tufail M, Jiang CH, Li N. Altered metabolism in cancer: insights into energy pathways and therapeutic targets. Mol Cancer. 2024;23(1):203.
27. Du J, Qin H. Lipid metabolism dynamics in cancer stem cells: potential targets for cancers. Front Pharmacol [Internet]. 2024 [cited 2025 Oct 8];15. Available from: https://www.frontiersin.org/journals/pharmacology/articles/10.3389/fphar.2024.1367981/full
28. Stephenson DJ, Hoeferlin LA, Chalfant CE. Lipidomics in translational research and the clinical significance of lipid-based biomarkers. Transl Res J Lab Clin Med. 2017;189:13–29.
29. Wang B, Wu L, Chen J, Dong L, Chen C, Wen Z, et al. Metabolism pathways of arachidonic acids: mechanisms and potential therapeutic targets. Signal Transduct Target Ther. 2021;6(1):1–30.
30. Greenlee JD, Subramanian T, Liu K, King MR. Rafting down the metastatic cascade: the role of lipid rafts in cancer metastasis, cell death, and clinical outcomes. Cancer Res. 2021;81(1):5–17.
31. Balijepalli P, Sitton CC, Meier KE. Lysophosphatidic acid signaling in cancer cells: what makes LPA so special? Cells. 2021;10(8):2059.
32. Martin-Perez M, Urdiroz-Urricelqui U, Bigas C, Benitah SA. The role of lipids in cancer progression and metastasis. Cell Metab. 2022;34(11):1675–99.
33. Garcia C, Andersen CJ, Blesso CN. The role of lipids in the regulation of immune responses. Nutrients. 2023;15(18):3899.
34. Zhao H, Wu L, Yan G, Chen Y, Zhou M, Wu Y, et al. Inflammation and tumor progression: signaling pathways and targeted intervention. Signal Transduct Target Ther. 2021;6(1):263.
35. Hoy AJ, Nagarajan SR, Butler LM. Tumour fatty acid metabolism in the context of therapy resistance and obesity. Nat Rev Cancer. 2021;21(12):753–66.
36. Liu X, Kang X, Kang H, Yan H. The immunosuppressive role of MDSCs in HCC: mechanisms and therapeutic opportunities. Cell Commun Signal. 2025;23(1):155.
37. Zekanovic S, Achaiber Sing P, Leenstra S, Lamfers MLM. Cut the fat: targeting cholesterol and lipid metabolism in glioblastoma. Cell Death Dis. 2025;16(1):717.
38. Kim JW, Lee JY, Oh M, Lee EW. An integrated view of lipid metabolism in ferroptosis revisited via lipidomic analysis. Exp Mol Med. 2023;55(8):1620–31.
39. Ogretmen B. Sphingolipid metabolism in cancer signalling and therapy. Nat Rev Cancer. 2018;18(1):33–50.
40. Quinville BM, Deschenes NM, Ryckman AE, Walia JS. A comprehensive review: sphingolipid metabolism and implications of disruption in sphingolipid homeostasis. Int J Mol Sci. 2021;22(11):5793.
41. Sasset L, Zhang Y, Dunn TM, Di Lorenzo A. Sphingolipid *De Novo* biosynthesis: a rheostat of cardiovascular homeostasis. Trends Endocrinol Metab. 2016;27(11):807–19.
42. Parashuraman S, D'Angelo G. Visualizing sphingolipid biosynthesis in cells. Chem Phys Lipids. 2019;(218):103–11.
43. Wajapeyee N, Beamon TC, Gupta R. Roles and therapeutic targeting of ceramide metabolism in cancer. Mol Metab. 2024;83:101936.
44. Coleman O, Ecker M, Haller D. Dysregulated lipid metabolism in colorectal cancer. Curr Opin Gastroenterol. 2022;38(2):162.
45. Li B, Mi J, Yuan Q. Fatty acid metabolism-related enzymes in colorectal cancer metastasis: from biological function to molecular mechanism. Cell Death Discov. 2024;10(1):350.
46. Wan M, Pan S, Shan B, Diao H, Jin H, Wang Z, et al. Lipid metabolic reprograming: the unsung hero in breast cancer progression and tumor microenvironment. Mol Cancer. 2025;24:61.
47. Scott DA, Drake RR. Glycosylation and its implications in breast cancer. Expert Rev Proteomics. 2019;16(8):665–80.

48. Wang J, Zhang W, Liu C, Wang L, Wu J, Sun C, et al. Reprogramming of lipid metabolism mediates crosstalk, remodeling, and intervention of microenvironment components in breast cancer. Int J Biol Sci. 2024;20(5):1884–904.
49. Giuliani S, Accetta C, di Martino S, De Vitis C, Messina E, Pescarmona E, et al. Metabolic reprogramming in melanoma: an epigenetic point of view. Pharmaceuticals. 2025;18(6):853.
50. Xiong L, Cheng J. Rewiring lipid metabolism to enhance immunotherapy efficacy in melanoma: a frontier in cancer treatment. Front Oncol. 2025;15:1519592.
51. Eltayeb K, La Monica S, Tiseo M, Alfieri R, Fumarola C. Reprogramming of lipid metabolism in lung cancer: an overview with focus on EGFR-mutated non-small cell lung cancer. Cells. 2022;11(3):413.
52. Merino Salvador M, Gómez de Cedrón M, Moreno Rubio J, Falagán Martínez S, Sánchez Martínez R, Casado E, et al. Lipid metabolism and lung cancer. Crit Rev Oncol Hematol. 2017;112:31–40.
53. Kotrikadze N, Alibegashvili M, Ramishvili L, Mikaia N, Khazaradze A, Sepiashvili B, et al. The role of lipids and fatty acid metabolism in the development of prostate cancer. Indian J Biochem Biophys IJBB. 2022;59(9):873–8.
54. Zeković M, Bumbaširević U, Živković M, Pejčić T. Alteration of lipid metabolism in prostate cancer: multifaceted oncologic implications. Int J Mol Sci. 2023;24(2):1391.
55. Zhang W, Wang P, Yuan G, Liu F, Jin G, Zhang J. Fatty acid metabolic reprogramming in the tumor microenvironment: unraveling mechanisms and therapeutic prospects. Genes Dis. 2025:101772.
56. Terry AR, Hay N. Emerging targets in lipid metabolism for cancer therapy. Trends Pharmacol Sci. 2024;45(6):537–51.
57. Lei G, Zhuang L, Gan B. Targeting ferroptosis as a vulnerability in cancer. Nat Rev Cancer. 2022;22(7):381–96.
58. El Omari N, El Fessikh M, Aboulaghras S, Bakrim S, Khalid A, Abdalla AN, et al. The role of inflammation in colorectal cancer and the preventive potential of natural compounds. J Funct Foods. 2025;129:106857.
59. Lagunas-Rangel FA. Cholesterol effects on the tumor immune microenvironment: from fundamental concepts to mechanisms and implications. Front Oncol [Internet]. 2025 [cited 2025 Oct 9];15. Available from: https://www.frontiersin.org/journals/oncology/articles/10.3389/fonc.2025.1579054/full
60. Ma H, Liu C, Li X, Zuo L, Li C, Xu X, et al. Lipid metabolites as biomarkers and therapeutic targets in oral squamous cell carcinoma. BMC Oral Health. 2025;25:1390.
61. Fhu CW, Ali A. Fatty acid synthase: an emerging target in cancer. Molecules. 2020;25(17):3935.

5 The Role of Oxidative Stress and Redox Regulation in Cancer

Nahid Nafissi, Pedram Fadavi, and Farzad Taghizadeh-Hesary

5.1 Introduction

Cellular homeostasis depends on an intricate balance between energy production and biosynthesis. In general, cells rely on energy-carrying biomolecules to support their functions and proliferation. However, metabolic activity and various biosynthetic pathways inevitably generate reactive oxygen species (ROS) as byproducts. Because ROS are inherently reactive and potentially toxic, normal cells maintain tightly regulated antioxidant systems to keep ROS levels low and prevent molecular damage [1]. Disruption of this redox balance is increasingly recognized as a marker of cancer biology [2]. Among the many regulatory mechanisms within cells, ROS generation and redox regulation play central roles in both normal physiology and disease. Redox imbalance has been shown not only to contribute to cancer initiation but also to promote tumor progression through multiple mechanisms [2]. This chapter introduces the fundamental and practical concepts necessary to understand the complex interplay between oxidative stress, redox biology, and cancer.

Nahid Nafissi and Pedram Fadavi contributed equally with all other contributors.

N. Nafissi
Breast Cancer Research Center, Iran University of Medical Sciences, Tehran, Iran

P. Fadavi
Breast Cancer Research Center, Iran University of Medical Sciences, Tehran, Iran

Department of Radiation Oncology, School of Medicine, Iran University of Medical Sciences, Tehran, Iran

F. Taghizadeh-Hesary (✉)
Breast Cancer Research Center, Iran University of Medical Sciences, Tehran, Iran

ENT and Head and Neck Research Center and Department, The Five Senses Health Institute, School of Medicine, Iran University of Medical Sciences, Tehran, Iran
e-mail: taghizadeh_hesary.f@iums.ac.ir

S. Ashique et al. (eds.), *Cancer Metabolism*, Cancer Treatment and Research 195, https://doi.org/10.1007/978-3-032-21861-2_5

5.1.1 What Is Cellular Metabolism?

Cellular metabolism encompasses the biochemical reactions that sustain life by converting nutrients into energy and macromolecules, while maintaining cellular integrity and function. It is broadly categorized into: (1) catabolism: breakdown of carbohydrates, lipids, and proteins to generate adenosine triphosphate (ATP, the main cellular energy carrier) and reducing equivalents (reduced form of nicotinamide adenine dinucleotide [NADH] and reduced form of flavin adenine dinucleotide [$FADH_2$]); and (2) anabolism: biosynthesis of macromolecules like nucleotides, amino acids, and lipids, essential for cell growth and division [3].

Metabolism is integrated with signaling networks that respond to nutrient availability, energy demand, oxygen levels, and environmental stress. Mitochondria are primary metabolic hubs, conducting oxidative phosphorylation (OXPHOS) to generate ATP. However, metabolism also generates byproducts, including ROS, which must be tightly regulated to prevent cellular damage [3]. Figure 5.1 illustrates the catabolism of glucose, as the main source of energy, in human cells.

5.1.2 What Are Reactive Oxygen Species?

Reactive oxygen species (ROS) are highly reactive molecules derived from molecular oxygen (O_2). They include free radicals (e.g., $O_2{\cdot}^-$, ·OH, ROO·) and non-radical derivatives (H_2O_2, HOCl) capable of oxidizing lipids, proteins, and nucleic acids. Table 5.1 summarizes various types of ROS in cells [4]. ROS molecules may not be considered only as destructive components; at physiological levels, ROS can act as second messengers in intracellular signaling, regulating gene expression, cell proliferation, differentiation, redox signaling, DNA repair, circadian rhythm regulation, and even immune responses [5].

5.1.3 How ROS Originates from Cellular Metabolism: Main Sources

ROS are inevitable products of aerobic metabolism. Their primary cellular sources include: (1) Mitochondria: About 90% of intracellular ROS is produced in mitochondria. The majority of mitochondrial ROS is generated through OXPHOS. During this process, electrons may derail from the electron transport chain (ETC) and leak through ETC Complexes, mainly Complexes I and III. The leaked single electrons then react with oxygen molecules, and generate superoxide [6]; (2) Peroxisomes: These organelles oxidize very-long-chain fatty acids and generate hydrogen peroxide (H_2O_2) as a byproduct mediated by acyl-CoA oxidase [7]; (3) endoplasmic reticulum (ER): ranked three among the organelles in producing ROS, ER mainly generate ROS during the process of oxidative protein folding [8]; (4) NADPH oxidases (NOX): these enzymes are transmembrane enzymes specifically devoted to generate ROS [9]; (5) Other sources: there are several other intracellular enzymes

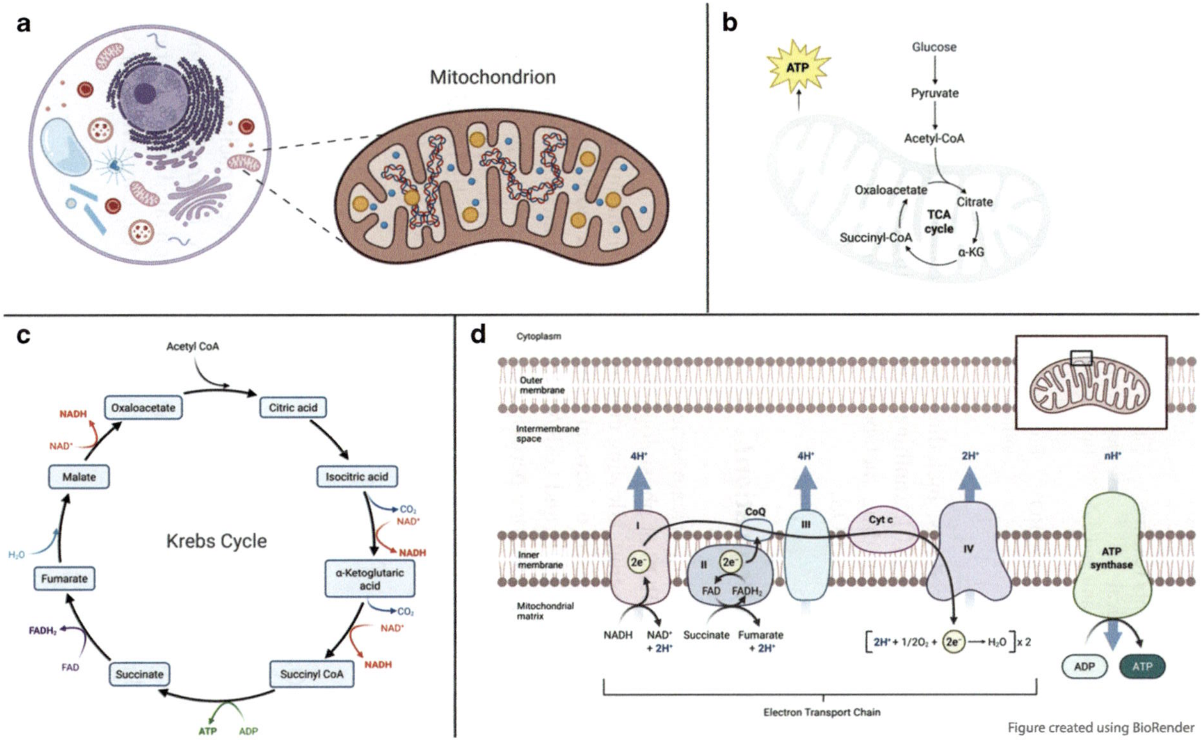

Fig. 5.1 Overview of cellular energy metabolism and mitochondrial function. (**a**) Schematic representation of a eukaryotic cell highlighting the mitochondrion as the major site of energy production. (**b**) Integration of glucose metabolism with mitochondrial function: glucose is converted to pyruvate through glycolysis, which is transported into mitochondria and converted to acetyl-CoA to enter the tricarboxylic acid (TCA) cycle. (**c**) The TCA (Krebs) cycle oxidizes acetyl-CoA to generate reducing equivalents in the form of NADH and $FADH_2$, along with ATP. (**d**) The electron transport chain (ETC), located in the inner mitochondrial membrane, utilizes NADH and $FADH_2$ to drive proton pumping across the membrane via complexes I–IV, generating a proton gradient used by ATP synthase (complex V) to produce ATP. Together, these processes form the core of mitochondrial oxidative phosphorylation, which provides the majority of cellular ATP and plays a central role in metabolism and redox balance. (Figure created using BioRender)

Table 5.1 Common reactive oxygen species subtypes

Type	Chemical nature	Notes
Superoxide ($O_2 \cdot^-$)	Oxygen free radical	Primary ROS generated in mitochondria
Hydrogen peroxide (H_2O_2)	Non-radical ROS	Membrane-permeable; acts as signaling molecule
Hydroxyl radical (·OH)	Highly reactive radical	Causes biomolecular damage; generated via Fenton reaction
Peroxyl radicals (ROO·)	Organic radicals	Involved in lipid peroxidation
Hypochlorous acid (HOCl)	Non-radical ROS	Produced by neutrophil myeloperoxidase during inflammation

that generate ROS as byproducts, including cyclooxygenases and lipoxygenases during eicosanoids synthesis [10], xanthine oxidase during purine synthesis [11], and Cytochrome P450 during drug metabolism [12]. This section demonstrated various sources of intracellular ROS.

5.1.4 What Is Redox Regulation?

Redox regulation refers to an intricate series of oxidation–reduction (redox) reactions to keep intracellular ROS at physiologic levels. It ensures a balance between ROS generation and scavenging, allowing controlled ROS signaling. Common cellular redox system is composed of several components, including redox couples ($NADH/NAD^+$, $NADPH/NADP^+$, and GSH/GSSG), antioxidant enzymes (superoxide dismutases, catalase, glutathione peroxidases), redox-regulating proteins (thioredoxins, peroxiredoxins, and glutaredoxins), and nonenzymatic small molecules (ascorbate [vitamin C] and α-tocopherol [vitamin E]) [13]. Cells benefit from a complex interaction among these biomolecules to maintain their ROS level at physiologic levels.

5.1.5 What Is Oxidative Stress?

Oxidative stress arises when the production of ROS exceeds the capacity of cellular antioxidant defenses, resulting in oxidative damage to DNA, organelles, and other biomolecules. It plays a significant role in aging and is implicated in a wide range of diseases, including neurodegenerative disorders, diabetes, cardiovascular disease, and cancer [14].

5.2 Oxidative Stress and Cancer Formation

5.2.1 Burden of Cancer

Cancer remains one of the most significant global health challenges of the twenty-first century, imposing a substantial burden on individuals, families, and healthcare systems worldwide. According to recent estimates from the GLOBOCAN, cancer is the second leading cause of death globally, responsible for nearly ten million deaths annually, approximately one in every six deaths [15]. The burden of cancer continues to rise due to aging populations, urbanization, and the increasing prevalence of risk factors such as tobacco use, obesity, sedentary lifestyles, environmental pollutants, and chronic infections. Beyond its physical toll, cancer has profound psychological, social, and economic consequences. Patients often experience long-term disability and reduced quality of life, while caregivers face emotional and financial strain. The cost of cancer care has escalated sharply, particularly with the emergence of advanced diagnostics and targeted therapies, creating disparities in access to care. Despite progress in early detection and treatment, the growing incidence of cancer highlights an urgent need for integrated prevention strategies, equitable access to healthcare, and continued research to improve outcomes and reduce the global cancer burden [16].

5.2.2 How Oxidative Stress Can Lead to Cancer Formation?

Oxidative stress can lead to carcinogenesis through a series of interrelated mechanisms that disrupt genomic integrity, alter cellular metabolism, and impair immune surveillance. This section outlines how oxidative stress can increase the risk of carcinogenesis through multiple interrelated mechanisms, as follows:

5.2.2.1 Direct ROS-Induced DNA Damage and Cancer Initiation

ROS readily interact with nucleic acids, causing chemical modifications that lead to genomic instability, an early and critical step in cancer formation. ROS attack DNA bases, which mispair during replication and cause point mutations. In addition to base modifications, ROS induce single- and double-strand DNA breaks, DNA cross-linking, and chromosomal rearrangements [17]. When these lesions accumulate beyond the capacity of DNA repair systems, they trigger mutations in key genes that regulate cell proliferation and apoptosis. For example, oxidative DNA damage can activate proto-oncogenes (e.g., RAS, MYC) or inactivate tumor suppressor genes (e.g., TP53, RB1) [17], pushing normal cells toward malignant transformation. Persistent oxidative stress, therefore, acts as a mutagenic force, driving the stepwise genetic alterations required for cancer initiation and progression.

5.2.2.2 Immune Cell Dysfunction Under Oxidative Stress

The immune system is pivotal in identifying and eliminating transformed cells through immune surveillance mechanisms mediated by cytotoxic T lymphocytes and natural killer (NK) cells. However, chronic oxidative stress disrupts normal immune function in several ways: (1) High ROS levels impair T-cell receptor signaling and reduce cytokine production, weakening antitumor responses [18]; (2) oxidative stress induces T-cell exhaustion, characterized by reduced effector function and increased expression of inhibitory receptors such as PD-1, Tim-3, Lag-3, and TIGIT [19]; (3) NK cell cytotoxicity decreases under oxidative conditions [20]; and (4) oxidative stress promotes the expansion of immunosuppressive cells such as myeloid-derived suppressor cells (MDSCs) and regulatory T cells (Tregs) both of which facilitate tumor immune evasion [21]. Consequently, oxidative stress not only initiates genetic damage but also suppresses the immune system's ability to eliminate early cancer cells, allowing them to survive and proliferate.

5.2.2.3 Mitochondrial Dysfunction, Energy Failure, and Genetic Instability

Mitochondria are major intracellular sources and targets of ROS. Excessive ROS generation damages mitochondrial DNA (mtDNA), ETC proteins, and membrane lipids, ultimately leading to mitochondrial dysfunction. It has been well established that various cancer risk factors (aging [22], smoking [23], lack of exercise [24], poor sleep [25], alcohol intake [26], and obesity [27]) can negatively affect mitochondrial function. As mitochondrial function declines, ATP production is reduced, impairing energy-dependent DNA repair mechanisms. Consequently, ATP-dependent DNA repair enzymes become inefficient, preventing the correction of ROS-induced DNA damage. This results in the accumulation of genetic mutations over time, promoting genomic instability and increasing the risk of malignant transformation [28]. Figure 5.2 illustrates how mitochondrial ATP depletion contributes to cancer development through impaired DNA repair and mutation accumulation. Future steps in the cancer journey are outlined in Chap. 6.

5.2.3 Cancer Risk Factors from the Scope of Oxidative Stress

Numerous lifestyle and environmental factors contribute to the development of oxidative stress. For instance, poor nutrition (high in fat and sugar but low in fiber) can disrupt gut microbiota and promote ROS generation [29]; inadequate sleep may impair antioxidant defense mechanisms [30]; obesity can increase oxidative stress through ROS released by adipose tissue [31]; smoking can lead to oxidative stress through releasing ROS and reactive nitrogen species (RNS) [32]; and ethanol consumption can also contribute oxidative stress through enhancing ROS generation and impairing antioxidants system [33]. On the other hand, it has been demonstrated that exercise and a high-fiber diet can alleviate oxidative stress [34, 35]. Consequently, unhealthy lifestyle habits place individuals at a higher risk of oxidative stress and related diseases.

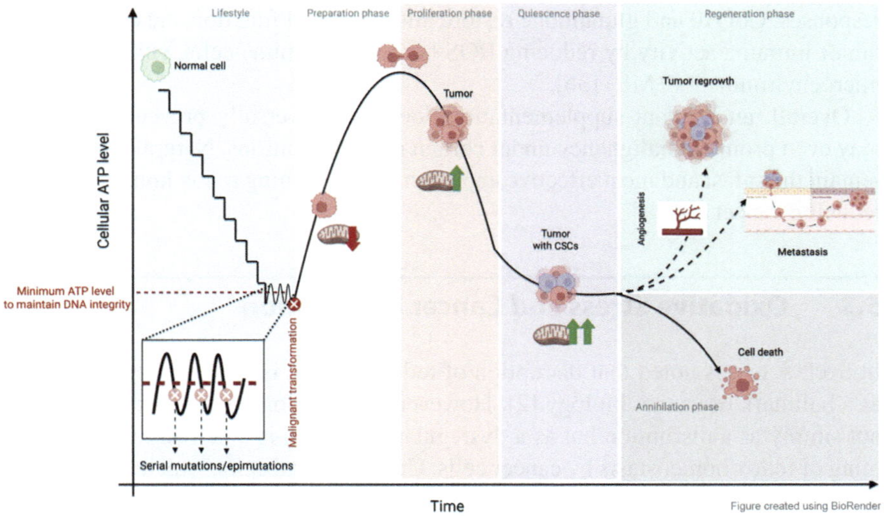

Fig. 5.2 Steps in cancer formation and progression based on the *Cell Energy* hypothesis [28]. According to this hypothesis, cancer arises from normal cells following lifestyle-induced or genetically induced mitochondrial dysfunction, which leads to progressive genomic instability and the accumulation of mutations, ultimately resulting in malignant transformation. (Figure created using BioRender)

5.2.4 The Role of Antioxidants in Cancer Formation and Prevention

Antioxidants counterbalance ROS and have therefore been proposed as a preventive strategy against cancer. However, the role of supplementary antioxidants in cancer prevention is complex, context-dependent, and in some cases harmful. Here, we present a practical summary of our recently published review on this topic [36].

Natural antioxidants obtained from fruits, vegetables, and whole foods are consistently associated with reduced cancer risk due to their synergistic effects and balanced redox regulation. In contrast, synthetic antioxidant supplements often fail to reproduce these benefits. For example, β-carotene, when consumed in high supplemental doses, has been shown to increase lung cancer risk, especially in smokers. Oxidative degradation of β-carotene generates breakdown products that impair mitochondrial ATP production and compromise ATP-dependent DNA repair enzymes, leading to mutation accumulation and cancer development. Similarly, vitamin E supplementation in high doses has been linked to increased prostate cancer risk by disrupting essential ROS-mediated signaling and generating prooxidant tocopheroxyl radicals. Other antioxidants, such as vitamin C, selenium, and folic acid, show no meaningful preventive effect when administered as supplements, despite strong protective associations when sourced from the diet. In contrast, zinc, coenzyme Q10 (CoQ10), and glutathione demonstrate potential beneficial effects in specific conditions. Zinc supports genomic stability and anti-inflammatory responses. CoQ10 and glutathione restore mitochondrial function and enhance antitumor immune activity by reducing ROS burden in immune cells within the tumor microenvironment (TME) [36].

Overall, antioxidant supplementation does not universally prevent cancer and may even promote malignancy under certain redox conditions. Natural antioxidants remain the safest and most effective approach to maintaining redox homeostasis and reducing cancer risk.

5.3 Oxidative Stress and Cancer Progression

In Sect. 5.1, it is noted that disruption of redox balance is increasingly recognized as a hallmark of cancer biology [2]. However, this phenomenon is better described not simply as a disruption but as a dysregulation, which is a deliberate reprogramming of redox homeostasis by cancer cells. Unlike normal cells, which tightly maintain low ROS levels, cancer cells elevate their ROS levels to the upper threshold of the physiological range. This controlled increase supports tumor growth, metabolic reprogramming, and survival signaling while avoiding excessive oxidative damage that would trigger cell death. In essence, cancer cells establish a new redox equilibrium at a higher ROS setpoint compared to normal cells. This section explores how cancer cells reorder the setpoint of ROS to a higher level responding to their metabolism and progression, and how elevated ROS levels contribute to cancer cell proliferation and progression.

5.3.1 ROS Regulation in Cancer Cells

As noted earlier, unlike normal cells that maintain ROS at low physiological levels, cancer cells depend on moderately elevated ROS to sustain their altered metabolism and malignant progression. To prevent oxidative damage while still benefiting from ROS-driven signaling, cancer cells employ redox-adaptive mechanisms that maintain ROS within a controlled range, high enough to promote proliferation and oncogenic pathways, yet low enough to avoid apoptosis. This finely tuned redox balance is achieved through the coordinated regulation of ROS production and detoxification systems [2].

Within the TME, cancer cells activate multiple oncogenic pathways, including Ras, Myc, and PI3K/Akt, which enhance mitochondrial activity and increase ROS generation [37, 38]. At the same time, they compensate for elevated ROS by upregulating antioxidant defenses, such as the glutathione and thioredoxin systems, to prevent excessive oxidative stress [39]. This dual strategy allows cancer cells to maintain ROS at prosurvival levels, enabling persistent activation of redox-sensitive signaling cascades that drive tumor growth, survival, and metastasis.

In contrast, cancer stem cells (CSCs) maintain low intracellular ROS levels to preserve genomic stability, retain stemness properties, and enhance therapeutic resistance. CSCs achieve this by activating a robust antioxidant network controlled by redox-regulated pathways such as Nrf2, HIF-1, and BACH1 [40]. Additionally, under hypoxic conditions common in the TME, CSCs stabilize hypoxia-inducible factor-1 (HIF-1), which promotes a metabolic shift from oxidative phosphorylation (OXPHOS) to glycolysis [41]. This metabolic reprogramming reduces mitochondrial ROS generation and offers further protection against oxidative damage.

5.3.2 Positive Effects of Elevated ROS Levels for Cancer Cells

5.3.2.1 Cancer Proliferation

One of the key hallmarks of cancer is sustained proliferative signaling, which enables continuous and uncontrolled cell division [42]. To achieve this, cancer cells activate growth-promoting pathways and bypass normal cell-cycle regulation. Elevated ROS contributes directly to this process by functioning as a secondary messenger in oncogenic signaling networks. For example, increased intracellular ROS levels can activate the PI3K/Akt and MAPK/ERK pathways, both of which are central to promoting cell survival, proliferation, and tumor growth [37, 43]. Through oxidative modification of signaling proteins, ROS enhance mitogenic signaling and drive cancer cell proliferation.

5.3.2.2 DNA Mutation and Genomic Instability

Genomic instability, a hallmark of cancer, drives tumor progression by generating new phenotypic traits that promote malignancy. Within the hypoxic and oxidative TME, cancer cells exploit elevated ROS to accumulate genetic mutations that progressively transform them into poorly differentiated and more aggressive phenotypes. These mutations enhance the ability of cancer cells to survive under hostile conditions, interact dynamically with TME components, and evade immune surveillance [44]. As noted earlier, ROS readily react with DNA bases, leading to a spectrum of oxidative DNA lesions, including base modifications, single- and double-strand breaks, cross-linking, and chromosomal rearrangements [17]. Consequently, elevated ROS levels support cancer evolution by inducing genomic instability while selecting for clones with growth and survival advantages.

5.3.2.3 Epithelial-Mesenchymal Transition: A Strategy to Enhance Treatment Resistance

Epithelial-mesenchymal transition (EMT) is a prelude of metastasis, during which cancer cells lose their epithelial characteristics and obtain mesenchymal features to depart from the colony and migrate to another body compartment [45]. It has been demonstrated that intracellular ROS can serve as a stimulator of EMT by activating various intracellular signaling cascades, including PI3K/Akt/mTOR, MAPK, and VEGFA/SOX2/SNAI2 axis [46, 47]. A recent study on breast cancer cells demonstrated that blocking ROS production by Complex III of ETC could effectively reverse the EMT process in cancer cells [48]. It has been demonstrated that EMT can effectively enhance cancer resistance against various treatments, including radiotherapy [49], cytotoxic chemotherapy [50], and immunotherapy [51]. This section outlined how elevated ROS levels can improve cancer cells' resistance against various cancer treatments by inducing EMT.

5.3.2.4 Immune Evasion

The immune system plays a central role in recognizing and eliminating malignant cells. However, cancer cells develop multiple mechanisms to evade immune surveillance, a process known as immune evasion. Elevated intracellular and microenvironmental ROS are key contributors to this phenomenon. High ROS levels in cancer cells upregulate immune checkpoint molecules, such as programmed death-ligand 1 (PD-L1), which bind to PD-1 receptors on activated T cells and suppress their cytotoxic function, promoting immune tolerance [52]. Furthermore, cancer cells release ROS into the TME, where they impair macrophage activation and $CD8^+$ cytotoxic T-cell function, while simultaneously promoting the expansion and activity of regulatory T cells (Tregs) [53]. These coordinated redox-mediated immune suppressive mechanisms enable cancer cells to escape immune destruction and promote tumor progression.

5.4 Conclusions

Oxidative stress is pivotal in cancer biology. As shown in this chapter, a persistent imbalance between ROS generation and antioxidants dysregulates cellular homeostasis and is the key driver of carcinogenesis. Elevated ROS levels induce genomic instability, mitochondrial dysfunction, and immune evasion, all facilitating cancer initiation and progression. In this chapter, we outlined how a controlled level of ROS acts as an important signaling mediators that support metabolic reprogramming, cell survival, angiogenesis, and proliferation of cancer cells. In addition, this chapter demonstrated how cancer cells adapt to oxidative challenges by establishing a new redox equilibrium, allowing them to maintain ROS levels within a range that is high enough to support oncogenic signaling yet below the threshold of cytotoxicity. This redox adaptation is achieved through intricate and delicate regulation of ROS generation and detoxification. Meanwhile, CSCs exhibit a distinct redox phenotype, characterized by low ROS levels, which enable them to preserve stemness and resist therapy.

Understanding ROS dynamics in cancer has significant diagnostic and therapeutic implications. Redox biomarkers are being explored as noninvasive tools for early detection and disease monitoring [54]. In addition, ROS-modulating strategies are also gaining attention in current practice for cancer treatment [55]. Future research should aim to extend our understanding of redox heterogeneity within tumors and its implications for personalized medicine.

References

1. Yang S, Lian G. ROS and diseases: role in metabolism and energy supply. Mol Cell Biochem. 2020;467(1–2):1–12. https://doi.org/10.1007/s11010-019-03667-9.
2. Ma N, Wang Y, Li X, Xu M, Tan D. Reactive oxygen species in cancer: mechanistic insights and therapeutic innovations. Cell Stress Chaperones. 2025;30(5):100108. https://doi.org/10.1016/j.cstres.2025.100108.

3. Judge A, Dodd MS. Metabolism. Essays Biochem. 2020;64(4):607–47. https://doi.org/10.1042/EBC20190041.
4. Nakamura H, Takada K. Reactive oxygen species in cancer: current findings and future directions. Cancer Sci. 2021;112(10):3945–52. https://doi.org/10.1111/cas.15068.
5. Hong Y, Boiti A, Vallone D, Foulkes NS. Reactive oxygen species signaling and oxidative stress: transcriptional regulation and evolution. Antioxidants. 2024;13(3):312. https://doi.org/10.3390/antiox13030312.
6. Zhang W, Hu X, Shen Q, Xing D. Mitochondria-specific drug release and reactive oxygen species burst induced by polyprodrug nanoreactors can enhance chemotherapy. Nat Commun. 2019;10(1):1704. https://doi.org/10.1038/s41467-019-09566-3.
7. Pascual-Ahuir A, Manzanares-Estreder S, Proft M. Pro- and antioxidant functions of the peroxisome-mitochondria connection and its impact on aging and disease. Oxidative Med Cell Longev. 2017;2017(1):9860841. https://doi.org/10.1155/2017/9860841.
8. Cao SS, Kaufman RJ. Endoplasmic reticulum stress and oxidative stress in cell fate decision and human disease. Antioxid Redox Signal. 2014;21(3):396–413. https://doi.org/10.1089/ars.2014.5851.
9. Reis J, et al. Targeting ROS production through inhibition of NADPH oxidases. Nat Chem Biol. 2023;19(12):1540–50. https://doi.org/10.1038/s41589-023-01457-5.
10. Liu X, Davis CM, Alkayed NJ. P450 eicosanoids and reactive oxygen species interplay in brain injury and neuroprotection. Antioxid Redox Signal. 2018;28(10):987–1007. https://doi.org/10.1089/ars.2017.7056.
11. Han C, Wu Y, Rong J, Xia Q, Du D. Unveiling the emerging role of xanthine oxidase in acute pancreatitis: beyond reactive oxygen species. Antioxidants. 2025;14(1):95. https://doi.org/10.3390/antiox14010095.
12. Veith A, Moorthy B. Role of cytochrome P450s in the generation and metabolism of reactive oxygen species. Curr Opin Toxicol. 2018;7:44–51. https://doi.org/10.1016/j.cotox.2017.10.003.
13. Xiao W, Loscalzo J. Metabolic responses to reductive stress. Antioxid Redox Signal. 2020;32(18):1330–47. https://doi.org/10.1089/ars.2019.7803.
14. Korovesis D, Rubio-Tomás T, Tavernarakis N. Oxidative stress in age-related neurodegenerative diseases: an overview of recent tools and findings. Antioxidants (Basel). 2023;12(1):131. https://doi.org/10.3390/antiox12010131.
15. Bray F, et al. Global cancer statistics 2022: GLOBOCAN estimates of incidence and mortality worldwide for 36 cancers in 185 countries. CA A Cancer J Clinicians. 2024;74(3):229–63. https://doi.org/10.3322/caac.21834.
16. Essue BM, Iragorri N, Fitzgerald N, de Oliveira C. The psychosocial cost burden of cancer: a systematic literature review. Psychooncology. 2020;29(11):1746–60. https://doi.org/10.1002/pon.5516.
17. Srinivas US, Tan BWQ, Vellayappan BA, Jeyasekharan AD. ROS and the DNA damage response in cancer. Redox Biol. 2019;25:101084. https://doi.org/10.1016/j.redox.2018.101084.
18. Larbi A, Kempf J, Pawelec G. Oxidative stress modulation and T cell activation. Exp Gerontol. 2007;42(9):852–8. https://doi.org/10.1016/j.exger.2007.05.004.
19. Rivadeneira DB, et al. Oxidative-stress-induced telomere instability drives T cell dysfunction in cancer. Immunity. 2025;58(10):2524–2540.e5. https://doi.org/10.1016/j.immuni.2025.08.008.
20. Poznanski SM, et al. Metabolic flexibility determines human NK cell functional fate in the tumor microenvironment. Cell Metab. 2021;33(6):1205–1220.e5. https://doi.org/10.1016/j.cmet.2021.03.023.
21. Ohl K, Tenbrock K. Reactive oxygen species as regulators of MDSC-mediated immune suppression. Front Immunol. 2018;9:2499. https://doi.org/10.3389/fimmu.2018.02499.
22. Srivastava S. The mitochondrial basis of aging and age-related disorders. Genes (Basel). 2017;8(12):398. https://doi.org/10.3390/genes8120398.
23. Fetterman JL, Sammy MJ, Ballinger SW. Mitochondrial toxicity of tobacco smoke and air pollution. Toxicology. 2017;391:18–33. https://doi.org/10.1016/j.tox.2017.08.002.
24. Memme JM, Erlich AT, Phukan G, Hood DA. Exercise and mitochondrial health. J Physiol. 2021;599(3):803–17. https://doi.org/10.1113/JP278853.

25. Han S, Kim D-K, Jun S-E, Kim N. Association of sleep quality and mitochondrial DNA copy number in healthy middle-aged adults. Sleep Med. 2024;113:19–24. https://doi.org/10.1016/j.sleep.2023.11.011.
26. Hoek JB, Cahill A, Pastorino JG. Alcohol and mitochondria: a dysfunctional relationship. Gastroenterology. 2002;122(7):2049–63. https://doi.org/10.1053/gast.2002.33613.
27. de Mello AH, Costa AB, Engel JDG, Rezin GT. Mitochondrial dysfunction in obesity. Life Sci. 2018;192:26–32. https://doi.org/10.1016/j.lfs.2017.11.019.
28. Akbari H, Taghizadeh-Hesary F, Heike Y, Bahadori M. Cell energy: a new hypothesis in decoding cancer evolution. Arch Iran Med. 2019;22(12):733–5.
29. Bailén M, et al. Microbiota features associated with a high-fat/low-fiber diet in healthy adults. Front Nutr. 2020;7:583608. https://doi.org/10.3389/fnut.2020.583608.
30. Vaccaro A, et al. Sleep loss can cause death through accumulation of reactive oxygen species in the gut. Cell. 2020;181(6):1307–1328.e15. https://doi.org/10.1016/j.cell.2020.04.049.
31. Furukawa S, et al. Increased oxidative stress in obesity and its impact on metabolic syndrome. J Clin Invest. 2004;114(12):1752–61. https://doi.org/10.1172/JCI21625.
32. Caliri AW, Tommasi S, Besaratinia A. Relationships among smoking, oxidative stress, inflammation, macromolecular damage, and cancer. Mutat Res Rev Mutat Res. 2021;787:108365. https://doi.org/10.1016/j.mrrev.2021.108365.
33. Tsermpini EE, Plemenitaš Ilješ A, Dolžan V. Alcohol-induced oxidative stress and the role of antioxidants in alcohol use disorder: a systematic review. Antioxidants (Basel). 2022;11(7):1374. https://doi.org/10.3390/antiox11071374.
34. Simioni C, et al. Oxidative stress: role of physical exercise and antioxidant nutraceuticals in adulthood and aging. Oncotarget. 2018;9(24):17181–98. https://doi.org/10.18632/oncotarget.24729.
35. Zhang Y, Dong A, Xie K, Yu Y. Dietary supplementation with high fiber alleviates oxidative stress and inflammatory responses caused by severe sepsis in mice without altering microbiome diversity. Front Physiol. 2018;9:1929. https://doi.org/10.3389/fphys.2018.01929.
36. Fadavi P, Taghizadeh-Hesary F. Supplementary antioxidants for preventing cancer: beneficial or detrimental? Asian Pac J Cancer Care. 2025;10(3):1083–8. https://doi.org/10.31557/apjcc.2025.10.3.1083-1088.
37. Koundouros N, Poulogiannis G. Phosphoinositide 3-kinase/Akt signaling and redox metabolism in cancer. Front Oncol. 2018;8:160. https://doi.org/10.3389/fonc.2018.00160.
38. Xian D, Lai R, Song J, Xiong X, Zhong J. Emerging perspective: role of increased ROS and Redox imbalance in skin carcinogenesis. Oxidative Med Cell Longev. 2019;2019:1–11. https://doi.org/10.1155/2019/8127362.
39. Tanaka G, Inoue K-I, Shimizu T, Akimoto K, Kubota K. Dual pharmacological inhibition of glutathione and thioredoxin systems synergizes to kill colorectal carcinoma stem cells. Cancer Med. 2016;5(9):2544–57. https://doi.org/10.1002/cam4.844.
40. Du M, Zhang J, Wicha MS, Luo M. Redox regulation of cancer stem cells: biology and therapeutic implications. MedComm Oncol. 2024;3(4):e70005. https://doi.org/10.1002/mog2.70005.
41. Ciavardelli D, et al. Breast cancer stem cells rely on fermentative glycolysis and are sensitive to 2-deoxyglucose treatment. Cell Death Dis. 2014;5(7):e1336. https://doi.org/10.1038/cddis.2014.285.
42. Hanahan D. Hallmarks of cancer: new dimensions. Cancer Discov. 2022;12(1):31–46. https://doi.org/10.1158/2159-8290.CD-21-1059.
43. Son Y, Cheong Y-K, Kim N-H, Chung H-T, Kang DG, Pae H-O. Mitogen-activated protein kinases and reactive oxygen species: how can ROS activate MAPK pathways? J Signal Transduct. 2011;2011:792639. https://doi.org/10.1155/2011/792639.
44. Taghizadeh-Hesary F, Akbari H, Bahadori M, Behnam B. Targeted anti-mitochondrial therapy: the future of oncology. Genes. 2022;13(10):1728. https://doi.org/10.3390/genes13101728.
45. Yang J, et al. Guidelines and definitions for research on epithelial–mesenchymal transition. Nat Rev Mol Cell Biol. 2020;21(6):341–52. https://doi.org/10.1038/s41580-020-0237-9.

46. Wang Z, Li Y, Sarkar FH. Signaling mechanism(s) of reactive oxygen species in epithelial-mesenchymal transition reminiscent of cancer stem cells in tumor progression. Curr Stem Cell Res Ther. 2010;5(1):74–80. https://doi.org/10.2174/157488810790442813.
47. Kim M, et al. VEGFA links self-renewal and metastasis by inducing Sox2 to repress miR-452, driving slug. Oncogene. 2017;36(36):5199–211. https://doi.org/10.1038/onc.2017.4.
48. Monti E, Mancini A, Marras E, Gariboldi MB. Targeting mitochondrial ROS production to reverse the epithelial-mesenchymal transition in breast cancer cells. CIMB. 2022;44(11):5277–93. https://doi.org/10.3390/cimb44110359.
49. Qiao L, et al. Targeting epithelial-to-mesenchymal transition in radioresistance: cross-linked mechanisms and strategies. Front Oncol. 2022;12:775238. https://doi.org/10.3389/fonc.2022.775238.
50. Dart A. EMT in chemoresistance. Nat Rev Cancer. 2023;23(6):349. https://doi.org/10.1038/s41568-023-00581-7.
51. Gu Y, Zhang Z, Ten Dijke P. Harnessing epithelial-mesenchymal plasticity to boost cancer immunotherapy. Cell Mol Immunol. 2023;20(4):318–40. https://doi.org/10.1038/s41423-023-00980-8.
52. Glorieux C, et al. Regulation of PD-L1 expression in K-ras-driven cancers through ROS-mediated FGFR1 signaling. Redox Biol. 2021;38:101780. https://doi.org/10.1016/j.redox.2020.101780.
53. Chen X, Song M, Zhang B, Zhang Y. Reactive oxygen species regulate T cell immune response in the tumor microenvironment. Oxidative Med Cell Longev. 2016;2016:1580967. https://doi.org/10.1155/2016/1580967.
54. Fuloria S, et al. Comprehensive review of methodology to detect reactive oxygen species (ROS) in mammalian species and establish its relationship with antioxidants and cancer. Antioxidants (Basel). 2021;10(1):128. https://doi.org/10.3390/antiox10010128.
55. Narayanan D, Ma S, Özcelik D. Targeting the redox landscape in cancer therapy. Cancers (Basel). 2020;12(7):1706. https://doi.org/10.3390/cancers12071706.

Mitochondrial Metabolism and Dynamics in Cancer Cells

6

Pedram Fadavi and Farzad Taghizadeh-Hesary

6.1 Introduction

Cancer remains one of the leading causes of morbidity and mortality worldwide. In 2023 alone, it accounted for 10.4 million deaths globally [1]. One of the major challenges in cancer therapy is the disease's intrinsic tendency to develop resistance against various treatments, including cytotoxic chemotherapy, targeted molecular therapy, immunotherapy, and even radiotherapy [2]. Understanding the unique metabolic features of cancer cells and how these differ from those of normal cells can greatly aid efforts to identify novel therapeutic strategies to overcome treatment resistance.

Since the early-1900s, it has been recognized that the metabolism of cancer cells differs fundamentally from that of normal human cells. In 1924, Otto Warburg demonstrated that cancer cells do not rely primarily on mitochondrial respiration for their energy production. Instead, they generate adenosine triphosphate (ATP) predominantly through an enhanced glycolytic pathway, even in the presence of oxygen, a phenomenon later termed "aerobic glycolysis" or the Warburg effect [3]. Subsequent studies supported Warburg's observations [4]. However, more recent investigations have revealed that this explanation is not complete. Well-designed experimental studies have shown that many cancer cells also utilize mitochondrial oxidative phosphorylation (OXPHOS). In other words, functional mitochondria

P. Fadavi
Breast Cancer Research Center, Iran University of Medical Sciences, Tehran, Iran

Department of Radiation Oncology, School of Medicine, Iran University of Medical Sciences, Tehran, Iran

F. Taghizadeh-Hesary (✉)
Breast Cancer Research Center, Iran University of Medical Sciences, Tehran, Iran

ENT and Head and Neck Research Center and Department, The Five Senses Health Institute, School of Medicine, Iran University of Medical Sciences, Tehran, Iran
e-mail: taghizadeh_hesary.f@iums.ac.ir

S. Ashique et al. (eds.), *Cancer Metabolism*, Cancer Treatment and Research 195, https://doi.org/10.1007/978-3-032-21861-2_6

remain essential for the survival and proliferation of cancer cells [5]. Supporting this view, experimental evidence indicates that cancer cells exhibit higher temperatures than surrounding normal tissues, reflecting elevated mitochondrial metabolic activity, as the main source of cellular temperature [6]. In essence, cancer cells depend on mitochondria not only to generate additional ATP through the tricarboxylic acid (TCA) cycle and OXPHOS but also to supply biosynthetic precursors for proliferation through alternative pathways, such as the pentose phosphate pathway [7].

In Sect. 6.2, we discuss whether Warburg's classical theory fully explains these metabolic adaptations or whether the recent experimental findings provide a more comprehensive understanding. This chapter aims to offer a concise yet comprehensive overview of mitochondrial metabolism in cancer cells, encompassing intrinsic metabolic pathways, calcium homeostasis, and mitochondrial dynamics.

6.2 Glucose Metabolism in Cancer: Focusing on Mitochondria

6.2.1 Warburg's Theory

During normal physiological conditions, glucose is metabolized through glycolysis. The resulting pyruvates then enter the TCA cycle, where they are oxidized to generate reducing equivalents in the form of NADH and $FADH_2$. These molecules subsequently donate electrons to the electron transport chain (ETC), located in the inner mitochondrial membrane. As electrons flow through the ETC, protons (H^+) are pumped into the intermembrane space, creating an electrochemical gradient. The accumulated protons then flow back through the final component of the ETC (i.e., ATP synthase), driving the phosphorylation of ADP to form ATP. At the same time, the transferred electrons combine with molecular oxygen (O_2) to produce water (H_2O). Overall, each molecule of glucose yields 2 ATPs via glycolysis and approximately 36 ATPs through the combined TCA and OXPHOS processes [8].

In 1924, Otto Warburg demonstrated that cancer cells deviate from this normal metabolic pathway. He observed that pyruvate derived from glycolysis does not enter the TCA cycle; instead, it undergoes fermentation to form lactate, even in the presence of sufficient oxygen. Warburg attributed this metabolic shift to impaired mitochondrial function, proposing that mitochondrial dysfunction prevents pyruvate from entering the TCA–OXPHOS system [3]. However, the precise mechanism underlying this mitochondrial impairment in cancer cells remained unclear.

This metabolic reprogramming, characterized by a high glycolytic flux, provides several advantages to cancer cells. First, glycolysis produces far fewer reactive oxygen species (ROS) than OXPHOS, thereby maintaining ROS levels within a moderate, nontoxic range conducive to rapid cell proliferation [9]. Second, glycolytic intermediates can be diverted into biosynthetic pathways to generate the molecular building blocks required for cell division, including nucleotides, fatty acids, and amino acids [10].

Subsequent studies confirmed Warburg's observations, showing that glycolysis remains highly active in cancer cells even under normoxic conditions, a phenomenon now known as "aerobic glycolysis" [11]. This raises an intriguing question: why do rapidly proliferating cancer cells rely on glycolysis, which yields only 2 ATP molecules per glucose, instead of the more efficient OXPHOS pathway that produces 36 ATPs? The answer lies in metabolic compensation: cancer cells increase glucose uptake and glycolytic flux to sustain sufficient ATP levels despite the lower energy yield [12]. This metabolic characteristic forms the basis for FDG-PET imaging, which detects elevated glucose uptake in tumors [13].

The regulation of this enhanced glycolysis involves several key mechanisms. Two major determinants are (1) the availability of glucose, governed by glucose transporter 1 (GLUT1), and (2) the activity of hexokinase 2 (HK2), the rate-limiting enzyme of glycolysis. The expression of both GLUT1 and HK2 in cancer cells is controlled primarily by two regulatory systems: (A) the hypoxia-inducible factor-1 (HIF-1) pathway, and (B) oncogenic signaling pathways involving Myc, Ras, and Akt. Moreover, loss of p53 function also leads to overexpression of GLUT1 and HK2. Under normal conditions, HIF-1 is degraded in the presence of oxygen, becoming active only during hypoxia to promote glycolysis. However, in cancer cells, HIF-1 can be aberrantly stabilized and activated even under normoxic conditions through pathways involving Akt, Ras, and mTOR [5]. These findings highlight the complexity and distinct metabolic adaptations of cancer cells compared with their normal counterparts.

6.2.2 Warburg's Theory: False or True?

In 1951, Sidney Weinhouse, using isotope tracing experiments, discovered that mitochondrial metabolism in cancer cells is as active as in normal cells [14]. This observation challenged the validity of Warburg's theory, which proposed that cancer cells rely primarily on glycolysis even under normoxic conditions due to mitochondrial dysfunction [3]. A recent study by Wang et al. helps explain this apparent discrepancy. Using the NCI-60 panel, which includes nine different cancer cell line types, the researchers showed that in rapidly proliferating cells, saturation of mitochondrial NADH shuttles, specifically the malate–aspartate shuttle and the glycerol 3-phosphate shuttle, forces cells to activate a backup metabolic pathway, namely glycolysis. This shift leads to lactate accumulation. In other words, cancer cells normally depend on mitochondrial OXPHOS for energy production, but when the NADH-shuttle capacity becomes saturated, they are compelled to redirect metabolism toward aerobic glycolysis [15].

While Warburg's findings established that glycolysis is a dominant energy-producing pathway in cancer cells, subsequent studies have shown that this dominance is most pronounced under hypoxic conditions, such as those commonly found in the tumor core [16]. In other words, the tumor microenvironment (TME) is inherently heterogeneous in oxygen availability—some regions are normoxic, whereas others are hypoxic. More recent investigations have revealed that certain subpopulations of cancer cells can express mitochondria-related genes and maintain oxidative metabolism even under hypoxia [17]. The following section discusses the metabolic paradigm shift that occurs during cancer progression and how this metabolic flexibility supports tumor survival and adaptation.

Consequently, it is unlikely that a single, universal metabolic model applies to all cancer cells within a tumor. In other words, Warburg's theory can only address a metabolic characteristic of a subpopulation of cancer cells within a tumor colony. The next section outlines how cancer metabolism is changing during its natural progression.

6.2.3 Dynamic Cancer Cells with Dynamic Metabolic Paradigms

In reality, cancer cells should not be viewed as a uniform population with fixed characteristics. Instead, they are highly dynamic, continually acquiring new properties as they progress and interact with their surrounding microenvironment. Consequently, cancer cells may rely on OXPHOS-dependent metabolism during one stage and shift toward glycolysis under different conditions. In oncology, this adaptive process is captured by the concept of cancer progression, which emphasizes that cancer cells are not static but evolve over successive generations, gaining new traits in response to environmental pressures. Figure 6.1 summarizes the principal metabolic and cellular events that drive malignant transformation:

In the early stages of tumor development, cancer cells reside in a nutrient-rich and well-oxygenated environment, relying primarily on OXPHOS to produce biosynthetic precursors—such as amino acids, fatty acids, and nucleotides—required for rapid proliferation. As the tumor mass expands, the imbalance between increasing metabolic demands and limited nutrient and oxygen supply gives rise to hypoxia, acidosis, and metabolic stress within the TME. To adapt and survive under these stressful conditions, cancer cells undergo a metabolic shift toward aerobic glycolysis (the Warburg effect), enabling continued growth despite reduced oxygen availability. This adaptive reprogramming is largely mediated by HIF-1, which activates transcriptional programs promoting glycolysis, angiogenesis, and cell survival. With further progression, subsets of tumor cells experience an epithelial–mesenchymal transition (EMT), acquiring the invasive and migratory characteristics necessary for metastasis—one of the classical hallmarks of cancer. EMT is regulated by transcription factors such as Snail, Twist, and ZEB, many of which are induced by HIF-1, thereby linking metabolic stress to metastatic potential. In addition, EMT contributes to the formation of cancer stem cells (CSCs), a subpopulation endowed with enhanced self-renewal capacity and resistance to therapy. These CSCs exhibit remarkable metabolic plasticity, switching between glycolysis and OXPHOS in response to environmental changes, ensuring their survival under fluctuating nutrient and oxygen conditions [18]. It has been demonstrated that CSCs downregulate their metabolic rates to sustain their survival and improve their resistance against various anticancer treatments [19].

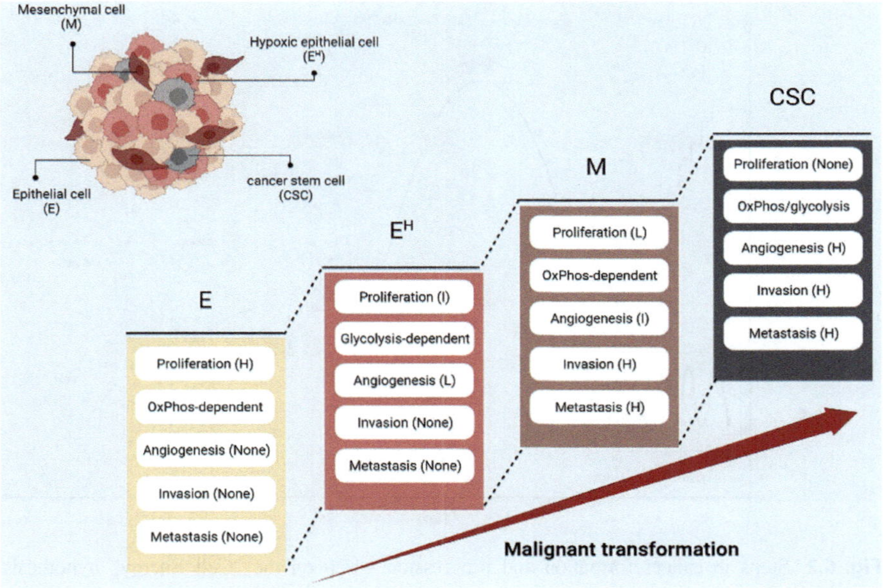

Fig. 6.1 Evolution of cancer metabolism and capabilities during malignant transformation. CSC indicates cancer stem cells, E epithelial cancer cells at normoxia, EH epithelial cancer cells at hypoxia, H high-level, I intermediate-level, L low-level, M mesenchymal cancer cells. (Source: [18] under CC BY 4.0)

6.2.4 Cancer Evolution Through the Lens of Mitochondria

In Chap. 5, we discussed how mitochondrial dysfunction can serve as a foundation for cancer initiation. According to our "Cell Energy hypothesis" [20], diverse cancer risk factors—such as obesity, aging, and smoking—can impair mitochondrial ATP production, ultimately promoting nuclear DNA mutations that drive malignant transformation. In this section, we continue to trace the journey of cancer cells through the mitochondrial lens. Figure 6.2 illustrates how cellular ATP levels (as a proxy for "cell energy") fluctuate during cancer progression [20].

After tumor initiation, cancer cells enter the "Preparation Phase," during which mitochondrial dysfunction—often caused by prior exposure to risk factors—forces the cells to rely predominantly on glycolysis. This metabolic shift allows cancer cells to accumulate ATP, NADH, and essential biosynthetic intermediates, including fatty acids, amino acids, and nucleotides, required for future proliferation.

Once sufficient resources are collected, cancer cells transition into the "Proliferation Phase," during which they consume the stored ATP, NADH, and building blocks to support active cell division. At this stage, cancer cells require functional mitochondria to sustain rapid proliferation. As demonstrated by Wang et al., during this phase, cancer cells may experience NADH shuttle saturation, which forces a compensatory switch back to glycolysis as a backup energy pathway [15]. Cancer cells located deep within the tumor mass often experience limited

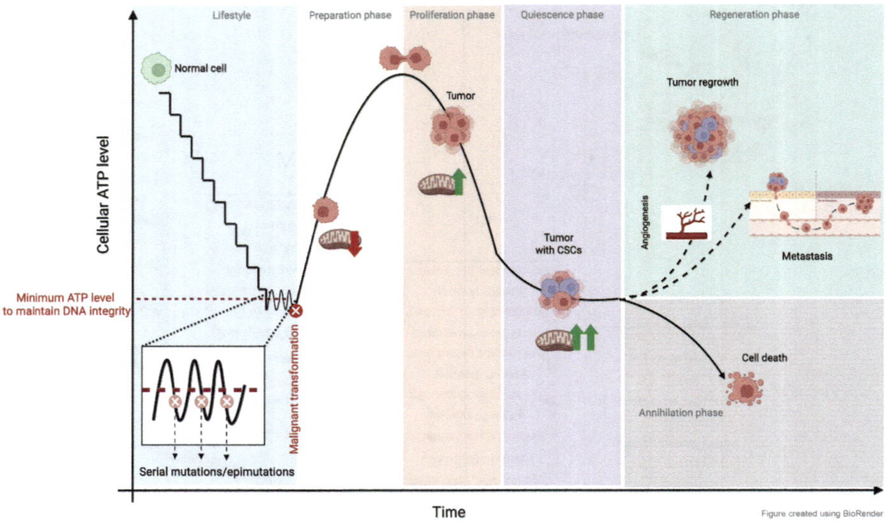

Fig. 6.2 Steps in cancer formation and progression based on the "Cell Energy" hypothesis. According to this hypothesis, cancer arises from normal cells following lifestyle- or genetic-induced mitochondrial dysfunction, which leads to progressive genomic instability and the accumulation of mutations, ultimately resulting in malignant transformation. (Figure created using BioRender)

oxygen availability, making glycolysis the dominant means of survival [16]. At this phase, cancer cells provide their mitochondrial content by hijacking from adjacent immune cells [21] or receiving from surrounding cancer cells [22], cancer-associated fibroblasts [23], and tumor-infiltrating nerves [24]. In addition, they can improve their mitochondrial content by activating upregulators of mitochondrial metabolism, including PGC-1 [25] and mitofusin-2 [26].

As proliferation proceeds and ATP reserves become depleted, intracellular energy levels begin to decline—a potentially lethal state for cancer cells. Cells unable to maintain sufficient ATP enter the "Quiescence Phase," characterized by reduced metabolic activity to preserve viability [27]. This state resembles the phenotype of CSCs (as described in Sect. 6.2.3) [19]. The Cell Energy hypothesis thus offers a plausible rationale for the emergence of stem-like features within a subset of cancer cells. CSCs have been shown to possess higher mitochondrial content, which enhances their metabolic flexibility and antioxidant capacity, enabling them to withstand intrinsic and therapy-induced oxidative stress [28]. Meanwhile, cancer cells that fail to adapt to low-ATP conditions—or cannot increase mitochondrial capacity to meet metabolic demands—undergo cell death due to excessive intracellular ROS accumulation. In contrast, cells that gain access to new energy sources, such as through local invasion or distant metastasis, can progress to the "Regeneration Phase," where metabolic activity and proliferation resume [20].

Taken together, this multistep schematic highlights how fluctuations in cellular energy and mitochondrial content shape the evolutionary journey of cancer cells from initiation to metastasis. The following two sections outline the importance of calcium regulation by mitochondria and mitochondrial dynamics in cancer cells' pathogenesis.

6.3 Mitochondrial Calcium Metabolism in Cancer Cells

As a second messenger, intracellular calcium (Ca^{2+}) plays a critical role in regulating cell survival, metabolism, and growth by modulating numerous enzymes, transcription factors, and ion channels [29]. While extracellular Ca^{2+} concentrations range from 1 to 4 mM, basal intracellular Ca^{2+} levels are tightly maintained at approximately 100 nM [30]. Even slight deviations from this physiological range can adversely affect cellular metabolism, survival, and proliferation. To prevent such disturbances, intracellular Ca^{2+} homeostasis is precisely controlled through coordinated interactions among various organelles, with the mitochondria–endoplasmic reticulum (ER) axis playing a central role. Excess Ca^{2+} is either extruded across the plasma membrane or sequestered into the ER, the principal intracellular Ca^{2+} storage compartment [29].

Mitochondrial Ca^{2+} functions as a key metabolic regulator. Elevated intramitochondrial Ca^{2+} enhances mitochondrial OXPHOS by stimulating several rate-limiting enzymes within the TCA cycle and ETC [31]. The primary regulator of mitochondrial Ca^{2+} uptake is the mitochondrial calcium uniporter (MCU) complex, located in the inner mitochondrial membrane [32]. Experimental studies have shown that MCU upregulation correlates with larger tumor size, increased metastatic potential, and poorer patient survival [32]. Elevated mitochondrial Ca^{2+} levels can promote cancer progression by increasing mitochondrial ROS production, which in turn activates HIF-1 and supports a protumorigenic phenotype [33]. Moreover, MCU overexpression has been shown to enhance resistance to chemotherapeutic agents, an effect demonstrated in ovarian cancer models [34].

Given the central role of mitochondrial Ca^{2+} in sustaining OXPHOS activity, these findings support our hypothesis that cancer cells with higher mitochondrial content exhibit more aggressive behavior and worse prognosis [35].

6.4 Mitochondrial Dynamics in Cancer Cells

Mitochondria in human cells are highly dynamic organelles. They can undergo fusion in response to hypoxia or nutrient depletion and fission during cellular stress or nutrient repletion [36]. These processes allow mitochondria to adopt a range of morphologies—from elongated, interconnected networks to small, fragmented, or swollen forms [37]. In addition, the number and structure of mitochondrial cristae can change depending on the cell's metabolic state [36]. Mitochondrial dynamics is an intricate process regulated by multiple factors. In mitochondrial fusion, two major groups of proteins are involved: mitofusins (MFN1 and MFN2) and OPA1. The mitofusins mediate outer mitochondrial membrane tethering and fusion, whereas OPA1 regulates inner mitochondrial membrane fusion. On the other hand, the primary protein responsible for mitochondrial fission is dynamin-related protein 1 (DRP1) [38].

During periods of heightened mitochondrial activity, mitochondrial proteins can become damaged, and mitochondrial DNA (mtDNA) may accumulate mutations due to exposure to ROS. Over time, this gradual accumulation of damage reduces mitochondrial quality and contributes to mitochondrial dysfunction. Mitochondrial dynamics offer a critical quality-control mechanism that allows mitochondria to restore function through coordinated cycles of fusion and fission. Mitochondrial fusion enables the mixing of mitochondrial contents, allowing damaged proteins or mutated mtDNA from an impaired mitochondrion to be diluted by merging with a healthier one. Conversely, mitochondrial fission facilitates the segregation of dysfunctional mitochondria from the healthy network, thereby marking them for mitophagy, a selective degradation pathway that recycles defective mitochondria and promotes the regeneration of functional mitochondrial units. The finely tuned balance between fusion and fission is essential for maintaining mitochondrial integrity and sustaining overall cellular homeostasis. Cancer cells are no exception; they also rely on this sophisticated mitochondrial quality-control system to support their survival, metabolic flexibility, and continued progression [36].

In cancer cells, mitochondrial fission provides several additional advantages. For instance, fission is required during cell division to ensure the proper distribution of mitochondria between daughter cells [39]. Moreover, mitochondrial fission–related proteins are frequently upregulated in highly invasive and metastatic tumors. Zhao et al. reported that DRP1, a key regulator of mitochondrial fission, is elevated in invasive and metastatic breast cancer cells [40]. Supporting this finding, Ghosh et al. demonstrated that DRP1 promotes EMT, a critical step in the metastatic cascade [41]. Mitochondrial fission has also been implicated in immune evasion, as it can downregulate MHC-I, thereby reducing antigen presentation to cytotoxic T cells [42]. In contrast, mitochondrial fusion supports OXPHOS activity, cellular dedifferentiation, and the quiescent state characteristic of CSCs [39, 43]. In a nutshell, mitochondrial fusion predominates in CSCs to preserve stemness, whereas mitochondrial fission dominates in proliferative cancer cells, facilitating their invasion and migration.

6.5 The Importance of Mitochondria for Cancer Cells

So far, we have established that, contrary to Warburg's original assumption, mitochondria in cancer cells remain functional. In other words, cancer cells actively depend on mitochondrial activity to sustain their metabolic demands. In this section, we highlight that the advantages provided by mitochondria extend far beyond metabolism alone. As summarized in our previous review [35], mitochondria are essential for enabling cancer cells to survive in the harsh tumor microenvironment, evade immune surveillance, acquire more aggressive phenotypes, and develop resistance to chemotherapy, radiotherapy, and immunotherapy (Fig. 6.3). Many of the

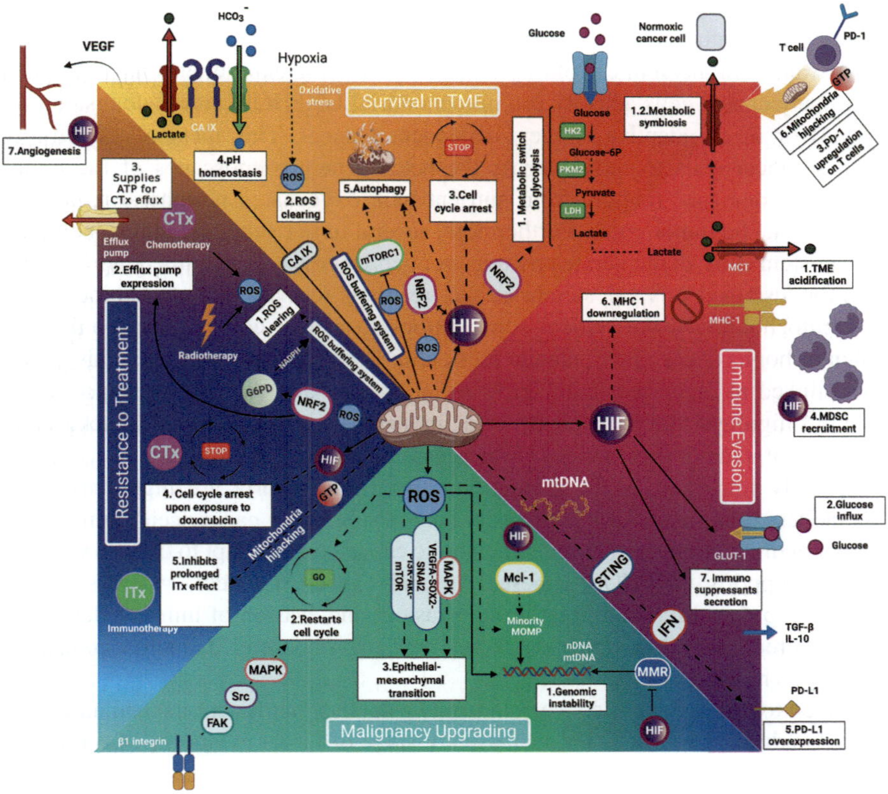

Fig. 6.3 Mitochondria as master regulators of cancer metabolism, progression, immune evasion, and therapy resistance. The titles of the benefits of mitochondria for cancer cells are shown in while boxes. (Source: [35] under CC BY 4.0)

protumorigenic effects of mitochondria are mediated by mitochondrial ROS and the resulting stabilization of HIF-1 [44], which serves as a central regulator of cancer cell adaptation and progression. For details of how mitochondria mediate these benefits for cancer cells, please refer to our published review articles [35, 45].

6.6 Conclusions

For nearly a century, cancer metabolism has been viewed through the lens of Otto Warburg's pioneering observations. Warburg concluded that mitochondria in cancer cells were dysfunctional, forcing malignant cells to rely on aerobic glycolysis for ATP generation. Although his work fundamentally shaped the field, accumulating evidence now indicates that this interpretation is incomplete. Modern experimental studies have demonstrated that mitochondria in cancer cells are not only functional but also indispensable for tumor growth, progression, and survival. Rather than being passive or damaged bystanders, mitochondria serve as central hubs for bioenergetics, biosynthesis, redox balance, and signaling in malignant tissues.

Advances in metabolic profiling and isotope-tracing experiments have revealed that many cancer cells actively use mitochondrial OXPHOS, either alongside glycolysis or in an adaptive, context-dependent manner. This metabolic flexibility allows cancer cells to thrive across the heterogeneous landscapes of the tumor microenvironment—ranging from nutrient-rich, oxygenated peripheral regions to hypoxic, acidic tumor cores. Furthermore, several tumor subpopulations, including cancer stem cells, demonstrate an even stronger dependence on mitochondrial function for sustained survival, stemness, and treatment resistance. Beyond bioenergetics, mitochondria make critical contributions to cancer cell physiology through calcium homeostasis and organelle cross talk. Dysregulation of MCU activity has been linked to increased tumor growth, metastasis, and therapy resistance. Such findings highlight that mitochondrial calcium signaling is not merely a background process but a major determinant of malignant behavior.

Equally important is the recognition that mitochondria are highly dynamic organelles. Continuous cycles of fusion and fission allow cancer cells to maintain mitochondrial quality, redistribute metabolic capacity, and adapt to diverse stresses. Fusion supports OXPHOS, quiescence, and cancer stemness, whereas fission enables rapid proliferation, migration, invasion, and evasion of immune detection. This bidirectional plasticity underscores how mitochondrial dynamics contribute directly to hallmark cancer traits.

Taken together, the collective data firmly establish that functional and adaptable mitochondria are essential for nearly every stage of tumor evolution—from initiation and metabolic reprogramming to immune evasion, metastasis, and therapy resistance. Warburg's observations remain historically and conceptually important, but the modern view of cancer biology recognizes mitochondria not as defective components but as powerful drivers of malignancy. Understanding these mitochondrial mechanisms opens new avenues for targeted oncology, where disrupting mitochondrial metabolism, calcium regulation, or organelle dynamics may offer promising therapeutic strategies for future cancer treatment.

References

1. Luo Q, Smith DP. Global cancer burden: progress, projections, and challenges. Lancet. 2025;406(10512):1536–7. https://doi.org/10.1016/S0140-6736(25)01570-3.
2. Li Q, et al. Radiotherapy/chemotherapy-immunotherapy for cancer management: from mechanisms to clinical implications. Oxidative Med Cell Longev. 2023;2023:7530794. https://doi.org/10.1155/2023/7530794.
3. Warburg O. Über den Stoffwechsel der Carcinomzelle. Naturwissenschaften. 1924;12(50):1131–7. https://doi.org/10.1007/BF01504608.
4. Carew JS, Huang P. Mitochondrial defects in cancer. Mol Cancer. 2002;1(1):9. https://doi.org/10.1186/1476-4598-1-9.
5. Bose S, Zhang C, Le A. Glucose metabolism in cancer: the Warburg effect and beyond. In: Le A, editor. The heterogeneity of cancer metabolism, Advances in experimental medicine

and biology, vol. 1311. Cham: Springer International Publishing; 2021. p. 3–15. https://doi.org/10.1007/978-3-030-65768-0_1.
6. Dou R, et al. Precision nanomedicines: targeting hot mitochondria in cancer cells. ACS Appl Bio Mater. 2022; https://doi.org/10.1021/acsabm.2c00641.
7. De Preter G, et al. Inhibition of the pentose phosphate pathway by dichloroacetate unravels a missing link between aerobic glycolysis and cancer cell proliferation. Oncotarget. 2016;7(3):2910–20. https://doi.org/10.18632/oncotarget.6272.
8. Wilson DF. Oxidative phosphorylation: regulation and role in cellular and tissue metabolism. J Physiol. 595(23):7023–38. https://doi.org/10.1113/JP273839.
9. Zheng J. Energy metabolism of cancer: glycolysis versus oxidative phosphorylation (Review). Oncol Lett. 2012;4(6):1151–7. https://doi.org/10.3892/ol.2012.928.
10. Liberti MV, Locasale JW. The Warburg effect: how does it benefit cancer cells? Trends Biochem Sci. 2016;41(3):211–8. https://doi.org/10.1016/j.tibs.2015.12.001.
11. Sciacovelli M, Gaude E, Hilvo M, Frezza C. The metabolic alterations of cancer cells. Methods Enzymol. 2014;542:1–23. Elsevier. https://doi.org/10.1016/B978-0-12-416618-9.00001-7.
12. Demetrius L, Tuszynski JA. Quantum metabolism explains the allometric scaling of metabolic rates. J R Soc Interface. 2010;7(44):507–14. https://doi.org/10.1098/rsif.2009.0310.
13. Avril N. GLUT1 expression in tissue and (18)F-FDG uptake. J Nucl Med. 2004;45(6):930–2.
14. Weinhouse S. Studies on the fate of isotopically labeled metabolites in the oxidative metabolism of tumors. Cancer Res. 1951;11(8):585–91.
15. Wang Y, et al. Saturation of the mitochondrial NADH shuttles drives aerobic glycolysis in proliferating cells. Mol Cell. 2022;82(17):3270–3283.e9. https://doi.org/10.1016/j.molcel.2022.07.007.
16. Hay N. Reprogramming glucose metabolism in cancer: can it be exploited for cancer therapy? Nat Rev Cancer. 2016;16(10):635–49. https://doi.org/10.1038/nrc.2016.77.
17. Le A, et al. Tumorigenicity of hypoxic respiring cancer cells revealed by a hypoxia-cell cycle dual reporter. Proc Natl Acad Sci USA. 2014;111(34):12486–91. https://doi.org/10.1073/pnas.1402012111.
18. Taghizadeh-Hesary F, Ghadyani M, Kashanchi F, Behnam B. Exploring TSGA10 function: a crosstalk or controlling mechanism in the signaling pathway of carcinogenesis? Cancer. 2024;16(17):3044. https://doi.org/10.3390/cancers16173044.
19. Masoudi M, et al. Metabolic adaptations in cancer stem cells: a key to therapy resistance. Biochim Biophys Acta (BBA) - Mol Basis Dis. 2024;1870(5):167164. https://doi.org/10.1016/j.bbadis.2024.167164.
20. Akbari H, Taghizadeh-Hesary F, Heike Y, Bahadori M. Cell energy: a new hypothesis in decoding cancer evolution. Arch Iran Med. 2019;22(12):733–5.
21. Saha T, et al. Intercellular nanotubes mediate mitochondrial trafficking between cancer and immune cells. Nat Nanotechnol. 2022;17(1):98–106. https://doi.org/10.1038/s41565-021-01000-4.
22. Lu J, et al. Tunneling nanotubes promote intercellular mitochondria transfer followed by increased invasiveness in bladder cancer cells. Oncotarget. 2017;8(9):15539–52. https://doi.org/10.18632/oncotarget.14695.
23. Goliwas KF, et al. Mitochondrial transfer from cancer-associated fibroblasts increases migration in aggressive breast cancer. J Cell Sci. 2023;136(14):jcs260419. https://doi.org/10.1242/jcs.260419.
24. Hoover G, et al. Nerve-to-cancer transfer of mitochondria during cancer metastasis. Nature. 2025;644(8075):252–62. https://doi.org/10.1038/s41586-025-09176-8.
25. Andrzejewski S, et al. PGC-1α promotes breast cancer metastasis and confers bioenergetic flexibility against metabolic drugs. Cell Metab. 2017;26(5):778–787.e5. https://doi.org/10.1016/j.cmet.2017.09.006.
26. Purohit PK, Edwards R, Tokatlidis K, Saini N. MiR-195 regulates mitochondrial function by targeting mitofusin-2 in breast cancer cells. RNA Biol. 2019;16(7):918–29. https://doi.org/10.1080/15476286.2019.1600999.

27. Lindell E, Zhong L, Zhang X. Quiescent cancer cells-A potential therapeutic target to overcome tumor resistance and relapse. Int J Mol Sci. 2023;24(4):3762. https://doi.org/10.3390/ijms24043762.
28. Fontana F, Macchi C, Anselmi M, Rizzuto AS, Ruscica M, Limonta P. PGC1-α-driven mitochondrial biogenesis contributes to a cancer stem cell phenotype in melanoma. Biochim Biophys Acta (BBA) - Mol Basis Dis. 2024;1870(1):166897. https://doi.org/10.1016/j.bbadis.2023.166897.
29. Garbincius JF, Elrod JW. Mitochondrial calcium exchange in physiology and disease. Physiol Rev. 2022;102(2):893–992. https://doi.org/10.1152/physrev.00041.2020.
30. Raffaello A, Mammucari C, Gherardi G, Rizzuto R. Calcium at the center of cell signaling: interplay between endoplasmic reticulum, mitochondria, and lysosomes. Trends Biochem Sci. 2016;41(12):1035–49. https://doi.org/10.1016/j.tibs.2016.09.001.
31. Giorgi C, Marchi S, Pinton P. The machineries, regulation and cellular functions of mitochondrial calcium. Nat Rev Mol Cell Biol. 2018;19(11):713–30. https://doi.org/10.1038/s41580-018-0052-8.
32. Weissenrieder JS, Kevin Foskett J. Mitochondrial Ca^{2+} in cancer growth and metabolism. J Cell Physiol. 2025;240(9):e70093. https://doi.org/10.1002/jcp.70093.
33. Tosatto A, et al. The mitochondrial calcium uniporter regulates breast cancer progression via HIF-1α. EMBO Mol Med. 2016;8(5):569–85. https://doi.org/10.15252/emmm.201606255.
34. Li L, et al. Long noncoding RNA RMRP contributes to paclitaxel sensitivity of ovarian cancer by regulating miR-580-3p/MICU1 signaling. J Oncol. 2022;2022:8301941. https://doi.org/10.1155/2022/8301941.
35. Taghizadeh-Hesary F, Akbari H, Bahadori M, Behnam B. Targeted anti-mitochondrial therapy: the future of oncology. Genes. 2022;13(10):1728. https://doi.org/10.3390/genes13101728.
36. Chen W, Zhao H, Li Y. Mitochondrial dynamics in health and disease: mechanisms and potential targets. Signal Transduct Target Ther. 2023;8(1):333. https://doi.org/10.1038/s41392-023-01547-9.
37. Quintana-Cabrera R, Scorrano L. Determinants and outcomes of mitochondrial dynamics. Mol Cell. 2023;83(6):857–76. https://doi.org/10.1016/j.molcel.2023.02.012.
38. Shaaban AH, Soliman Wadan A-H, El-Sadek MZ, Mostafa SA. Mitochondrial dynamics regulators in cancer metabolism and progression. Mitochondrial Commun. 2025:S2590279225000057. https://doi.org/10.1016/j.mitoco.2025.04.001.
39. Giannitti G, Marchesi S, Garavaglia R, Preosto I, Fontana F. Unraveling the role of mitochondrial dynamics in cancer stem cells: molecular basis and therapeutic implications. Biochim Biophys Acta BBA - Rev Cancer. 2025;1880(6):189450. https://doi.org/10.1016/j.bbcan.2025.189450.
40. Zhao J, et al. Mitochondrial dynamics regulates migration and invasion of breast cancer cells. Oncogene. 2013;32(40):4814–24. https://doi.org/10.1038/onc.2012.494.
41. Ghosh D, Pakhira S, Ghosh DD, Roychoudhury S, Roy SS. Ets1 facilitates EMT/invasion through Drp1-mediated mitochondrial fragmentation in ovarian cancer. iScience. 2023;26(9):107537. https://doi.org/10.1016/j.isci.2023.107537.
42. Lei X, et al. Mitochondrial fission induces immunoescape in solid tumors through decreasing MHC-I surface expression. Nat Commun. 2022;13(1):3882. https://doi.org/10.1038/s41467-022-31417-x.
43. Fan M, Shi Y, Zhao J, Li L. Cancer stem cell fate determination: mito-nuclear communication. Cell Commun Signal CCS. 2023;21(1):159. https://doi.org/10.1186/s12964-023-01160-x.
44. Van Gisbergen MW, et al. Mitochondrial dysfunction inhibits Hypoxia-Induced HIF-1α stabilization and expression of its downstream targets. Front Oncol. 2020;10:770. https://doi.org/10.3389/fonc.2020.00770.
45. Behnam B, Taghizadeh-Hesary F. Mitochondrial metabolism: a new dimension of personalized oncology. Cancer. 2023;15(16):4058. https://doi.org/10.3390/cancers15164058.

Metabolic Cross Talk in the Tumor Microenvironment

7

Chinmay Das, Somya Ranjan Dash, Biswajit Das, Subhajit Chatterjee, and Tithi Parija

7.1 Introduction

Cancer remains one of the most profound global health burdens, accounting for significant morbidity and mortality worldwide. It is defined not only by the uncontrolled proliferation of malignant cells but also by the intricate and adaptive niche in which these cells reside, the tumor microenvironment (TME). The TME is a highly dynamic and heterogeneous group of tumor resident cells, which includes both cellular and noncellular elements that communicate with cancer cells and vice versa; this significantly rewires the characteristics of both the cell types [1, 2]. Key components of the TME include malignant cells, immune cells such as T cells, B cells, natural killer (NK) cells, dendritic cells (DCs), and neutrophils, stromal components including tumor-associated macrophages (TAMs) and cancer-associated fibroblasts (CAFs), as well as supporting cells such as endothelial cells (ECs), pericytes, adipocytes, and nerve cells. The noncellular component includes extracellular matrix (ECM), cytokines, chemokines, growth factors, and other metabolites, all of

C. Das · T. Parija (✉)
School of Biotechnology, Kalinga Institute of Industrial Technology Deemed to be University, Bhubaneswar, Odisha, India
e-mail: tithi.parija@kiitbiotech.ac.in

S. R. Dash
Cancer Metastasis & Therapeutics Lab, Department of Biological Sciences, Indian Institute of Science Education and Research (IISER), Berhampur, Odisha, India

B. Das
Department of Molecular, Cell and Developmental Biology, University of California, Santa Cruz, CA, USA

S. Chatterjee
Laboratory of Cellular Oncology, National Cancer Institute, National Institutes of Health (NIH), Bethesda, MD, USA

S. Ashique et al. (eds.), *Cancer Metabolism*, Cancer Treatment and Research 195, https://doi.org/10.1007/978-3-032-21861-2_7

which collectively create a biochemical framework that supports tumor survival [2, 3].

Metabolism refers to the total reactions that occur throughout the body within each cell and that provide the body with energy. Metabolites are any intermediate or end products formed during metabolism-usually small molecules that serve various functions, such as providing energy, acting as structural components, functioning as signaling molecules, or regulating biochemical processes [4, 5]. Tumor cells have higher metabolic activity, resulting in the production of various oncometabolites in the TME, which promote cancer. Cancer cells possess reprogrammed energy metabolism, where they predominantly rely on aerobic glycolysis, also known as the Warburg effect. Even in the presence of oxygen, they produce a high amount of lactate and others metabolite [6, 7]. These secret metabolites in the TME suppress the activity of cytotoxic T cells and NK cells, thereby promoting immune escape, making it easier for cancer to evade the host's immunosurveillance detection. Similarly, some metabolites released by cancer cells, such as adenosine and kynurenine, act as signal molecules and bind to various components of the TME, thereby blocking immune cell activity and contributing to tumor survival [8]. Cancer cells also establish metabolic symbiosis with neighboring stromal components. Notably, TAMs and CAFs can undergo metabolic reprogramming upon interaction with tumor cells, exchanging metabolites that support cancer growth and drug resistance. For example, CAFs often display enhanced glycolytic activity and release lactate, which oxidative tumor cells then use for mitochondrial respiration, a process known as reverse Warburg effect. Similarly, TAMs shift toward fatty acid (FA) oxidation (FAO) and oxidative phosphorylation (OXPHOS), producing anti-inflammatory cytokines that facilitate tumor immune suppression and progression of therapy resistance [9]. Certain mutations in cancer cells can lead to the accumulation of oncometabolites (e.g., D-2-hydroxyglutarate, fumarate, succinate, etc.). These can interfere with enzymes that regulate gene expression, leading to changes in DNA and histone structure that make cancer more aggressive [10]. Oncometabolites also activate protumorigenic signaling pathways like HIF-1α, promoting angiogenesis, metabolic adaptation, and metastatic potential. The ECM is a crucial noncellular component that modulates the metabolic landscape of the TME. By influencing nutrient diffusion, metabolite retention, and drug penetration, ECM remodeling can contribute to tumor progression and chemoresistance [11].

This chapter explores the complex metabolic communication networks within the TME that drive cancer progression and therapeutic resistance. Intercellular metabolic communication within the TME occurs through multiple modes of signaling, categorized broadly into four types, i.e., (1) autocrine signaling, in which tumor cells produce and respond to their own metabolites (e.g., lactate, purines) to promote self-sustaining growth and survival, (2) paracrine signaling, involving metabolic exchange between tumor cells and neighboring stromal or immune cells, thereby creating a cooperative microenvironment that supports tumor adaptation, (3) juxtacrine signaling, characterized by direct metabolite transfer through gap junctions, exosomes, or membrane transporters under stress conditions, (4) endocrine-like signaling, where tumor-derived metabolites enter circulation to remodel systemic metabolism and establish premetastatic niches [12, 13].

A comprehensive understanding of the metabolic crosstalk within the TME is therefore essential for identifying novel therapeutic targets. Interventions aimed at disrupting tumor-specific metabolic dependencies, inhibiting metabolite-mediated signaling, or reprogramming immune cell metabolism hold immense promise in overcoming resistance and improving clinical outcomes. Furthermore, the identification of metabolic biomarkers offers new opportunities for early detection, treatment monitoring, and personalized therapy. Therefore, this chapter focuses on elucidating the multifaceted mechanisms of metabolic communication within the TME, including autocrine, paracrine, juxtacrine, and endocrine-like interactions. It explores their roles in driving tumor progression and therapy resistance. Understanding these complex networks provides a foundation for developing metabolism-based therapeutic strategies that can complement conventional and immunotherapeutic approaches, ultimately enhancing the efficacy of cancer treatment and improving patient survival [14].

7.2 Autocrine Metabolic Cross Talk of Cancer in TME

Autocrine metabolic cross talk in the TME refers to the ability of cancer cells to secrete metabolites and signaling molecules that act back upon the same cells through specific receptors and transporters, thereby reinforcing metabolic reprogramming, proliferation, and survival. The major metabolites and pathways implicated in autocrine-mediated metabolic communication include lactate, fatty acids (FAs), amino acids, nucleotides/adenosine, as well as cytokines/growth factors, which are discussed below (Fig. 7.1).

7.2.1 Lactate

Cancer cells predominantly depend on aerobic glycolysis, producing large amounts of lactate even in the presence of oxygen, a phenomenon known as the Warburg effect [15]. This metabolic adaptation enhances glucose uptake, leading to lactate accumulation and the subsequent acidification of the TME. Lactate is secreted via monocarboxylate transporter 4 (MCT4) to the TME, leading to an acidic microenvironment production where lactate concentrations reach 10–40 mM compared to 1.5–3 mM in that present in normal tissues [16, 17]. Lactate functions as an autocrine signaling molecule through two key mechanisms: (i) G-protein-coupled receptor 81 (GPR81) receptor-mediated signaling, where lactate binds GPR81 without being transported intracellularly, activating downstream oncogenic pathways, and (ii) MCT1-mediated reuptake for metabolic utilization, supporting the lactate shuttle [17, 18].

Activation of GPR81 induces the upregulation of glycolytic enzymes such as hexokinase 2 (HK2), phosphofructokinase 1(PFK1), and lactate dehydrogenase A

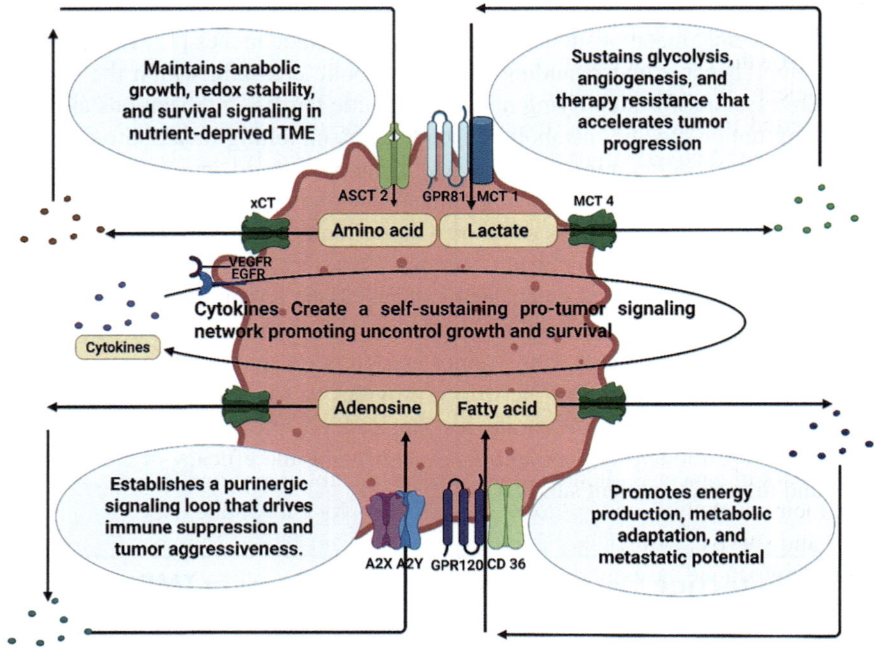

Fig. 7.1 Autocrine metabolic cross talk of cancer cells in the TME

(LDHA), enhances adenosine triphosphate (ATP) production, and promotes MCT4 expression, thereby creating a positive feedback loop that sustains glycolysis. Lactate signaling also stabilizes hypoxia-inducible factor 1 alpha (HIF-1α), upregulates vascular endothelial growth factor (VEGF), and stimulates angiogenesis to improve tumor vascularization. Moreover, lactate enhances epithelial–mesenchymal transition (EMT), invasion, and metastasis while promoting programmed death-ligand 1 (PD-L1) expression and suppressing antitumor immunity. Through mammalian target of rapamycin (mTOR) and nuclear factor-kappa B (NF-κB) activation, lactate contributes to drug resistance via acidic ion-trapping [18]. Clinically, GPR81 is highly elevated in stage II & III breast cancers, with high lactate levels correlating with poor prognosis, highlighting GPR81 as a promising therapeutic target to disrupt this self-reinforcing lactate signaling loop that drives cancer progression [18].

7.2.2 Fatty Acids

Cancer cells can release free fatty acids (FFAs) into the TME through enhanced lipolysis or de novo lipogenesis, often packaged in lipid-rich vesicles or exosomes. These extracellular FAs can rebind to cancer cells through autocrine mechanisms mediated by lipid transporters and receptors, including cluster of differentiation 36

(CD36) (FA translocase), FA-binding proteins (FABPs), and G-protein-coupled receptors (GPR40, GPR120) [19, 20].

Among these, CD36 serves as a key mediator of FA uptake and is highly expressed in several aggressive malignancies, including breast, ovarian, gastric, and prostate cancers [21]. CD36-driven FA uptake not only helps in energy production via enhanced β-oxidation but also activates Peroxisome proliferator-activated receptor (PPAR) -dependent transcriptional programs that rewire cellular metabolism to support growth and survival [22, 23]. Furthermore, CD36 and GPR120 signaling converge on oncogenic cascades involving STAT3, ERK1/2, and PI3K/Akt, promoting EMT, metastasis, and resistance to apoptosis under metabolic stress [21, 24].

7.2.3 Amino Acids

Unlike lactate and FA autocrine signaling, amino acid autocrine mechanisms also involve complex transporter systems, metabolic sensing pathways, and different cellular pathways. Cancer cells actively secrete amino acids, particularly glutamine and glutamate, where they are subsequently reabsorbed through high-affinity transporters to form a self-sustaining metabolic loop. The most well-characterized example is the xCT (SLC7A11) transporter system, which exports glutamate while importing cystine [25]. Alanine-Serine-Cysteine Transporter 2 (ASCT2) mediates glutamine uptake, which fuels biosynthetic processes and serves as an exchange substrate for LAT1 (SLC7A5), a transporter that imports leucine to activate mTORC1 signaling and drive protein synthesis and proliferation [26]. Similarly, xCT (SLC7A11) imports cystine in exchange for glutamate, supporting glutathione synthesis and redox balance, thereby promoting cancer therapy resistance [27]. Additionally, both SNAT1 (SLC38A1) and SNAT2 (SLC38A2) facilitate the uptake of neutral amino acids, including serine and glutamine, supporting nucleotide biosynthesis and maintaining mTORC1 activation during nutrient stress [28]. Through these transporter systems, cancer cells establish autocrine loops that sustain signaling pathways such as mTORC1, PI3K/Akt, and MAPK, enhancing proliferation, invasion, redox homeostasis, and therapy resistance within the TME [29].

7.2.4 Nucleotides and Adenosine

Cancer cells also release nucleotides and ATP into the extracellular space, functioning as autocrine signaling mediators. Extracellular ATP binds to purinergic P2X and P2Y receptors on tumor cells, triggering calcium signaling and activating downstream pathways that regulate cell proliferation, migration, and survival [30]. ATP is rapidly hydrolyzed to adenosine by the ectonucleotidases CD39 and CD73. Adenosine, in turn, binds to A2A and A2B receptors, activating cyclic adenosine monophosphate(cAMP) dependent signaling cascades that promote immune evasion, angiogenesis, and metabolic adaptation [30, 31]. Elevated extracellular ATP and adenosine levels have been associated with increased tumor aggressiveness and resistance to therapy. Targeting the CD39 and CD73 adenosine axis represents a promising therapeutic strategy to inhibit autocrine purinergic signaling and restore antitumor immunity [31].

7.2.5 Cytokines and Growth Factors

Cytokines and growth factors are key signaling molecules secreted by both cancer and stromal cells in the TME, regulating tumor growth, survival, angiogenesis, immune evasion, and metastasis [32]. Key cytokines, such as interleukin-6 (IL-6), tumor necrosis factor-alpha (TNF-α), and transforming growth factor-beta (TGF-β), as well as chemokines like C-X-C motif chemokine ligand 12 (CXCL12), exert their effects through specific receptors, including IL-6R/gp130, TNFR1/2, TGF-β receptors, and CXCR4/CXCR7 [32]. Engagement of these receptors activates major intracellular signaling cascades such as JAK/STAT, NF-κB, MAPK/ERK, PI3K/AKT, and SMAD pathways, leading to transcriptional reprogramming that promotes cell proliferation, survival, EMT, angiogenesis, and immune suppression [32, 33]. Similarly, growth factors such as epidermal growth factor (EGF), vascular endothelial growth factor (VEGF), fibroblast growth factor (FGF), and hepatocyte growth factor (HGF) act through their corresponding receptor tyrosine kinases, that are, epidermal growth factor eceptor (EGFR), vascular endothelial growth factor receptor (VEGFR), fibroblast growth factor receptor (FGFR), and cellular mesenchymal-epithelial transition factor (c-MET) respectively, to drive RAS/MAPK, PI3K/Akt, and STAT pathways [34]. These autocrine signaling loops contribute to metabolic reprogramming, uncontrolled proliferation, and vascular remodeling, creating a protumorigenic environment that supports progression and resistance to therapy.

7.3 Paracrine Metabolic Cross Talk in TME

7.3.1 Metabolic Cross Talk Between T Cells and Cancer Cells

In the TME, cancer cells and tumor-infiltrating T cells participate in immune negotiation via three interconnected mechanisms: substrate competition, metabolite signaling, and checkpoint-mediated metabolic reprogramming. Enhanced tumor glycolysis leads to local glucose depletion, suppressing T-cell mTOR activity, glycolytic function, and interferon-γ production. Mitigating this limitation either genetically or via immune checkpoint blockade restores T-cell effector function *in vivo* [35].

Tumors make lactic acid, which lowers the pH inside the tumor and stops T-cell growth, cytokine production, and cytotoxicity. Buffers that raise the pH inside the tumor enhance antitumor responses and improve checkpoint activity. Low pH also disrupts interleukin-2 (IL-2)/IL-2 receptor signaling, which lowers mTORC1 and c-Myc activity [36, 37]. Indoleamine-2,3-dioxygenase-1 (IDO1) and the tumor-specific enzyme tryptophan-2,3-dioxygenase (TDO) break down tryptophan to make kynurenine. This kynurenine attaches to the aryl hydrocarbon receptor (AhR) in T cells, which makes them exhausted. Inhibiting AhR with drugs can stop this IDO/TDO-mediated resistance [38, 39]. When myeloid arginases (ARG1/ARG2) use L-arginine in small amounts, activated T cells can't cycle as rapidly. On the other hand, when intracellular L-arginine levels rise, activated T cells are reprogrammed to oxidative phosphorylation (OXPHOS) and memory-like persistence. Tumors become more sensitive to antiprogrammed cell death protein-1 (PD-1) therapy, and blocking arginase increases the number of CD8+ T lymphocytes within the tumor [40, 41]. Under hypoxic conditions, HIF-1α is stabilized, leading to the upregulation of PD-L1 expression in both tumor and myeloid compartments, which in turn lowers T-cell activation. Inhibition of HIF-1α reduces PD-L1 levels and modulates the TME through context-dependent effects [42, 43]. Extracellular adenosine, generated from ATP by ectonucleotidases CD39 and CD73, transmits signals via the A2A adenosine receptor (A2AR) on T cells to inhibit effector functions. Disruption of the CD39/CD73/A2AR axis, whether through genetic or pharmacological interventions, reveals antitumor T-cell activity, while CD73 also supports tumor metabolism through enhanced respiration and aspartate biosynthesis, highlighting its dual immune-metabolic role [44, 45].

Glutamine antagonism, which can be both systemic and tumor-targeted (e.g., with JHU083), breaks down tumor bioenergetics, lowers suppressive myeloid populations, improves T-cell OXPHOS, and works synergistically with checkpoint treatment across models [46, 47]. The effector T cells also need the serine-glycine-one-carbon (SGOC) network to make nucleotides and to proliferate clonally; even when there is enough glucose, extracellular serine slows down the process of proliferative bursts [48]. Lipid stress is another checkpoint. The scavenger receptor CD36 takes in oxidized lipids, which leads to lipid peroxidation, ferroptosis-prone states, and the destruction of CD8+ T lymphocytes in tumors. This process can be targeted by genetic or drug-based methods and is important for treating cancer in the clinic [49]. In summary, immune checkpoints profoundly reshape T-cell metabolism, PD-1 signaling suppresses glycolysis while promoting lipolysis and FAO, providing a mechanistic rationale for combining metabolic modulators (targeting acidosis, arginase, adenosine, glutamine, or lipid peroxidation) with PD-1/PD-L1 or CTLA-4 blockade [50].

7.3.2 Metabolic Cross Talk Between B Cells and Cancer Cells

In the TME, cancer and B cells interact through intricate metabolic signaling networks that influence B-cell fate from antigen-presenting and antibody-secreting phenotypes (typically found in tertiary lymphoid structures) to immunosuppressive IL-10-producing regulatory B cells (Bregs). Recent evidence highlights the metabolic dependence and dual functional nature of tumor-infiltrating B cells [51, 52]. Lactate is a well-known tumor-secreted product shown to elevate glycolytic flux. In vivo, lactic acid absorbed by intratumoral B cells enhances histone H3 lysine-27 acetylation (H3K27ac) and influences them toward IL-10^{+} Bregs, establishing a direct connection between a cancer metabolite and B-cell epigenetic programming and immune suppression. Beyond serving as a carbon source, lactate and related protein "lactylation" act as instructive metabolic signals within the immune compartment [53, 54]. Adenosine signaling represents another major immunoregulatory pathway. Human B cells express CD39 (ENTPD1) and CD73 (NT5E), which hydrolyze extracellular ATP into adenosine. $CD39^{+}CD73^{+}$ Bregs, observed in head and neck squamous cell carcinoma, suppress immune responses via A2A adenosine receptor (A2AR) activation [55]. Tumors further influence B-cell function through tryptophan catabolism. IDO1 and TDO catalyze kynurenine synthesis, which activates the aryl hydrocarbon receptor (AhR). In lung cancer models, IDO1-kynurenine-AhR signaling drives Breg differentiation in vivo, and pharmacological inhibition of AhR disrupts this tolerance circuit [56, 57]. Concerning the intrinsic side of B cells, regulatory function depends on a unique bioenergetic basis: The process of Breg development and the synthesis of IL-10 necessitate mitochondrial electron transport and OXPHOS. Additionally, thioredoxin-dependent redox regulation serves as a metabolic rheostat that supports Bregs [58]. In hepatocellular carcinoma, TAMs enhance PD-L1 expression on B cells through the CXCL12/CXCR4 axis, linking stromal-derived stress signals to a $PD\text{-}L1^{+}$ Breg phenotype [59]. Collectively, multiple metabolic axes including the lactate/pH axis, the CD39/CD73–adenosine–A2AR pathway, the tryptophan–kynurenine–AhR axis, the OXPHOS/redox network, and hypoxia-driven PD-L1 signaling, constitute a coherent "metabolic language" that enables tumors to reshape B-cell behavior. These interactions skew B cells toward $IL\text{-}10^{+}/PD\text{-}L1^{+}$ Bregs that suppress antitumor immunity. Conversely, in nutrient-rich microenvironments such as tertiary lymphoid structures, B cells sustain antigen presentation and promote effective immune responses [51].

7.3.3 Metabolic Cross Talk Between NK Cells and Cancer Cells

The complex metabolic interaction between NK cells and malignant cells in the TME affects immune surveillance and cancer progression (Fig. 7.2). It is well known that malignant cells depend on aerobic glycolysis through the Warburg effect, glutamine, and dysfunctional lipid metabolism to fuel the energy needs for their growth [60]. This metabolic rewiring promotes intense competition for carbon sources such as glucose and glutamine, and produces metabolites that directly suppress NK cell function [61]. It is reported that cancer cells rapidly utilize glucose via glycolysis, thus depleting extracellular glucose in the TME and starving nearby NK cells. This glucose limitation restricts NK glycolytic flux required for survival and proliferation [62]. Moreover, lactate accumulation and acidification induce NK cell mTOR signaling and impair granzyme/perforin synthesis. Additionally, release a suppression that can be countered by targeting monocarboxylate transporters (MCTs) or buffering acidity [62]. In general, the core of the tumor experiences hypoxia, which stabilizes HIF-1α in malignant cells, which further stimulates metabolism toward glycolysis, FAO, and reductive carboxylation [63]. In contrast, hypoxia in NK cells induces mitochondrial dysfunction such as depolarization, fragmentation, and accumulation of ROS, thereby diminishing cytotoxicity. So, the

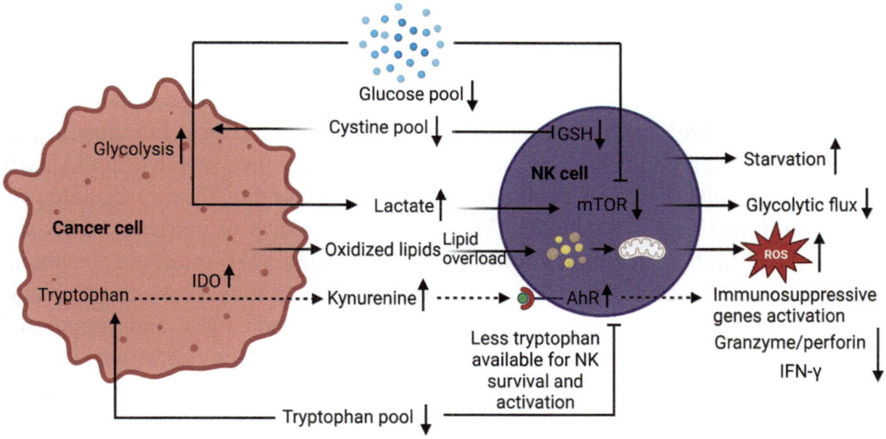

Fig. 7.2 Immunosuppressive metabolic interactions between cancer and NK cells in the TME

development of strategies that upregulate the expression of PGC-1α or mitochondrial-targeted antioxidants rescues the function of NK cells in a hypoxic environment [64]. Amino acid metabolism further defines this asymmetric interaction. The report suggested that most cancers express indoleamine 2,3-dioxygenase (IDO), depleting tryptophan while producing kynurenine, therefore directly impairing NK proliferation, IFN-γ production, and cytotoxicity potential [65]. Likewise, tumor uptake of arginine via arginase and lowered availability of cystine inhibit NK activation by limiting mTOR signaling and glutathione synthesis [62]. In contrast to that, NK cells that secrete IFN-γ can rewire the cancer cell metabolism. Thereby, suppressing glycolytic flux and promoting antigen presentation bidirectional feedback. Likewise, lipid metabolism is another important axis where tumors and surrounding stromal cells generate free fatty acids (FFAs) and oxidized lipids. NK cells uptake these metabolites via CD36 and other lipid transporters, due to which NK cells suffer from lipid overload and excess induction of mitochondrial ROS, resulting in NK cell dysfunction [66]. Previous studies have shown that pharmacologic blockade of FA uptake receptors, such as CD36, inhibits NK cells from lipid overload stress and protects their functional activity. For example, carnitine palmitoyl transferase 1A (CPT1A) mediated FAO can rescue the functional activity of NK cells [67]. Interestingly, it is reported that lactate and low pH in TME act as immunomodulators, inhibiting NK receptor proximal signaling and promoting histone acetylation in both NK and cancer cells, altering gene programs to support immune escape. Therefore, targeting lactate production with LDH inhibitors showed promising results in an experimental model [68]. Fundamentally, the interaction of NK cells closer to the blood vessels may have higher oxygen and glucose availability, which retain their functionality in contrast to the cells that are centrally located in hypoxic and nutrient-deprived niches that suppress NK cell functionality [69]. Hence, using systemic metabolic therapies such as glycolysis inhibitors can starve tumors but also impair NK cells. Instead of doing that, targeting metabolites such as lactate depletion and MCT inhibition may optimize outcomes. In vivo animal experiments showed that combining NK cells adoptive transfer along with metabolic modulation, such as IDO-kynurenine inhibitors, MCT blockers, FAO modulators, and mTOR pathway inhibitors, has shown synergistic tumor clearance potential in tumorigenic mouse models, though timing and dosing are critical to maintain NK fitness [70]. When NK cells were induced by the metabolites secreted in the TME by malignant cells, their energy utilization increased. Notably, they upregulate glycolysis and the OXPHOS pathway. The existence of a lack of nutrients, increased hypoxia, and higher accumulation of lactate, etc., in the TME promotes metabolic exhaustion that severely affects T-cell deregulation, which is characterized by attenuated glycolytic reserve, increased mitochondrial fragmentation, and suppressed calcium signaling [71]. Currently, researchers are investigating different ways to stimulate NK cells to enhance their survivability during treatment. One of the approaches is to induce the cells with IL-15 before they are given to the patients [72]. Likewise, another strategy is to rewire their metabolic energy, for example, elevating the expression of enzymes that help them use glucose or by increasing antioxidant proteins like MnSOD level to guard themselves from stress. Moreover, a potential possibility is to augment the number and efficiency of their mitochondria, which are the main energy producers. Next-generation technologies, such as single-cell metabolomics, spatial metabolic imaging, and isotope tracing experiments, are now unraveling various clues that explore valuable insights to remodel NK cells with tailored metabolic traits, such as engineering NK cells that are resistant to lactate and altered fuel preferences, such as ketone bodies or alternative amino acids.

7.3.4 Metabolic Cross Talk Between DCs and Cancer Cells

Similarly, metabolic cross talk between DCs and the malignant cells constitutes a complex, bidirectional dialogue within TME that influences the immune activation and the success of antitumor immunity (Fig. 7.3). Yet decoding its complexity has only recently begun to yield actionable insights [73]. Evidence shows that there is metabolic competition between DCs and the malignant cells for key nutrients. During the competition for nutrients, malignant cells secrete immunomodulatory metabolites that affect the DCs' function and impact the immune outcome. Malignant cells generally undergo aerobic glycolysis (the Warburg effect), where they utilize large amounts of glucose and convert it into lactate, which acidifies the TME [74]. Due to the consumption of a high amount of glucose, there is a shortage of glucose that prevents DCs from shifting to glycolysis after their toll-like receptors (TLRs) are activated. Due to this, mTORC1 and HIF-1α signals are inactivated in DCs. These inactivation affects the generation of costimulatory molecules such as CD80/CD86, interleukin-12 (IL-12), or express CCR7, which is required for DCs to migrate toward lymph nodes and trigger immune responses [75, 76].

In addition, tumors release the enzyme IDO, which catalyzes the conversion of tryptophan to kynurenine. Kynurenine activates aryl hydrocarbon receptor (AhR) in

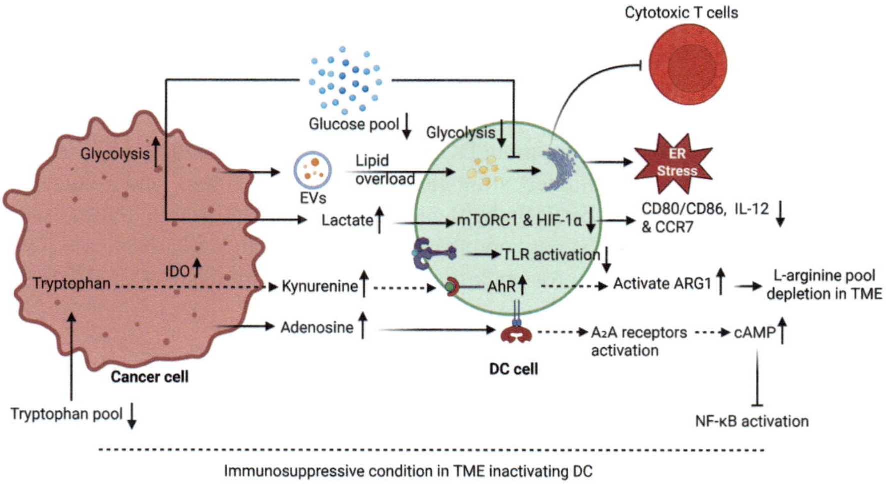

Fig. 7.3 Metabolic suppression of DC function by cancer cells within the TME

DCs, turning on genes that further upregulate the expression of immunosuppressive enzyme (i.e., ARG1). This promotes the development of regulatory T cells (Tregs) and weakens the ability of DCs to activate cytotoxic T cells [77, 78]. The dead cancer cells secrete ATP contained in exosomes, which are converted into adenosine by nearby cancer cells that express CD39 and CD73 on their surface. The accumulation of adenosine then binds to A_2A receptors on DCs and activates the cAMP pathway, which further blocks NF-κB pathway activation and disables the DCs from activating the immune system [79, 80]. Additionally, lipid metabolism also plays an important role in disabling the activity of DCs. Evidence shows that malignant cells secrete oxidized lipids such as LDLs and FA-rich vesicles that are taken up by DCs via scavenger receptors like CD36 and MSR1, therefore enhancing lipid droplet accumulation, inducing ER stress via activation of IRE1α-XBP1 pathways, and impairing MHC class I and II antigen cross-presentation through misrouting to the lysosomal compartments [81]. Notably, this effect can be reversed by using inhibitors like TOFA (acetyl-CoA carboxylase blocker) or etomoxir (CPT1 inhibitor), which rescue DC function and T-cell priming. Hypoxia in the TME makes these effects worse. In malignant cells, hypoxia stabilizes HIF-1α, which induces the cells to rely heavily on the glycolysis pathway and secrete VEGF, CCL2, CCL20, CXCL12, HMGB1, and other DAMPs, attracting immature DCs [82]. HIF-1α also forces DCs to rely on glycolysis. As a result, DCs lose their ability to process antigens properly as they reduce energy production through OXPHOS. Moreover, extracellular vesicles (EVs) produced by cancer cells further reprogram DC metabolism by delivering metabolic enzymes such as PKM2, LDH-A, microRNAs, and lipids that convert DCs into tolerogenic states [83]. DCs can also rewire tumor metabolism. When activated, DCs secrete cytokines like IL-12, IL-18, TNF-α, and type I interferons, which decrease tumor glycolysis, increase ROS production, and push cancer cells to depend more on oxidative metabolism [84]. Therapeutic agents like oxamate targeting LDH-A or lactate transporters inhibitors such as syrosingopine and VB253 free up glucose for DCs [85], inhibiting IDO1 by epacadostat, indoximod, navoximod, and linrodostat restore DC activity, or prevent lipid accumulation in DCs [86]. Metabolic modulators, such as 2-DG, mTOR activators, or AMPK modulators, can also promote DC energy use [87]. Combining DC vaccines along with the above-mentioned strategies may activate T-cells and reduce the tumor. Malignant cells hinder DCs by depleting nutrients and accumulating metabolic byproducts, yet DCs can counteract this, reshaping tumor metabolism. Deregulating this metabolic cross talk may enhance the effectiveness of DC-based cancer immunotherapy in the future.

7.3.5 Metabolic Cross Talk Between Neutrophils and Cancer Cells

Neutrophils, generally known as short-lived first responders in innate immunity, are now recognized as important players in the TME, where metabolic cross talk with malignant cells influences tumor progression, immune suppression, and development of therapeutic resistance [88]. Here also, nutrient competition between malignant cells and neutrophils reprograms the metabolic needs of each other (Fig. 7.4). For instance, tumor-derived metabolites such as lactate, adenosine, kynurenines, eicosanoids, succinate, etc., can rewire neutrophil phenotypes, and neutrophil-derived metabolites also influence tumor metabolism, which overall affects the immune outcomes [89].

Earlier reports suggested that acidified TME suppresses the immune functions of neutrophils, such as chemotaxis and degranulation, which impairs NADPH oxidase-driven ROS generation and promotes a protumoral N2-like tumor-associated

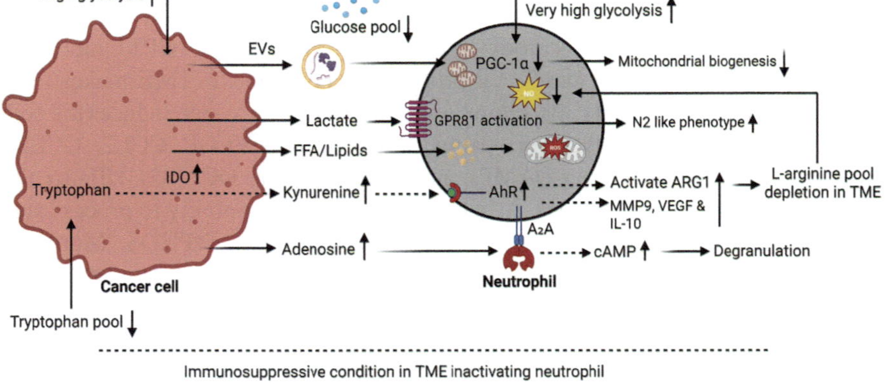

Fig. 7.4 Tumor-derived metabolites reprogram neutrophil functions to promote immunosuppression

neutrophils (TANs) phenotype through lactate receptor GPR81 signaling [89]. Notably, lactate also stabilizes HIF-1α in neutrophils, therefore, shifting them more toward glycolysis and away from mitochondrial respiration. This thing decreases phagocytic potentiality and induces the release of neutrophil extracellular traps (NETs), which can promote tumor metastasis and thrombosis [89]. In parallel, malignant cells exhaust arginine and tryptophan in the TME via upregulating the expression of arginase and IDO overexpression, depriving neutrophils of substrates required for iNOS and NAD production. Decreased arginine levels inhibited nitric oxide (NO) synthesis in neutrophils, which weakens their efficacy to kill malignant cells [90]. In addition, kynurenine secretion in the TME induces the increase of aryl hydrocarbon receptor (AhR) in neutrophils, activating an immunosuppressive state that releases MMP9, VEGF, and IL-10 [88]. Remarkably, lipid metabolism also constitutes a key axis where cancer cells secrete free fatty acids (FFAs) and oxidized lipids that are taken up by TANs via CD36 and FATP2 receptors, leading to FA accumulation, mitochondrial ROS production, and promoting immune suppression [91]. Inhibiting lipid uptake receptors such as CD36 and FATP2 reverts TANs to an N1-like phenotype with rescued antitumor activity. Adenosine secreted from malignant cells binds A_2A receptors on neutrophils, hence increasing cAMP, ROS, and decreasing degranulation. In contrast, using antagonizing A_2A rescued neutrophil antitumor functionality [92]. According to previous reports, EVs secreted from tumors contain metabolic enzymes such as ENO1, LDH-A, short-chain FA, and microRNAs (e.g., miR-23a) that reprogram neutrophil metabolism, therefore enhancing glycolysis and reducing mitochondrial biogenesis via downregulating PGC-1α [93]. On the other hand, neutrophils themselves influence the cancer cell metabolism by increasing neutrophil-derived ROS that can impair cancer cell mitochondrial function and induce metabolic stress. Along with that, it also shifts cancer cells more toward glycolysis. Furthermore, neutrophils secrete elastase and MMPs, which break down the extracellular matrix. This process frees stored lipids and growth factors such as VEGF, inducing tumor cells to take up lipids, stimulate FAO, and promote angiogenesis [88]. Moreover, neutrophil-released cytokines such as TNF-α and IL-1β can remodel malignant cell metabolism through NF-κB-dependent upregulation of glycolysis and glutaminolysis, initiating positive feedback loops that support both tumor growth and mobilization of protumoral neutrophils [94]. Therapeutic approaches targeting this metabolic axis are currently being developed. For example, the use of LDH inhibitors decreases lactate secretion by cancer cells in the TME, thus rescuing neutrophil ROS and cytotoxicity [95]. Interestingly, the use of arginase or IDO inhibitors preserves nutrient supply for neutrophils [96]. Notably, lipid uptake blockers or FATP2 inhibitors also stop neutrophil rewiring toward suppressive phenotypes [91]. Likewise, A_2A antagonists restore neutrophil function in adenosine-rich tumors [97]. Deregulating neutrophil metabolism by using mTOR inhibitors or metabolic adjuvants is being investigated to reprogram TANs toward antitumor N1 states and enhance the therapeutic response [89]. Thus, therapeutically targeting these metabolic axes can rescue neutrophil function in cancer, opening new avenues for immunometabolism therapy.

7.3.6 Metabolic Cross Talk Between TAMs and Cancer Cells

The intrinsic relationship between macrophages and malignant cells in the TME is a dynamic process that enhances tumor progression, immune suppression, and the development of drug resistance. TAMs, developed from circulating monocytes but can also derive from tissue-resident macrophages (Fig. 7.5). These tumor resident macrophages are activated by tumor-derived metabolites, which differentiate them into M1 (antitumor functionality) and M2 (protumor functionality) like characteristics. The key metabolites that are involved in TAM polarization have been listed in Table 7.1 [98–101].

Reports suggested that high rates of lactate production from the malignant cells promote acidification of the TME, which can be sensed by the macrophages and stimulate them toward the development of protumoral characteristics in TAMs [30]. Due to extensive nutrient competition between the stromal and cancer cells, the TME has been shown to harbor low levels of glucose and glycolysis intermediates that affect TAMs' metabolism. Literature suggested an increase in glycolysis in in vitro TAM models, but at the same time, it also increased mitochondrial respiration, which helps TAMs to survive under conditions of glucose unavailability. Interestingly, in a previous study, it was found that under hypoxic conditions TAMs upregulate the expression of Development and DNA Damage Response 1 (REDD1-stress-response protein) in lung and breast tumorigenic mice, which inhibits mTOR activation and thereby decreases glycolysis [37, 38]. Interestingly, REDD1 silencing in TAM allows them to compete for glucose with ECs, leading to better blood vessel growth and decreasing the chance of metastasis [37]. Notably, TAMs have been explored to oxidize more lactic acid than other cells within a Lewis lung cancer (LLC) mouse model [22], showing that a lack of REDD1 forces the TAMs to choose an alternative fuel source. Moreover, an increase in glutamine synthetase was observed in TAMs of LLC mouse models and glioblastoma patients due to glucose starvation, and it induced TAM polarization to a protumorigenic M2-like phenotype and reversed the polarization to an M1-like phenotype when glutamine

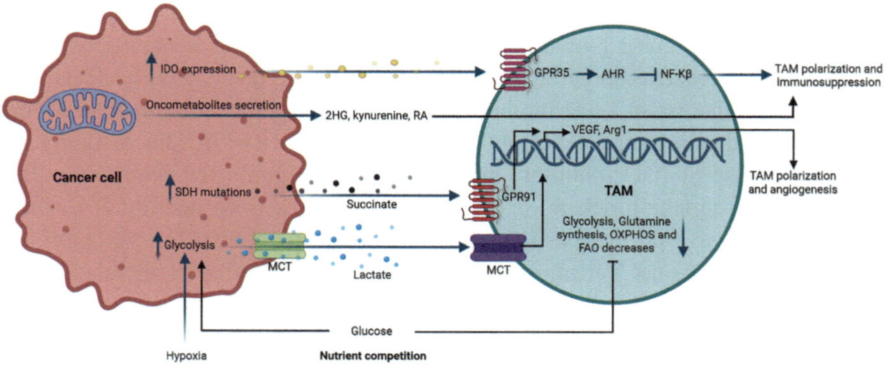

Fig. 7.5 Metabolic cross talk between cancer cells and TAM promotes immunosuppression and angiogenesis

Table 7.1 Key metabolites driving TAM polarization

Metabolites	Source in TME	Effect on TAMs	Phenotype
Lactate	Glycolytic tumor cells	HIF-1α activation, ARG1↑	M2-like
Adenosine	ATP breakdown (CD39/CD73)	A_2A/A_2B signaling, suppression	M2-like
Kynurenine (from Trp)	IDO/TDO-expressing tumors	AhR activation, tolerance	M2-like
Succinate	Tumor metabolism, TAMs	HIF-1α stabilization, IL-1β↑	M1-like
Hypoxia, Acidosis	Poor perfusion in tumor	HIF-driven angiogenesis, suppression	M2-like
Exosomal miRNAs (miR-21, miR-146a)	Tumor-derived vesicles	Epigenetic reprogramming	M2-like

synthetase was knocked out. Thus, it reduces cancer aggressiveness and promotes CD8+ T-cell infiltration at the tumor site. Likewise, lower levels of arginine and tryptophan have been found in the TME of most of the cancers as they overexpress the enzymes that metabolize these amino acids. Similarly, higher expression of Arg1 in TAMs also contributes to low arginine concentrations in TME, which is required for T-cell activation and survival. Similar to arginine deprivation, tryptophan starvation has also been found to stimulate a regulatory T-cell phenotype [47]. For instance, lactate also reprograms the macrophage metabolism. Notably, MCT4-mediated uptake of tumor-derived lactic acid enhances the secretion of VEGF and Arg1 expressions in murine TAMs, which significantly supports tumor growth. It was reported that lactate directly modulates the TAMs gene via histone acetylation, hence polarizing TAMs to secrete VEGF, FGF2, suppress cytotoxic T cells and NK cells, followed by ECM remodeling and promoting metastasis. In addition, lactate can also promote TAM differentiation from M1 to M2-like TAM differentiation through the activation of GPR132 signaling [64]. Another in vivo breast cancer study found that protumorigenic lactate signaling is mediated through extracellular signal-regulated kinase (ERK)/signal transducer and activator of STAT3, inhibition of which reduces TAM presence in the TME and decreases tumor size and angiogenesis [65]. Tumor-derived succinate was found to induce TAMs polarization and metastasis of human lung cancer through activation of succinate receptor (SUCNR1/GPR91) signaling. This activation enhances PI3K signaling.

Reports suggested that cancer cells metabolize vitamin A at high rates through upregulation of ALDH1A expression, converting retinol into retinoic acid (RA), a process linked to poor prognosis in several cancers (e.g., breast, prostate). Although RA was once viewed as antitumor due to its potency to induce cell cycle arrest, recent studies showed context-dependent effects. In the TME, T cell-derived IL-13 can promote RA generation by tumor cells, enhancing monocyte differentiation into M-2-like TAMs. Blocking of RA signaling promotes tumor sensitivity to PD-1 blockade, suggesting therapeutic potential. However, RA can also limit monocyte recruitment and macrophage IL-8/VEGF production in vitro. Moreover, exosomes serve as key mediators of metabolic cross talk between malignant cells and macrophages by delivering molecules such as miRNAs, proteins, lipids, metabolites, and enzymes. Their secretion and uptake are promoted in acidic, hypoxic, and nutrient-poor TME, contributing to cancer development. Tumor-derived exosomes influence TAM polarization and metabolism, enhancing M2-like phenotype. Notably, exosomes secreted by melanoma cells that include miR-125b-5p impair lipid catabolism in macrophages by blocking lysosomal acid lipase A, while hypoxic melanoma exosomes carrying let-7a promote $CD206^+$ TAMs and activate OXPHOS via REDD1–mTOR signaling. Additionally, exosomes secreted by breast cancers rearchitect the premetastatic niche by inhibiting stromal glycolysis. Although exosomes are known to contain metabolic components (e.g., lactate, amino acids, TCA intermediates), further studies are needed to determine how cancer cell-derived exosomes modulate TAMs' metabolism specifically.

Macrophage metabolic reprogramming is a key focus in cancer research. Metabolic and functional diversity among TAMs likely depends on the type of cancer and TME context. Rewiring TAMs from protumoral to antitumoral phenotypes could potentially decrease metastasis and promote immunity. Several metabolic pathway targets, such as lactate, lipid, glutamine, and tryptophan, have emerged as promising therapeutic targets. Inhibiting these metabolite uptakes by TAMs can restore $CD8^+$ T-cell activity, reduce tumor growth, and improve immunotherapy response. A major challenge remains in specifically targeting macrophages without impairing immune effector cells that share similar glycolytic profiles. Despite these hurdles, advancing our understanding of TAMs' metabolism and its interplay with tumor cells holds great potential for developing new cancer therapies.

7.3.7 Metabolic Cross Talk Between CAFs and Cancer Cells

Cancer-associated fibroblasts (CAFs) are not a monolithic type of stromal population in TME but a metabolically and functionally heterogeneous type of cells that show highly dynamic and reciprocal metabolic cross talk with malignant cells (Fig. 7.6) [102]. Tumor resident fibroblast, when stimulated by cancer cells, can be converted into Myofibroblastic CAF (myCAF), inflammatory CAF (iCAF), and antigen-presenting CAF (apCAF) (Table 7.2). The table below summarizes tumor-derived cytokines and their roles in converting resident fibroblasts into CAF subsets, and their characterization markers [102].

CAFs can be differentiated from localized fibroblasts, mesenchymal stem cells, endothelial cells, hepatic or pancreatic stellate cells, and adipocytes. Their heterogeneity indicates differences in origin, gene expression profile, and having both protumor and antitumor functionality [103]. CAFs are genetically stable, but sometimes they change phenotypic plasticity in response to tumor-derived factors such as TGF-β, IL-6, and oxidative stress [103]. This rewiring activates CAFs to secrete metabolites that remodel the ECM and develop a barrier that restricts drug penetration and immune invasion. It is well known that cancer cells often use glucose as the main carbon source for their metabolism to generate energy [104]. Notably, the malignant cells often exhibit the Warburg effect, characterized by enhanced aerobic glycolysis and lactate production even in oxygen-rich conditions in TME. Increased

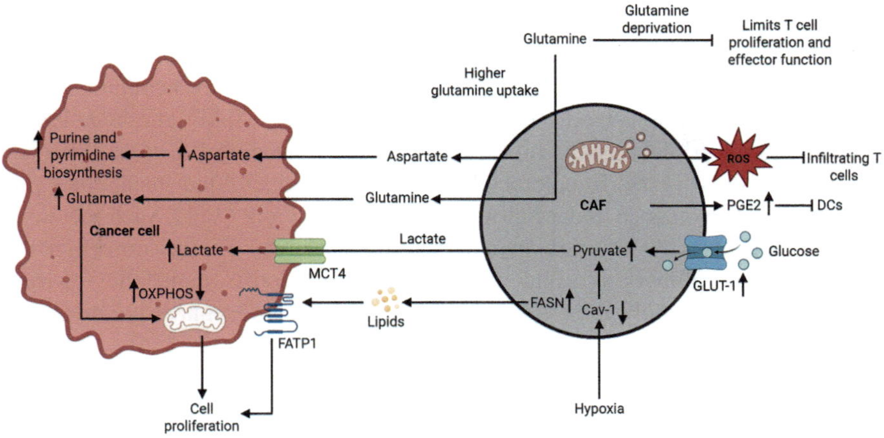

Fig. 7.6 Metabolic coupling between CAF and cancer cell promotes tumor growth and immune suppression

Table 7.2 Subsets of CAFs along with their defining tumor-derived factors and phenotypic characteristics

CAF subset	Key tumor-derived cytokines/factors	Resulting fibroblast phenotype
myCAF (myofibroblastic CAF)	TGF-β	High α-SMA expression, contractile, and ECM-producing, supports desmoplasia
iCAF (inflammatory CAF)	IL-1α, IL-6, TNF-α	Secretes inflammatory cytokines and chemokines, low α-SMA, promotes immunomodulation
apCAF (antigen-presenting CAF)	IFN-γ, IL-1β (TGF-β in some contexts)	Express MHC-II and CD74, can present antigens, limited co-stimulatory molecules, immunosuppressive effect

production of lactate and pyruvate in TME facilitates its uptake by the cancer cells through MCT1 and utilizes it for mitochondrial OXPHOS [105]. An increase in glycolytic enzymes such as HK2 and PFKL identifies glycolytic reprogramming. In contrast, the reduction of caveolin-1 (Cav-1) in CAFs further increases glycolysis and lactate secretion in the TME, facilitating cancer growth. Thus, glucose metabolism supports CAF-tumor metabolic symbiosis [106].

Moreover, amino acids are major players in retaining cancer anabolism. As previously reported, CAFs produce glutamine, which fuels the TCA cycle and promotes nucleotide and lipid biosynthesis in malignant cells. In addition, CAFs also enhance serine, glycine, and cysteine secretion in TME, driving one-carbon metabolism and increasing glutathione (GSH) synthesis, which is crucial for redox balance [107]. Interestingly, the usage of arginine by CAFs develops lower availability of arginine to T cells, which impairs their function [108]. Moreover, exosomes released from CAFs contain various amino acids and metabolites that reprogram malignant cell metabolism and affect immune cell function. In addition to that, lipids also indicate another axis of metabolic cross talk. CAFs go through lipidomic rewiring, aggregating FAs and phospholipids that are released into the TME [109]. They transfer FAs through FA transport proteins or via exosomes containing FAs, phospholipids, and lipid-modifying enzymes. For instance, CAFs stimulate FATP1 upregulation in triple-negative breast cancer cells, enhancing FA uptake and survival under stress [110]. In colorectal cancer, CAF-derived lipid metabolites promote cell migration even under nutrient-deprived conditions [111]. Such metabolic rewiring connects CAFs' metabolism to metastatic behavior. Furthermore, hypoxia, a well-known hallmark of solid tumors, further reinforces metabolic rewiring. HIF-1α triggers glycolysis in CAFs and increases immunosuppressive molecules like PD-L1 on myeloid-derived suppressor cells (MDSCs) [112]. CAFs also regulate angiogenesis and ECM deposition, creating hypoxic niches that restrict T-cell infiltration, thus decreasing localized antitumor activity [102].

In recent years, a lot of research on different therapeutic strategies has been developed, which aimed at disrupting CAF–immune metabolic cross talk in the TME, and is emerging as a promising avenue for cancer treatment. One strategy involves that is blocking monocarboxylate transporters such as MCT1/4 to prevent lactate uptake between CAFs and malignant cells, thereby reducing metabolic symbiosis [113]. Another promising way is to inhibit amino acid metabolism by targeting glutaminase (GLS) or arginase, which can help restore suppressed T-cell activity [114]. Likewise, lipid metabolism modulation via inhibition of FASN or FATP1 can restrict lipid fueling of tumors and reduce metastatic potential [115]. Beyond direct metabolic interventions, CAF-directed therapies targeting markers such as fibroblast activation protein (FAP), caveolin-1 (Cav-1), or exosome secretion are being explored to diminish CAF-mediated support of tumor progression [116]. Importantly, combination immunotherapy, where immune checkpoint blockade is paired with metabolic inhibitors, has the potential to overcome CAF-driven immunosuppression and enhance antitumor responses. However, due to the high degree of metabolic plasticity and redundancy in TME, single-agent approaches may be insufficient, highlighting the need for multitargeted interventions.

7.3.8 Metabolic Cross Talk Between ECs and Cancer Cells

Endothelial cells (ECs) generate the inner lining of the blood vessels and play a crucial role in maintaining vascular homeostasis, angiogenesis, as well as the exchange of nutrients (Fig. 7.7). In the TME, malignant cells depend on constant metabolic adaptation to sustain growth and invasion [117]. This adaptation is closely linked with the metabolic activity of surrounding stromal cells that also includes ECs. The metabolites mediated cross talk between ECs and malignant cells is not merely a consequence of proximity but also represents a bidirectional interaction that involves tumor progression, vascular remodeling, and therapeutic response [117]. ECs provide metabolic support to malignant tumors, while tumor cells in turn modulate ECs' metabolism to develop a vascular niche conducive to angiogenesis and tumor growth [117].

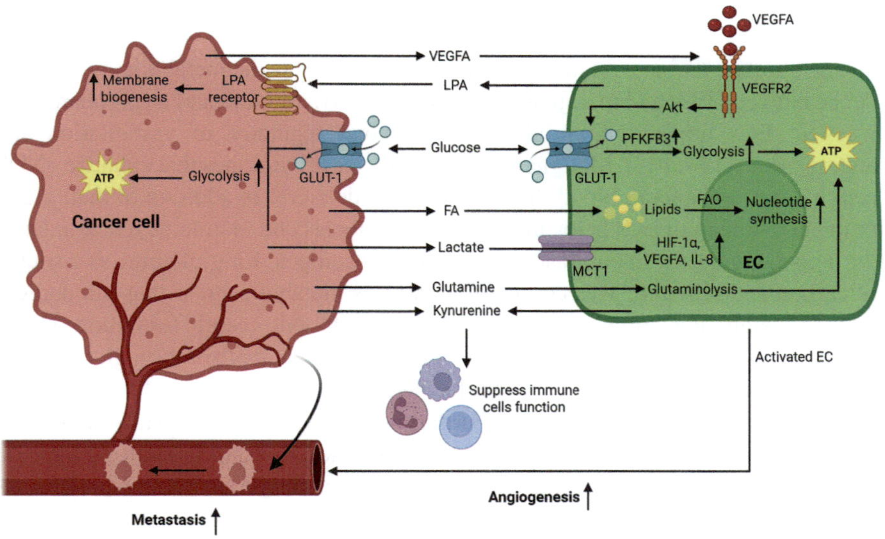

Fig. 7.7 Metabolic cross talk between cancer cells and EC promotes angiogenesis, immune suppression, and metastasis

ECs depend on glycolysis, controlled by phosphofructokinase-2/fructose-2,6-bisphosphatase 3 (PFKFB3) and induced by VEGF, released by the malignant cells. This rapid utilization of enhances ECs-mediated angiogenesis development, enriching tumors with oxygen and nutrients [118]. Studies found that increased glycolysis makes vessels abnormal and leaky, promoting cancer and immune cell evasion. This metabolic modulation helps EC proliferation and sprouting, thereby promoting tumor angiogenesis [119]. Notably, lactate secreted by cancer cells acts not only as a metabolic fuel for ECs but also as a signaling inducer molecule. For instance, lactate uptake by ECs through MCTs induces the expression of HIF-1α, thereby increasing the VEGF secretion in the TME and developing angiogenesis [120]. Likewise, ECs metabolize lactate through oxidative pathways to spare glucose for neighboring malignant cells, reinforcing a metabolic symbiosis. This "lactate shuttle" shows how cancer cell metabolism directly affects ECs' function. Furthermore, glutamine and FAs secreted by the cancer cells can also be exchanged with ECs, driving EC proliferation and lipid biosynthesis important for membrane expansion during vessel formation and sprouting [121]. Literature suggested that ECs utilize FAO for nucleotide biosynthesis, which supports proliferation but not ATP generation. For example, carnitine palmitoyl transferase 1a (CPT1a) dependent FAO in ECs provides acetyl-CoA for deoxyribonucleotide synthesis. As reported, malignant cells can also modulate FAO in ECs by releasing angiogenic signals like FGFs and VEGF, while also competing for circulating lipids [122]. At the same time, EC-derived lipids and lipid metabolites can diffuse back into cancer cells, fueling their membrane biogenesis and energy demands. For instance, lysophosphatidic acid (LPA) released by ECs acts as a metabolic intermediate that promotes tumor progression [123].

As reported, amino acid metabolism further highlights the metabolic interdependence between ECs and malignant cells. Specifically, arginine and tryptophan pathways in ECs impact NO production, a pivotal regulator of vasodilation and angiogenesis [124, 125]. Malignant cells often release cytokines that enhance eNOS activity, thus enhancing blood flow and nutrient delivery. In addition to that, glutamine metabolism in ECs helps in nucleotide synthesis and maintains redox balance during angiogenesis. In contrast, malignant cells compete for glutamine as a source of carbon and nitrogen. This competition induces metabolic stress that can deregulate EC signaling, often leading to aberrant blood vessel formation [126]. Additionally, kynurenine, a metabolite of tryptophan catabolism through IDO, can be secreted by both ECs and cancer cells, deregulate the immune cell functionality and angiogenesis in the TME [127]. Furthermore, it was reported that ECs increase glycolysis while reducing dependency on mitochondrial respiration during hypoxia and induce the expression of HIF-1α and HIF-2α signaling to increase VEGF secretion, angiogenic sprouting, and metabolic rewiring [128]. Interestingly, extracellular exosomes released by cancer cells add another dimension to metabolic communication between the cells. Exosomes contain metabolic enzymes, microRNAs, and metabolites that rewire EC metabolism. For example, cancer-derived miR-155 and miR-210 can deregulate glycolysis and mitochondrial respiration in ECs, promoting angiogenesis [129]. Conversely, EC-derived exosomes also deliver FAs, amino acids, or even mitochondrial components to cancer cells, directly providing fuel for their metabolic demands. This type of metabolite exchange exemplifies the complexity and specificity of metabolic cross talk between the cells in the TME. The effects of this metabolic symbiosis extend beyond angiogenesis to influence therapeutic outcome [130]. Anti-angiogenic interventions targeting VEGF or EC metabolism often encounter resistance due to metabolic flexibility. For example, blocking PFKFB3 affects ECs' glycolysis, which normalizes the tumor vessels, enhancing drug delivery and immune cell infiltration [131]. However, malignant cells can develop resistance to these interventions by channelizing alternative metabolic pathways in ECs. Likewise, inhibiting FAO in ECs disrupts angiogenesis but may indirectly promote vessel regression and hypoxia, which can promote metastatic dissemination [132]. Thus, a deeper understanding of the metabolic cross talk between ECs and cancer cells is crucial to developing therapeutic interventions that disrupt abnormal tumor angiogenesis without affecting normal vascular function.

7.4 Juxtacrine Metabolic Cross Talk in TME

Juxtacrine signaling represents a distinct mode of intercellular communication that depends on direct cell-cell contact between neighboring cells. Unlike autocrine or paracrine signaling, juxtacrine interactions occur through membrane-associated ligands and receptors, ensuring direct, highly localized, and specific cell-to-cell communication [133]. Within the TME, such signaling establishes intricate metabolic cross talk between cancer cells and surrounding stromal components, including CAFs, immune cells, and endothelial cells. This direct mode of communication allows tumors to finely regulate nutrient exchange, immune evasion, angiogenesis, and therapeutic resistance through contact-dependent metabolic reprogramming [133, 134].

7.4.1 Notch Signaling and Juxtacrine-Mediated Metabolic Cross Talk

The Notch signaling pathway exemplifies the profound metabolic influence exerted by juxtacrine interactions in the TME. Activation occurs when Delta-like ligands (DLL1, DLL4) or Jagged ligands (Jagged1, Jagged2) on adjacent cells bind to Notch receptors (Notch1–4), triggering proteolytic cleavage and nuclear translocation of the Notch intracellular domain (NICD) [135]. This pathway exhibits remarkable metabolic flexibility by both hyperactivation and hypoactivation of Notch, which can induce glycolytic switching through distinct mechanisms. Hyperactivated Notch enhances glycolysis by activating the PI3K/AKT pathway, which upregulates glucose transporters GLUT1 and GLUT3, as well as key glycolytic enzymes, including hexokinase 2 (HK2) and lactate dehydrogenase A (LDHA). Conversely, reduced Notch activity decreases mitochondrial respiratory activity while promoting glycolysis in a p53-dependent manner [136]. Recent studies have demonstrated that Notch1 directly regulates aerobic glycolysis through the TAZ (transcriptional coactivator with PDZ-binding motif) pathway in lung adenocarcinoma [137]. Patients with increased glucose uptake, as indicated by 18F-FDG PET scans, exhibit elevated Notch1 and TAZ expression. The Notch/TAZ axis emerges as a critical mediator of the Warburg effect, facilitating rapid tumor growth while maintaining metabolic flexibility [137]. In the TME context, hypoxic ECs upregulate Jagged ligands, which activate Notch in neighboring tumor cells, promoting their glycolytic adaptation. This juxtacrine interaction simultaneously promotes angiogenic sprouting in ECs and reprograms CAFs toward aerobic glycolysis, creating a coordinated metabolic network that sustains tumor progression [138].

7.4.2 Eph-Ephrin Bidirectional Metabolic Regulation

The Eph-ephrin system represents a unique juxtacrine pathway capable of transmitting bidirectional signals that coordinate metabolic reprogramming between adjacent cells. In tumor cells, EphA2 activation enhances GLUT1 expression and stimulates PI3K/AKT and MAPK pathways, thereby increasing glucose uptake and glycolytic flux under hypoxic conditions. This adaptation confers a metabolic advantage that supports tumor survival in oxygen-deprived conditions [139, 140]. The bidirectional nature of Eph-ephrin signaling ensures synchronized metabolic coordination across interacting cell types. For instance, endothelial cells engaged in ephrin-B2/EphB4 signaling shift their metabolism toward FAO, generating ATP and biosynthetic intermediates necessary for angiogenesis and vascular remodeling [141]. Meanwhile, reverse signaling in ephrin-expressing CAFs enhances their glycolytic activity and lactate secretion, which is subsequently utilized by tumor cells for OXPHOS. This reciprocal metabolic exchange underscores how juxtacrine pathways form intricate metabolic networks that support mutual cell survival and growth [142].

7.4.3 Integrin-Cadherin Adhesion-Dependent Metabolism

Cell adhesion molecules, particularly integrins and cadherins, serve dual roles as mechanical anchors and metabolic regulators. Integrin engagement with ECM components activates focal adhesion kinase (FAK), PI3K/AKT, and MAPK pathways, enhancing glucose transporter recruitment, lipid synthesis via acetyl-CoA carboxylase (ACC) and FASN, and mitochondrial metabolism. This adhesion-dependent metabolic rewiring supports rapid proliferation and survival in nutrient-deprived microenvironments [143]. Cadherins exhibit context-dependent metabolic effects. E-cadherin loss during EMT promotes metabolic plasticity and glycolytic switching. Paradoxically, recent evidence shows that E-cadherin can also enhance glycolytic behavior under hypoxic conditions, with its loss reducing HIF-1α expression and extracellular acidification. Integrin-cadherin cross talk creates a sophisticated regulatory network where physical cell-matrix and cell-cell interactions translate into coordinated metabolic adaptations [144]. Within the TME, CAFs activated via integrin signaling undergo autophagy and enhanced glycolysis, releasing metabolites such as alanine and lactate that fuel tumor cell OXPHOS. This adhesion-mediated metabolic coupling reinforces tumor–stroma interdependence and contributes to the persistence of a protumorigenic metabolic ecosystem phosphorylation [138].

7.4.4 Gap Junction-Mediated Metabolite Transfer

Gap junctions, formed by connexin proteins (Cx26, Cx32, Cx43), provide direct cytoplasmic channels between adjacent cells, permitting the free diffusion of metabolites, ions, and signaling molecules. This represents the most direct and continuous form of juxtacrine metabolic communication, creating a metabolic channel that redistributes cellular resources [145, 146].

In pancreatic cancer spheroids, Cx43-mediated gap junctions facilitate lactate transfer from hypoxic cores to normoxic peripheral cells, where it undergoes oxidative metabolism. This transfer creates an alkalinizing effect, increasing intracellular pH and generating favorable conditions for tumor growth. Similarly, in colorectal cancer, glucose trafficking from peripheral to central hypoxic cells occurs through gap junctions, with bicarbonate (HCO_3^-) diffusion maintaining pH homeostasis across the tumor mass [145]. The reverse Warburg effect further illustrates gap junction-mediated metabolic cooperation, where CAFs undergo glycolytic reprogramming and transfer metabolites to tumor cells through unidirectional connexin channels. Mesenchymal stem cells also transfer intact mitochondria and ATP to tumor cells via connexin-based connections, enhancing chemotherapy resistance. In the immune context, gap junctions facilitate transfer of immunosuppressive metabolites like adenosine and lactate from tumor cells to T lymphocytes, promoting T-cell exhaustion and metabolic dysfunction [147, 148]. Collectively, gap junction-mediated metabolite exchange exemplifies the direct and cooperative metabolic interplay that enables tumors to adapt, resist stress, and maintain a supportive microenvironment.

7.5 Endocrine-Like (Systemic) Metabolic Cross Talk

Endocrine-like metabolic cross talk in the TME refers to the systemic exchange of metabolites and signaling molecules that travel through circulation to influence both local tumor growth and distant tissues. Unlike autocrine or paracrine interactions that remain confined to tumor or stromal cells, endocrine-like signaling operates across the whole organism, reshaping systemic metabolism and creating a tumor-permissive environment [149, 150].

7.5.1 Systemic Regulation of Immune Metabolism

Tumors exert profound effects on systemic immunometabolism through the release of metabolites and extracellular vesicles into circulation. A prominent example involves tryptophan catabolism mediated by IDO and TDO, which generate the metabolite kynurenine, which acts as a potent immunosuppressant [151, 152]. Kynurenine suppresses T-cell activation, promotes regulatory T-cell (Treg) differentiation, and impairs effector T-cell function via activation of the AhR. Accumulation of kynurenine in plasma disrupts amino acid homeostasis by creating competition at System L transporters (LAT1/LAT2), which transport both tryptophan and kynurenine [153]. Elevated kynurenine levels outcompete tryptophan, effectively starving immune cells of this essential amino acid while simultaneously delivering immunosuppressive signals. This systemic tryptophan–kynurenine imbalance functions as a circulating metabolic "rheostat" that establishes a state of widespread immune suppression across the body [154].

7.5.2 Glutamine Depletion and Myeloid Dysregulation

Advanced tumors also disrupt systemic amino acid balance. Circulating glutamine, normally maintained at 0.6–0.9 mmol/L, becomes depleted due to high tumor demand [155]. However, the high metabolic demand of proliferating tumors leads to significant glutamine depletion in circulation. This systemic deficiency exerts dual effects: it deprives T cells of a critical substrate required for proliferation, effector differentiation, and cytokine production, while concurrently promoting the expansion and immunosuppressive polarization of MDSCs [47]. Experimental glutamine depletion using PEGylated glutaminase has shown that systemic deprivation enhances MDSC accumulation rather than providing therapeutic benefit [156].

7.5.3 Systemic Lipid Signaling

Tumor-derived lipid metabolites also act as systemic mediators of immune modulation. Circulating FAs and their derivatives influence both the inflammatory balance and immune cell fate [157]. Among them, omega-6 polyunsaturated FA–derived metabolites such as prostaglandin E_2 (PGE_2) and leukotrienes are key immunomodulators that drive MDSC differentiation and suppress dendritic cell maturation. This lipid-driven systemic signaling axis not only facilitates immune evasion but also promotes chronic inflammation, angiogenesis, and metastatic progression. By integrating metabolic and inflammatory pathways at the organismal level, endocrine-like signaling enables tumors to extend their metabolic influence far beyond the primary site, thereby sustaining systemic immune suppression and cancer progression [158].

Unlike autocrine, paracrine, or juxtacrine signaling, which act locally through direct or short-range interactions, endocrine-like signaling disseminates metabolites, cytokines, and extracellular vesicles through the bloodstream. This allows tumors to reprogram distant organs, modulate immune responses, and establish a body-wide metabolic and inflammatory state that favors cancer progression. Understanding these systemic metabolic interactions provides critical insights into how tumors manipulate host metabolism and opens new avenues for therapeutic interventions targeting cancer-induced systemic dysregulation.

7.6 Role of Metabolic Cross Talk in TME Toward the Development of Therapy Resistance

Therapy resistance remains one of the major challenges in oncology, leading to poor clinical outcomes, disease relapse, and metastasis. Despite substantial advances in chemotherapy, targeted therapy, radiotherapy, and immunotherapy, most tumors eventually develop resistance over time. A key driver of this phenomenon is the TME, a dynamic and heterogeneous ecosystem composed of malignant cells, stromal cells, ECs, immune cells, and ECM components. Within this complex milieu, metabolic cross talk, the exchange of metabolites, signaling molecules, and nutrients, plays a central role in driving tumor adaptation, metabolic plasticity, and therapeutic failure.

7.6.1 Glycolytic-Mediated Cross Talk and Drug Resistance

Cancer cells exhibit elevated glycolytic flux through the Warburg effect, producing substantial lactate even under normoxic conditions. Also, in the reverse Warburg effect, CAFs secrete lactate that tumor cells uptake via MCT1, fueling oxidative metabolism and providing ATP and biosynthetic precursors. This metabolic symbiosis significantly reduces the efficacy of cytotoxic drugs like cisplatin. Mechanistically, MCT1 stabilizes HIF-1α, which in turn activates downstream genes such as VEGF and GLUT1, promoting angiogenesis, glucose uptake, and survival under stress conditions. Additionally, enhanced NF-κB signaling further upregulates anti-apoptotic proteins such as Bcl-2 and survivin, directly counteracting cisplatin-induced apoptosis. Clinical studies demonstrate that MCT1 expression serves as a biomarker for poor prognosis across different cancer types, underscoring the importance of glycolytic crosstalk in therapy resistance [159].

7.6.2 Amino Acid-Mediated Cross Talk and Drug Resistance

Altered amino acid metabolism is another crucial driver of therapeutic resistance. Tumor cells exhibit heightened dependence on glutamine and serine, which provide carbon and nitrogen sources for nucleotide and amino acid biosynthesis. In the TME, CAFs secrete glutamine to support tumor proliferation and diminish the effectiveness of antimetabolite therapies such as cisplatin, methotrexate, and 5-fluorouracil (5-FU), all of which target nucleotide metabolism [160, 161]. Furthermore, glutamine activates mTORC1 signaling, which promotes protein translation and cell growth even under chemotherapeutic stress. It also contributes to redox balance, as glutamine-derived α-ketoglutarate supports NADPH production through the pentose phosphate pathway, helping neutralize the reactive oxygen species (ROS) generated by chemotherapeutic agents [160]. Elevated glutathione (GSH) levels are strongly associated with methotrexate resistance, as several genes involved in GSH metabolism correlate with both increased GSH concentrations and reduced drug sensitivity [161]. To counteract these effects, glutaminase inhibitors such as CB-839 are being tested clinically in combination with immune checkpoint inhibitors and mTOR inhibitors [160, 162]. However, cancer cells remain adaptable and can bypass glutamine dependency by upregulating alternative metabolic pathways, including enhanced tricarboxylic acid (TCA) cycle activity and FA oxidation, thereby sustaining growth and survival despite therapy.

7.6.3 Lipid-Mediated Cross Talk and Drug Resistance

Lipid metabolism within the TME plays a pivotal role in therapy resistance through CD36-mediated FA uptake from adipocytes and CAFs. By promoting lipid droplet formation, FA uptake shields tumor cells from drug-induced oxidative stress, thereby driving resistance to a wide range of therapies [21]. FAO further strengthens this resistance by activating PPARα/PGC-1α signaling, enhancing mitochondrial respiration and ATP production, thereby allowing cells to evade apoptosis even under EGFR-targeted treatments. In chronic myeloid leukemia, CD36-positive leukemic stem cells exhibit heightened chemoresistance, while CD36 knockout significantly reduces FA uptake and restores drug sensitivity. To counter this mechanism, therapeutic strategies are being developed to inhibit CD36, including blocking monoclonal antibodies and small-molecule inhibitors. Since enhanced lipid uptake through CD36 is a key contributor to resistance against both chemotherapy and targeted therapy, targeting this pathway holds significant promise in overcoming treatment failure [21].

7.7 Conclusion and Future Prospects

The TME represents a complex metabolic ecosystem where cancer cells orchestrate intricate communication networks through autocrine, paracrine, juxtacrine, and endocrine-like signaling mechanisms that fundamentally reshape cellular mechanisms to promote tumor progression and therapeutic resistance. Understanding the metabolic cross talk serves as a master regulator, where tumor cells modulate key metabolites such as lactate, adenosine, glutamine, cytokines, and FA. These metabolites act in an autocrine manner to influence various cellular signaling pathways, suppress immune responses, and remodel the surrounding microenvironment to promote tumor survival and progression. Similarly, the bidirectional metabolic exchanges between cancer cells and diverse stromal populations, including T cells, B cells, NK cells, DCs, neutrophils, TAMs, CAFs, and ECs, create self-reinforcing loops that enhance tumor survival, promote angiogenesis, facilitate metastasis, and drive resistance to conventional therapies through mechanisms such as hypoxia-induced metabolic switching, acid-mediated immune suppression, and FA-driven survival signaling. A comprehensive understanding of these metabolic networks provides valuable insights into the molecular basis of tumor plasticity and resistance. Advances in single-cell metabolomics, isotope tracing, and spatial imaging are expected to elucidate the temporal and spatial dynamics of these metabolic interactions. Future therapeutic strategies should focus on targeting metabolic dependencies and intercellular metabolite exchange, in combination with immune checkpoint or targeted therapies for better outcomes. Such integrated approaches hold the potential to reprogram the TME, overcome therapy resistance, and establish metabolism-based precision medicine strategies for effective and durable cancer treatment.

Acknowledgments The authors are very much thankful to the Council of Scientific & Industrial Research (CSIR), Government of India, for providing a senior research fellowship (File no.-09/1035(23652)/2025-EMR-I) to C. Das. The authors would like to acknowledge the Indian Council of Medical Research (ICMR) (File No- 5/13/59/2022/NCD-III), Government of India, for partly supporting the research of T. Parija. The figures have been created using Biorender (Created in BioRender. CNK, C. (2025)).

Conflict of Interest The authors declare that they have no known competing financial interests or personal relationships that could have appeared to influence the work reported in this chapter.

References

1. Yu H, Li J, Peng S, et al. Tumor microenvironment: nurturing cancer cells for immunoevasion and druggable vulnerabilities for cancer immunotherapy. Cancer Lett. 2025;611:217385.
2. Baghban R, Roshangar L, Jahanban-Esfahlan R, et al. Tumor microenvironment complexity and therapeutic implications at a glance. Cell Commun Signal. 2020;18:59. https://doi.org/10.1186/s12964-020-0530-4.
3. Wei R, Liu S, Zhang S, et al. Cellular and extracellular components in tumor microenvironment and their application in early diagnosis of cancers. Anal Cell Pathol. 2020;2020:1–13. https://doi.org/10.1155/2020/6283796.
4. Martínez-Reyes I, Chandel NS. Cancer metabolism: looking forward. Nat Rev Cancer. 2021;21:669–80.
5. Cortellino S, Longo VD. Metabolites and immune response in tumor microenvironments. Cancer. 2023;15:3898.
6. Elia I, Haigis MC. Metabolites and the tumour microenvironment: from cellular mechanisms to systemic metabolism. Nat Metab. 2021;3:21–32.
7. Yang J, Shay C, Saba NF, Teng Y. Cancer metabolism and carcinogenesis. Exp Hematol Oncol. 2024;13:10. https://doi.org/10.1186/s40164-024-00482-x.
8. Kim SK, Cho SW. The evasion mechanisms of cancer immunity and drug intervention in the tumor microenvironment. Front Pharmacol. 2022;13:868695.
9. Zhang F, Ma Y, Li D, et al. Cancer associated fibroblasts and metabolic reprogramming: unraveling the intricate crosstalk in tumor evolution. J Hematol Oncol. 2024;17:80. https://doi.org/10.1186/s13045-024-01600-2.
10. Sciacovelli M, Frezza C. Oncometabolites: unconventional triggers of oncogenic signalling cascades. Free Radic Biol Med. 2016;100:175–81.
11. Baryła M, Semeniuk-Wojtaś A, Róg L, et al. Oncometabolites—a link between cancer cells and tumor microenvironment. Biology. 2022;11:270.
12. Zhou JX, Taramelli R, Pedrini E, et al. Extracting intercellular signaling network of cancer tissues using ligand-receptor expression patterns from whole-tumor and single-cell transcriptomes. Sci Rep. 2017;7:8815.
13. Kay EJ, Zanivan S. The tumor microenvironment is an ecosystem sustained by metabolic interactions. Cell Rep. 2025;44:115432.
14. Luo Z, Eichinger KM, Zhang A, Li S. Targeting cancer metabolic pathways for improving chemotherapy and immunotherapy. Cancer Lett. 2023;575:216396.
15. Kocianova E, Piatrikova V, Golias T. Revisiting the Warburg effect with focus on lactate. Cancer. 2022;14:6028.
16. Gao Y, Zhou H, Liu G, et al. Tumor microenvironment: lactic acid promotes tumor development. J Immunol Res. 2022;2022:1–8. https://doi.org/10.1155/2022/3119375.
17. Li Z, Wang Q, Huang X, et al. Lactate in the tumor microenvironment: a rising star for targeted tumor therapy. Front Nutr. 2023;10:1113739.
18. Ishihara S, Hata K, Hirose K, et al. The lactate sensor GPR81 regulates glycolysis and tumor growth of breast cancer. Sci Rep. 2022;12:6261.
19. Gyamfi J, Yeo JH, Kwon D, et al. Interaction between CD36 and FABP4 modulates adipocyte-induced fatty acid import and metabolism in breast cancer. NPJ Breast Cancer. 2021;7:129.
20. Cui Z, Liu J, Sun Q, et al. GPR120 promotes radiation resistance in esophageal cancer via regulating AKT and apoptosis pathway. Anti-Cancer Drugs. 2021;32:53–60.
21. Guerrero-Rodriguez SL, Mata-Cruz C, Perez-Tapia SM, Velasco-Velazquez MA. Role of CD36 in cancer progression, stemness, and targeting. Front Cell Dev Biol. 2022;10:1079076.

22. Zhao J, Xie F, Yang Y, Wang S. Reprogramming of fatty acid metabolism in breast cancer: a narrative review. Transl Breast Cancer Res. 2021;2:5.
23. Griffiths A, Wang J, Song Q, et al. ATF4-mediated CD36 upregulation contributes to palmitate-induced lipotoxicity in hepatocytes. Am J Physiol-Gastrointest Liver Physiol. 2023;324:G341–53. https://doi.org/10.1152/ajpgi.00163.2022.
24. Zaidi NE, Shazali NAH, Leow T-C, et al. CD36-fatty acid-mediated metastasis via the bidirectional interactions of cancer cells and macrophages. Cells. 2022;11:3556.
25. Jyotsana N, Ta KT, DelGiorno KE. The role of cystine/glutamate antiporter SLC7A11/xCT in the pathophysiology of cancer. Front Oncol. 2022;12:858462.
26. Lopes C, Pereira C, Medeiros R. ASCT2 and LAT1 contribution to the hallmarks of cancer: from a molecular perspective to clinical translation. Cancer. 2021;13:203.
27. Saito Y, Soga T. Amino acid transporters as emerging therapeutic targets in cancer. Cancer Sci. 2021;112:2958–65. https://doi.org/10.1111/cas.15006.
28. Gauthier-Coles G, Bröer A, McLeod MD, et al. Identification and characterization of a novel SNAT2 (SLC38A2) inhibitor reveals synergy with glucose transport inhibition in cancer cells. Front Pharmacol. 2022;13:963066.
29. Chen J, Cui L, Lu S, Xu S. Amino acid metabolism in tumor biology and therapy. Cell Death Dis. 2024;15:42.
30. Ai Y, Wang H, Liu L, et al. Purine and purinergic receptors in health and disease. MedComm. 2023;4:e359. https://doi.org/10.1002/mco2.359.
31. Gardani CFF, Diz FM, Dondé LB, et al. The potential role of purinergic signaling in cancer therapy: perspectives on anti-CD73 strategies for prostate cancer. Front Immunol. 2024;15:1455469.
32. Qu R, Zhao Y, Zhang Y. The mechanism of cytokine regulation of cancer occurrence and development in the tumor microenvironment and its application in cancer treatment: a narrative review. Transl Cancer Res. 2024;13:5649.
33. Yi M, Li T, Niu M, et al. Targeting cytokine and chemokine signaling pathways for cancer therapy. Signal Transduct Target Ther. 2024;9:176.
34. Zhang N, Li Y. Receptor tyrosine kinases: biological functions and anticancer targeted therapy. MedComm. 2023;4:e446. https://doi.org/10.1002/mco2.446.
35. Chang C-H, Qiu J, O'Sullivan D, et al. Metabolic competition in the tumor microenvironment is a driver of cancer progression. Cell. 2015;162:1229–41. https://doi.org/10.1016/j.cell.2015.08.016.
36. Fischer K, Hoffmann P, Voelkl S, et al. Inhibitory effect of tumor cell–derived lactic acid on human T cells. Blood. 2007;109:3812–9. https://doi.org/10.1182/blood-2006-07-035972.
37. Pilon-Thomas S, Kodumudi KN, El-Kenawi AE, et al. Neutralization of tumor acidity improves antitumor responses to immunotherapy. Cancer Res. 2016;76:1381–90. https://doi.org/10.1158/0008-5472.CAN-15-1743.
38. Opitz CA, Litzenburger UM, Sahm F, et al. An endogenous tumour-promoting ligand of the human aryl hydrocarbon receptor. Nature. 2011;478:197–203. https://doi.org/10.1038/nature10491.
39. Campesato LF, Budhu S, Tchaicha J, et al. Blockade of the AHR restricts a Treg-macrophage suppressive axis induced by L-Kynurenine. Nat Commun. 2020;11:4011. https://doi.org/10.1038/s41467-020-17750-z.
40. Geiger R, Rieckmann JC, Wolf T, et al. L-arginine modulates T cell metabolism and enhances survival and anti-tumor activity. Cell. 2016;167:829–842.e13. https://doi.org/10.1016/j.cell.2016.09.031.
41. Menjivar RE, Nwosu ZC, Du W, et al. Arginase 1 is a key driver of immune suppression in pancreatic cancer. eLife. 2023;12:e80721. https://doi.org/10.7554/eLife.80721.
42. Noman MZ, Desantis G, Janji B, et al. PD-L1 is a novel direct target of HIF-1α, and its blockade under hypoxia enhanced MDSC-mediated T cell activation. J Exp Med. 2014;211:781–90. https://doi.org/10.1084/jem.20131916.

43. Bailey CM, Liu Y, Liu M, et al. Targeting HIF-1α abrogates PD-L1–mediated immune evasion in tumor microenvironment but promotes tolerance in normal tissues. J Clin Invest. 2022;132 https://doi.org/10.1172/JCI150846.
44. Ohta A, Gorelik E, Prasad SJ, et al. A2A adenosine receptor protects tumors from antitumor T cells. Proc Natl Acad Sci. 2006;103:13132–7. https://doi.org/10.1073/pnas.0605251103.
45. Allard B, Longhi MS, Robson SC, Stagg J. The ectonucleotidases CD39 and CD73: novel checkpoint inhibitor targets. Immunol Rev. 2017;276:121–44. https://doi.org/10.1111/imr.12528.
46. Leone RD, Zhao L, Englert JM, et al. Glutamine blockade induces divergent metabolic programs to overcome tumor immune evasion. Science. 2019;366:1013–21. https://doi.org/10.1126/science.aav2588.
47. Oh M-H, Sun I-H, Zhao L, et al. Targeting glutamine metabolism enhances tumor-specific immunity by modulating suppressive myeloid cells. J Clin Invest. 2020;130:3865–84. https://doi.org/10.1172/JCI131859.
48. Ma EH, Bantug G, Griss T, et al. Serine is an essential metabolite for effector T cell expansion. Cell Metab. 2017;25:345–57. https://doi.org/10.1016/j.cmet.2016.12.011.
49. Xu S, Chaudhary O, Rodríguez-Morales P, et al. Uptake of oxidized lipids by the scavenger receptor CD36 promotes lipid peroxidation and dysfunction in CD8+ T cells in tumors. Immunity. 2021;54:1561–1577.e7. https://doi.org/10.1016/j.immuni.2021.05.003.
50. Patsoukis N, Bardhan K, Chatterjee P, et al. PD-1 alters T-cell metabolic reprogramming by inhibiting glycolysis and promoting lipolysis and fatty acid oxidation. Nat Commun. 2015;6:6692. https://doi.org/10.1038/ncomms7692.
51. Hegoburu A, Amer M, Frizelle F, Purcell R. B cells and tertiary lymphoid structures in cancer therapy response. BJC Rep. 2025;3:40. https://doi.org/10.1038/s44276-025-00146-1.
52. Liu C, Cao J. The pivotal role of tertiary lymphoid structures in the tumor immune microenvironment. Front Oncol. 2025;15 https://doi.org/10.3389/fonc.2025.1616904.
53. Muraoka S, Baba T, Akazawa T, et al. Tumor-derived lactic acid promotes acetylation of histone H3K27 and differentiation of IL-10-producing regulatory B cells through direct and indirect signaling pathways. Int J Cancer. 2025;156:840–52. https://doi.org/10.1002/ijc.35229.
54. Chen J, Huang Z, Chen Y, et al. Lactate and lactylation in cancer. Signal Transduct Target Ther. 2025;10:38. https://doi.org/10.1038/s41392-024-02082-x.
55. Jeske SS, Brand M, Ziebart A, et al. Adenosine-producing regulatory B cells in head and neck cancer. Cancer Immunol Immunother. 2020;69:1205–16. https://doi.org/10.1007/s00262-020-02535-6.
56. Tousif S, Wang Y, Jackson J, et al. Indoleamine 2, 3-dioxygenase promotes aryl hydrocarbon receptor-dependent differentiation of regulatory B cells in lung cancer. Front Immunol. 2021;12 https://doi.org/10.3389/fimmu.2021.747780.
57. Abd El-Fattah EE. IDO/kynurenine pathway in cancer: possible therapeutic approaches. J Transl Med. 2022;20:347. https://doi.org/10.1186/s12967-022-03554-w.
58. Bradford HF, McDonnell TCR, Stewart A, et al. Thioredoxin is a metabolic rheostat controlling regulatory B cells. Nat Immunol. 2024;25:873–85. https://doi.org/10.1038/s41590-024-01798-w.
59. Lian S-L, Lu Y-T, Lu Y-J, et al. Tumor-associated macrophages promoting PD-L1 expression in infiltrating B cells through the CXCL12/CXCR4 axis in human hepatocellular carcinoma. Am J Cancer Res. 2024;14:832–53. https://doi.org/10.62347/ZIAX8828.
60. Zhang H, Liu S, Fu S, et al. Novel insight into the Warburg effect: sweet temptation. Crit Rev Oncol Hematol. 2025;214:104844. https://doi.org/10.1016/j.critrevonc.2025.104844.
61. Lim SA. Metabolic reprogramming of the tumor microenvironment to enhance immunotherapy. BMB Rep. 2024;57:388–99. https://doi.org/10.5483/BMBRep.2024-0031.
62. Terrén I, Orrantia A, Vitallé J, et al. NK cell metabolism and tumor microenvironment. Front Immunol. 2019;10:2278. https://doi.org/10.3389/fimmu.2019.02278.

63. Infantino V, Santarsiero A, Convertini P, et al. Cancer cell metabolism in hypoxia: role of HIF-1 as key regulator and therapeutic target. Int J Mol Sci. 2021;22:5703. https://doi.org/10.3390/ijms22115703.
64. Portale F, Di Mitri D. NK cells in cancer: mechanisms of dysfunction and therapeutic potential. Int J Mol Sci. 2023;24:9521. https://doi.org/10.3390/ijms24119521.
65. Song X, Si Q, Qi R, et al. Indoleamine 2,3-dioxygenase 1: a promising therapeutic target in malignant tumor. Front Immunol. 2021;12:800630. https://doi.org/10.3389/fimmu.2021.800630.
66. Corn KC, Windham MA, Rafat M. Lipids in the tumor microenvironment: from cancer progression to treatment. Prog Lipid Res. 2020;80:101055. https://doi.org/10.1016/j.plipres.2020.101055.
67. Wißfeld J, Werner A, Yan X, et al. Metabolic regulation of immune responses to cancer. Cancer Biol Med. 2022;19:1528–42. https://doi.org/10.20892/j.issn.2095-3941.2022.0381.
68. Gu X-Y, Yang J-L, Lai R, et al. Impact of lactate on immune cell function in the tumor microenvironment: mechanisms and therapeutic perspectives. Front Immunol. 2025;16:1563303. https://doi.org/10.3389/fimmu.2025.1563303.
69. Garcés-Lázaro I, Kotzur R, Cerwenka A, Mandelboim O. NK cells under hypoxia: the two faces of vascularization in tumor and pregnancy. Front Immunol. 2022;13:924775. https://doi.org/10.3389/fimmu.2022.924775.
70. Melaiu O, Lucarini V, Cifaldi L, Fruci D. Influence of the tumor microenvironment on NK cell function in solid tumors. Front Immunol. 2020;10:3038. https://doi.org/10.3389/fimmu.2019.03038.
71. Poznanski SM, Singh K, Ritchie TM, et al. Metabolic flexibility determines human NK cell functional fate in the tumor microenvironment. Cell Metab. 2021;33:1205–1220.e5. https://doi.org/10.1016/j.cmet.2021.03.023.
72. Robinson TO, Schluns KS. The potential and promise of IL-15 in immuno-oncogenic therapies. Immunol Lett. 2017;190:159–68. https://doi.org/10.1016/j.imlet.2017.08.010.
73. Peng X, He Y, Huang J, et al. Metabolism of dendritic cells in tumor microenvironment: for immunotherapy. Front Immunol. 2021;12:613492. https://doi.org/10.3389/fimmu.2021.613492.
74. Xia L, Oyang L, Lin J, et al. The cancer metabolic reprogramming and immune response. Mol Cancer. 2021;20:28. https://doi.org/10.1186/s12943-021-01316-8.
75. Zhang H, Li S, Wang D, et al. Metabolic reprogramming and immune evasion: the interplay in the tumor microenvironment. Biomark Res. 2024;12:96. https://doi.org/10.1186/s40364-024-00646-1.
76. Lawless SJ, Kedia-Mehta N, Walls JF, et al. Glucose represses dendritic cell-induced T cell responses. Nat Commun. 2017;8:15620. https://doi.org/10.1038/ncomms15620.
77. Mor A, Tankiewicz-Kwedlo A, Pawlak D. Kynurenines as a novel target for the treatment of malignancies. Pharmaceuticals. 2021;14:606. https://doi.org/10.3390/ph14070606.
78. Proietti E, Rossini S, Grohmann U, Mondanelli G. Polyamines and kynurenines at the intersection of immune modulation. Trends Immunol. 2020;41:1037–50. https://doi.org/10.1016/j.it.2020.09.007.
79. Kayhan M, Koyas A, Akdemir I, et al. adenosine receptor signaling targets both PKA and Epac pathways to polarize dendritic cells to a suppressive phenotype. J Immunol (Baltim Md 1950). 2019;203:3247–55. https://doi.org/10.4049/jimmunol.1900765.
80. Da M, Chen L, Enk A, et al. The multifaceted actions of CD73 during development and suppressive actions of regulatory T cells. Front Immunol. 2022;13 https://doi.org/10.3389/fimmu.2022.914799.
81. Wang D, Ye Q, Gu H, Chen Z. The role of lipid metabolism in tumor immune microenvironment and potential therapeutic strategies. Front Oncol. 2022;12:984560. https://doi.org/10.3389/fonc.2022.984560.
82. Abou Khouzam R, Zaarour RF, Brodaczewska K, et al. The effect of hypoxia and hypoxia-associated pathways in the regulation of antitumor response: friends or foes? Front Immunol. 2022;13:828875. https://doi.org/10.3389/fimmu.2022.828875.

83. Tran CW, Gold MJ, Garcia-Batres C, et al. Hypoxia-inducible factor 1 alpha limits dendritic cell stimulation of CD8 T cell immunity. PLoS One. 2020;15:e0244366. https://doi.org/10.1371/journal.pone.0244366.
84. Giovanelli P, Sandoval TA, Cubillos-Ruiz JR. Dendritic cell metabolism and function in tumors. Trends Immunol. 2019;40:699–718. https://doi.org/10.1016/j.it.2019.06.004.
85. Verma S, Budhu S, Serganova I, et al. Pharmacologic LDH inhibition redirects intratumoral glucose uptake and improves antitumor immunity in solid tumor models. J Clin Invest. 2024;134:e177606. https://doi.org/10.1172/JCI177606.
86. Tang K, Wu Y-H, Song Y, Yu B. Indoleamine 2,3-dioxygenase 1 (IDO1) inhibitors in clinical trials for cancer immunotherapy. J Hematol Oncol. 2021;14:68. https://doi.org/10.1186/s13045-021-01080-8.
87. Guerra L, Bonetti L, Brenner D. Metabolic modulation of immunity: a new concept in cancer immunotherapy. Cell Rep. 2020;32:107848. https://doi.org/10.1016/j.celrep.2020.107848.
88. Wang Z, Hu H, Bao Y, et al. Neutrophils in cancer: from immune defense to tumor promotion. Cancer Biol Med. 2025;22:598–617. https://doi.org/10.20892/j.issn.2095-3941.2025.0023.
89. Lin J, He X-L, Zhang W-W, Mo C-F. Metabolic reprogramming of tumor-associated neutrophils in tumor treatment and therapeutic resistance. Front Cell Dev Biol. 2025;13:1584987. https://doi.org/10.3389/fcell.2025.1584987.
90. Xiong S, Dong L, Cheng L. Neutrophils in cancer carcinogenesis and metastasis. J Hematol Oncol. 2021;14:173. https://doi.org/10.1186/s13045-021-01187-y.
91. Veglia F, Tyurin VA, Blasi M, et al. Fatty acid transporter 2 reprograms neutrophils in cancer. Nature. 2019;569:73–8. https://doi.org/10.1038/s41586-019-1118-2.
92. Yang Y, Zhu L, Xu Y, et al. The progress and prospects of targeting the adenosine pathway in cancer immunotherapy. Biomark Res. 2025;13:75. https://doi.org/10.1186/s40364-025-00784-0.
93. Tan S, Yang Y, Yang W, et al. Exosomal cargos-mediated metabolic reprogramming in tumor microenvironment. J Exp Clin Cancer Res. 2023;42:59. https://doi.org/10.1186/s13046-023-02634-z.
94. Feng Y, Liu G, Li H, Cheng L. Target neutrophil heterogeneity and plasticity in cancer. J Hematol OncolJ Hematol Oncol. 2025;18:79. https://doi.org/10.1186/s13045-025-01731-0.
95. Ma M, Hu R, Huang Q, et al. Decoding the metabolic-immune Axis: neutrophil glycolysis-driven tumor niche remodeling and its therapeutic exploitation. Pharmacol Res. 2025;217:107811. https://doi.org/10.1016/j.phrs.2025.107811.
96. Caldwell RW, Rodriguez PC, Toque HA, et al. Arginase: a multifaceted enzyme important in health and disease. Physiol Rev. 2018;98:641–65. https://doi.org/10.1152/physrev.00037.2016.
97. Sounbuli K, Mironova N, Alekseeva L. Diverse neutrophil functions in cancer and promising neutrophil-based cancer therapies. Int J Mol Sci. 2022;23:15827. https://doi.org/10.3390/ijms232415827.
98. Mehla K, Singh PK. Metabolic regulation of macrophage polarization in cancer. Trends Cancer. 2019;5:822–34. https://doi.org/10.1016/j.trecan.2019.10.007.
99. Chen S, Saeed AFUH, Liu Q, et al. Macrophages in immunoregulation and therapeutics. Signal Transduct Target Ther. 2023;8:207. https://doi.org/10.1038/s41392-023-01452-1.
100. Bai R, Li Y, Jian L, et al. The hypoxia-driven crosstalk between tumor and tumor-associated macrophages: mechanisms and clinical treatment strategies. Mol Cancer. 2022;21:177. https://doi.org/10.1186/s12943-022-01645-2.
101. Ren W, Hou J, Yang C, et al. Extracellular vesicles secreted by hypoxia pre-challenged mesenchymal stem cells promote non-small cell lung cancer cell growth and mobility as well as macrophage M2 polarization via miR-21-5p delivery. J Exp Clin Cancer Res. 2019;38:62. https://doi.org/10.1186/s13046-019-1027-0.
102. Jia H, Chen X, Zhang L, Chen M. Cancer associated fibroblasts in cancer development and therapy. J Hematol Oncol. 2025;18:36. https://doi.org/10.1186/s13045-025-01688-0.

103. Guo T, Xu J. Cancer-associated fibroblasts: a versatile mediator in tumor progression, metastasis, and targeted therapy. Cancer Metastasis Rev. 2024;43:1095–116. https://doi.org/10.1007/s10555-024-10186-7.
104. Li Z, Sun C, Qin Z. Metabolic reprogramming of cancer-associated fibroblasts and its effect on cancer cell reprogramming. Theranostics. 2021;11:8322–36. https://doi.org/10.7150/thno.62378.
105. De Leon-Oliva D, González-Prieto P, De Castro-Martinez P, et al. Revisiting the biological role of the Warburg effect: evolving perspectives on cancer metabolism. Pathol – Res Pract. 2025;273:156151. https://doi.org/10.1016/j.prp.2025.156151.
106. Liang C, Qin Y, Zhang B, et al. Metabolic plasticity in heterogeneous pancreatic ductal adenocarcinoma. Biochim Biophys Acta BBA – Rev Cancer. 2016;1866:177–88. https://doi.org/10.1016/j.bbcan.2016.09.001.
107. Li X, Zhu H, Sun W, et al. Role of glutamine and its metabolite ammonia in crosstalk of cancer-associated fibroblasts and cancer cells. Cancer Cell Int. 2021;21:479. https://doi.org/10.1186/s12935-021-02121-5.
108. Niu F, Yu Y, Li Z, et al. Arginase: An emerging and promising therapeutic target for cancer treatment. Biomed Pharmacother. 2022;149:112840. https://doi.org/10.1016/j.biopha.2022.112840.
109. Peng Z, Tong Z, Ren Z, et al. Cancer-associated fibroblasts and its derived exosomes: a new perspective for reshaping the tumor microenvironment. Mol Med. 2023;29:66. https://doi.org/10.1186/s10020-023-00665-y.
110. Brogna MR, Varone V, DelSesto M, Ferrara G. The role of CAFs in therapeutic resistance in triple negative breast cancer: an emerging challenge. Front Mol Biosci. 2025;12:1568865. https://doi.org/10.3389/fmolb.2025.1568865.
111. Peng S, Li Y, Huang M, et al. Metabolomics reveals that CAF-derived lipids promote colorectal cancer peritoneal metastasis by enhancing membrane fluidity. Int J Biol Sci. 2022;18:1912–32. https://doi.org/10.7150/ijbs.68484.
112. Corzo CA, Condamine T, Lu L, et al. HIF-1α regulates function and differentiation of myeloid-derived suppressor cells in the tumor microenvironment. J Exp Med. 2010;207:2439–53. https://doi.org/10.1084/jem.20100587.
113. Payen VL, Mina E, Van Hée VF, et al. Monocarboxylate transporters in cancer. Mol Metab. 2019;33:48–66. https://doi.org/10.1016/j.molmet.2019.07.006.
114. Lukey MJ, Katt WP, Cerione RA. Targeting amino acid metabolism for cancer therapy. Drug Discov Today. 2017;22:796–804. https://doi.org/10.1016/j.drudis.2016.12.003.
115. Fhu CW, Ali A. Fatty acid synthase: An emerging target in cancer. Molecules. 2020;25:3935. https://doi.org/10.3390/molecules25173935.
116. Cao Z, Quazi S, Arora S, et al. Cancer-associated fibroblasts as therapeutic targets for cancer: advances, challenges, and future prospects. J Biomed Sci. 2025;32:7. https://doi.org/10.1186/s12929-024-01099-2.
117. García-Caballero M, Sokol L, Cuypers A, Carmeliet P. Metabolic reprogramming in tumor endothelial cells. Int J Mol Sci. 2022;23:11052. https://doi.org/10.3390/ijms231911052.
118. Xu Y, An X, Guo X, et al. Endothelial 6-phosphofructo-2-kinase (PFKFB3) plays a critical role in angiogenesis. Arterioscler Thromb Vasc Biol. 2014;34:1231–9. https://doi.org/10.1161/ATVBAHA.113.303041.
119. Kane K, Edwards D, Chen J. The influence of endothelial metabolic reprogramming on the tumor microenvironment. Oncogene. 2025;44:51–63. https://doi.org/10.1038/s41388-024-03228-5.
120. Sonveaux P, Copetti T, Saedeleer CJD, et al. Targeting the lactate transporter MCT1 in endothelial cells inhibits lactate-induced HIF-1 activation and tumor angiogenesis. PLoS One. 2012;7:e33418. https://doi.org/10.1371/journal.pone.0033418.
121. Huang H, Vandekeere S, Kalucka J, et al. Role of glutamine and interlinked asparagine metabolism in vessel formation. EMBO J. 2017;36:2334–52. https://doi.org/10.15252/embj.201695518.

122. Liu B, Dai Z. Fatty acid metabolism in endothelial cell. Genes. 2022;13:2301. https://doi.org/10.3390/genes13122301.
123. Mukherjee A, Wu J, Barbour S, Fang X. Lysophosphatidic acid activates Lipogenic pathways and de novo lipid synthesis in ovarian cancer cells. J Biol Chem. 2012;287:24990–5000. https://doi.org/10.1074/jbc.M112.340083.
124. Liu X, Ren B, Ren J, et al. The significant role of amino acid metabolic reprogramming in cancer. Cell Commun Signal. 2024;22:380. https://doi.org/10.1186/s12964-024-01760-1.
125. Keshet R, Erez A. Arginine and the metabolic regulation of nitric oxide synthesis in cancer. Dis Model Mech. 2018;11:dmm033332. https://doi.org/10.1242/dmm.033332.
126. Nan D, Yao W, Huang L, et al. Glutamine and cancer: metabolism, immune microenvironment, and therapeutic targets. Cell Commun Signal. 2025;23:45. https://doi.org/10.1186/s12964-024-02018-6.
127. Gouasmi R, Ferraro-Peyret C, Nancey S, et al. The kynurenine pathway and cancer: why keep it simple when You can make it complicated. Cancer. 2022;14:2793. https://doi.org/10.3390/cancers14112793.
128. Bakleh MZ, Al Haj Zen A. The distinct role of HIF-1α and HIF-2α in hypoxia and angiogenesis. Cells. 2025;14:673. https://doi.org/10.3390/cells14090673.
129. Fridman ES, Ginini L, Gil Z. The role of extracellular vesicles in metabolic reprogramming of the tumor microenvironment. Cells. 2022;11:1433. https://doi.org/10.3390/cells11091433.
130. Carles-Fontana R, Heaton N, Palma E, Khorsandi SE. Extracellular vesicle-mediated mitochondrial reprogramming in cancer. Cancer. 2022;14:1865. https://doi.org/10.3390/cancers14081865.
131. Cantelmo AR, Conradi L-C, Brajic A, et al. Inhibition of the glycolytic activator PFKFB3 in endothelium induces tumor vessel normalization, impairs metastasis, and improves chemotherapy. Cancer Cell. 2016;30:968–85. https://doi.org/10.1016/j.ccell.2016.10.006.
132. Chen Z, Han F, Du Y, et al. Hypoxic microenvironment in cancer: molecular mechanisms and therapeutic interventions. Signal Transduct Target Ther. 2023;8:70. https://doi.org/10.1038/s41392-023-01332-8.
133. Yang W-H, Cha J-H, Xia W, et al. Juxtacrine signaling inhibits antitumor immunity by upregulating PD-L1 expression. Cancer Res. 2018;78:3761–8.
134. Clay R, Li K, Jin L. Metabolic signaling in the tumor microenvironment. Cancer. 2025;17:155.
135. Li X, Yan X, Wang Y, et al. The notch signaling pathway: a potential target for cancer immunotherapy. J Hematol Oncol. 2023;16:45. https://doi.org/10.1186/s13045-023-01439-z.
136. Landor SK-J, Mutvei AP, Mamaeva V, et al. Hypo- and hyperactivated Notch signaling induce a glycolytic switch through distinct mechanisms. Proc Natl Acad Sci. 2011;108:18814–9. https://doi.org/10.1073/pnas.1104943108.
137. Xie M, Fu X, Jiang K. Notch1/TAZ axis promotes aerobic glycolysis and immune escape in lung cancer. Cell Death Dis. 2021;12:832.
138. Zhu Y, Li X, Wang L, et al. Metabolic reprogramming and crosstalk of cancer-related fibroblasts and immune cells in the tumor microenvironment. Front Endocrinol. 2022;13:988295.
139. Pasquale EB. Eph receptors and ephrins in cancer: bidirectional signalling and beyond. Nat Rev Cancer. 2010;10:165–80.
140. Falivelli G, Lisabeth EM, de la Torre ER, et al. Attenuation of eph receptor kinase activation in cancer cells by coexpressed ephrin ligands. PLoS One. 2013;8:e81445.
141. Jensen PL. Eph receptors and ephrins. Stem Cells. 2000;18:63–4. https://doi.org/10.1634/stemcells.18-1-63.
142. Ieguchi K, Maru Y. Eph/Ephrin signaling in the tumor microenvironment. In: Birbrair A, editor. Tumor microenvironment. Cham: Springer International Publishing; 2021. p. 45–56.
143. Sousa B, Pereira J, Paredes J. The crosstalk between cell adhesion and cancer metabolism. Int J Mol Sci. 2019;20:1933.
144. Chu K, Boley KM, Moraes R, et al. The paradox of E-cadherin: role in response to hypoxia in the tumor microenvironment and regulation of energy metabolism. Oncotarget. 2013;4:446.
145. Zhou M, Zheng M, Zhou X, et al. The roles of connexins and gap junctions in the progression of cancer. Cell Commun Signal. 2023;21:8. https://doi.org/10.1186/s12964-022-01009-9.

146. Jones JC, Bodenstine TM. Connexins and glucose metabolism in cancer. Int J Mol Sci. 2022;23:10172.
147. Nakajima EC, Van Houten B. Metabolic symbiosis in cancer: refocusing the Warburg lens. Mol Carcinog. 2013;52:329–37. https://doi.org/10.1002/mc.21863.
148. Li C, Cheung MK, Han S, et al. Mesenchymal stem cells and their mitochondrial transfer: a double-edged sword. Biosci Rep. 2019;39:BSR20182417.
149. Nong S, Han X, Xiang Y, et al. Metabolic reprogramming in cancer: mechanisms and therapeutics. MedComm. 2023;4:e218. https://doi.org/10.1002/mco2.218.
150. You M, Xie Z, Zhang N, et al. Signaling pathways in cancer metabolism: mechanisms and therapeutic targets. Signal Transduct Target Ther. 2023;8:196.
151. Platten M, von Knebel Doeberitz N, Oezen I, et al. Cancer immunotherapy by targeting IDO1/TDO and their downstream effectors. Front Immunol. 2015;5:673.
152. Stone TW, Williams RO. Tryptophan metabolism as a 'reflex' feature of neuroimmune communication: sensor and effector functions for the indoleamine-2, 3-dioxygenase kynurenine pathway. J Neurochem. 2024;168:3333–57. https://doi.org/10.1111/jnc.16015.
153. Rad Pour S, Morikawa H, Kiani NA, et al. Exhaustion of CD4+ T-cells mediated by the kynurenine pathway in melanoma. Sci Rep. 2019;9:12150.
154. Sinclair LV, Neyens D, Ramsay G, et al. Single cell analysis of kynurenine and system L amino acid transport in T cells. Nat Commun. 2018;9:1981.
155. Hensley CT, Wasti AT, DeBerardinis RJ. Glutamine and cancer: cell biology, physiology, and clinical opportunities. J Clin Invest. 2013;123:3678–84.
156. Kumar M, Leekha A, Nandy S, et al. Enzymatic depletion of circulating glutamine is immunosuppressive in cancers. IScience. 2024;27:109817.
157. Pascual G, Benitah SA. Lipids in the tumor microenvironment: immune modulation and metastasis. Front Oncol. 2024;14:1435480.
158. Hicks KC, Tyurina YY, Kagan VE, Gabrilovich DI. Myeloid cell–derived oxidized lipids and regulation of the tumor microenvironment. Cancer Res. 2022;82:187–94.
159. Yan C, Yang F, Zhou C, et al. MCT1 promotes the cisplatin-resistance by antagonizing Fas in epithelial ovarian cancer. Int J Clin Exp Pathol. 2015;8:2710.
160. Yoo H-C, Han J-M. Amino acid metabolism in cancer drug resistance. Cells. 2022;11:140.
161. Canevarolo RR, de Melo CPS, Cury NM, et al. Glutathione levels are associated with methotrexate resistance in acute lymphoblastic leukemia cell lines. Front Oncol. 2022;12:1032336.
162. Varghese S, Pramanik S, Williams LJ, et al. The glutaminase inhibitor CB-839 (telaglenastat) enhances the antimelanoma activity of T-cell–mediated immunotherapies. Mol Cancer Ther. 2021;20:500–11.

Metabolic Reprogramming in Cancer Stem Cells

8

Gaurav Ranjan, Srijani Dasgupta, Uttam Kumar Mishra, Priyashree Sunita, and Shakti Prasad Pattanayak

8.1 Introduction

Cancer is a multifaceted disease, including genetic and epigenetic alterations that allow for cells to circumvent growth restraints, avoid apoptosis, and maintain unrestrained proliferation. The rarity and long latency are due to the low odds of acquiring the mutations in question. Tissue stem cells are the most common site of these mutations because they can regenerate themselves. Nevertheless, early progenitor cells may also give rise to cells of origin if they acquire self-renewal properties [1]. Research confirms that both stem cells and progenitor cells can act as tumor initiators in hematological and solid cancers. Within tumors, a subset of cells exhibits stem-like properties and is known as cancer stem cells (CSCs). These CSCs are key drivers of therapeutic resistance and increasing tumor progression. CSCs can survive throughout the course of cancer development. Their persistence contributes to

G. Ranjan
Department of Pharmacy, School of Health Science, Central University of South Bihar, Gaya, Bihar, India
e-mail: gauravranjan@cusb.ac.in

S. Dasgupta
Department of Pharmaceutical Sciences, Jharkhand Rai University, Rajaulatu, Namkum, Ranchi, India

U. K. Mishra
Department of Chemistry, Birla Institute of Technology, Mesra, Ranchi, India

P. Sunita
Department of Surgery, Case Comprehensive Cancer Centre, Case Western Reserve University, Wolstein Research Building, Cleveland, OH, USA
e-mail: pxs854@case.edu

S. P. Pattanayak (✉)
Department of Biochemistry, School of Medicine, Case Western Reserve University, Euclid Ave, Cleveland, OH, USA
e-mail: sxp1286@case.edu

S. Ashique et al. (eds.), *Cancer Metabolism*, Cancer Treatment and Research 195, https://doi.org/10.1007/978-3-032-21861-2_8

tumor recurrence and increased aggressiveness, even after initial treatment. Over the years, the CSC concept has gained prominence for its role in resistance, relapse, and metastasis, reforming our understanding of cancer biology.

8.1.1 Cancer Stem Cells in Tumor Initiation and Progression

The origin of cancer stem cells (CSCs) remains unclear. It is debated whether they develop from normal stem cells or from differentiated non-stem cells [2]. The exact phenotypes and functions of CSCs are not completely defined. They may resist therapy by staying quiescent or via active resistance mechanisms in proliferating cells [3]. Current evidence suggests that CSCs may exist as dynamic states, acquiring stem-like traits that promote tumor progression and therapeutic resistance (Fig. 8.1). The tumor microenvironment (TME) plays a critical role in influencing CSC behavior, including their survival, progression, and metastasis [4]. Tumor growth results from genetic and epigenetic alterations that transform normal cells. This process advances through initiation, promotion, and progression, each involving dynamic cellular events. These phases involve dynamic cellular events and continual changes in tumor structure. Evidence indicates that CSCs adapt to these shifts for survival, showing their role in tumor heterogeneity progression and resistance to therapy [5]. This chapter examines CSC behavior, regulatory pathways, and their phenotypic outcomes throughout cancer phases, highlighting the importance of understanding their microenvironmental interactions to design more effective therapeutic strategies.

The discovery of CSCs has reformed our understanding of cancer biology, revealing that not all cancer cells equally drive disease advancement and relapse. CSCs possess self-renewal and metabolic adaptability, along with enhanced drug efflux and efficient DNA repair. They also exhibit epithelial-to-mesenchymal transition (EMT) potential and niche-forming ability, supporting their proliferation and tumorigenic capacity. They also facilitate metastasis by detaching from primary tumors and establishing secondary tumors that are often more aggressive. CSCs can evade conventional chemotherapy and radiotherapy because these treatments mainly target actively dividing cells. Quiescent CSCs survive, contributing to tumor relapse and disease progression. Therapies should specifically target CSC characteristics, including their signaling pathways and metabolic adaptations. This can be achieved by blocking their self-renewal and survival mechanisms or promoting their differentiation. By selectively eradicating CSCs, such approaches hold promise for reducing tumor recurrence, limiting metastasis, and improving long-term patient outcomes.

CSCs are abnormal stem-like cells with the capacity for both self-renewal and differentiation. They may remain quiescent under therapeutic stress or divide symmetrically to sustain their pool, fueling tumor growth. Through asymmetric division, they also generate diverse tumor cell populations, maintaining intratumoral heterogeneity (Table 8.1).

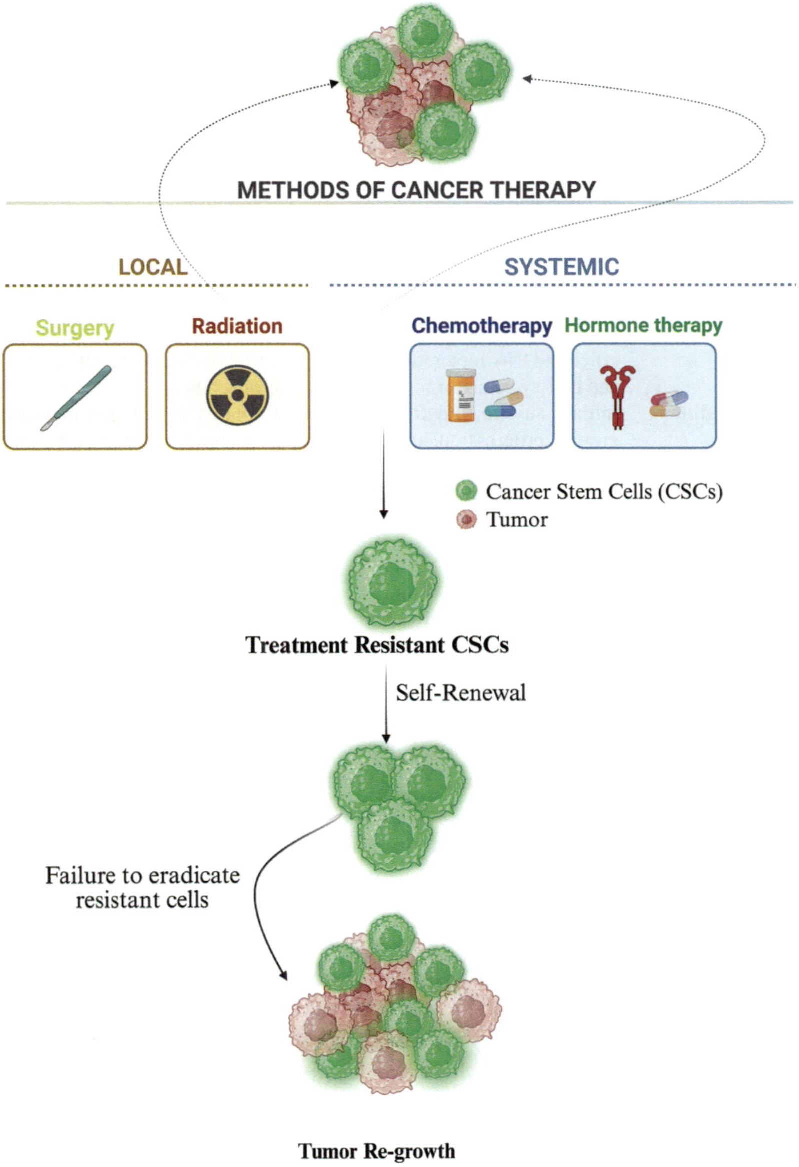

Fig. 8.1 Characteristics of cancer stem cells (CSCs). (Figure created using BioRender)

Research on cancer stem cells (CSCs has transformed the view of tumor biology, overturning the traditional belief that all cancer cells contribute equally to tumor initiation, progression, and relapse. This shift highlights CSCs as the root drivers of therapeutic resistance and relapse, making them a prime focus for novel treatment opportunities for targeted interventions. By mapping their distinct properties,

Table 8.1 Distinctive features of cancer stem cells (CSCs) compared to regular cancer cells

Characteristic	Cancer stem cells (CSCs)	Progeny cancer cells
Self-renewal	Capable of continuous self-renewal through symmetric or asymmetric division, sustaining their population	Lacks true self-renewal capacity; exhibits restricted growth capacity
Differentiation	Generate multiple cancer cell lineages, driving cellular heterogeneity	Limited differentiation ability often forms a more uniform cell population
Transdifferentiation	Can convert into specialized cell types (e.g., endothelial cells), supporting angiogenesis and tumor growth	Rarely undergo transdifferentiation; generally, they do not form specialized cell types
Chemotherapy resistance	Exhibit strong resistance via efficient DNA repair, drug efflux, and cell-cycle arrest in quiescence	More vulnerable to chemotherapy, particularly during active proliferation
Tumor formation	Initiate, sustain, and drive tumor growth, progression, and metastasis	Primarily form tumor mass but play a minor role in initiation and sustained growth
Tumor progression	Persist after therapy, leading to recurrence and aggressive progression	More likely eliminated by conventional therapies; limited role in recurrence

signaling pathways, and metabolic behaviors, researchers aim to design precision-based therapy approaches that specifically eradicate CSCs. This approach marks a turning point in oncology, with the potential to develop more durable and effective treatments. CSCs differ markedly from the bulk of tumor cells through their capacity for self-renewal, and underpin their roles in tumor growth, metastasis, and resistance to therapy. These include multilineage differentiation and a heightened ability to survive conventional treatments. A deeper understanding of these hallmarks is essential for developing therapies that can effectively eliminate CSCs and improve treatment success. CSCs sustain tumor growth through their hallmark ability of self-renewal, achieved by symmetric division to expand their pool or asymmetric division to generate non-CSC progeny [6]. Experimental studies have shown that CSCs isolated from patient tumors can initiate new tumors when transplanted into immunodeficient mice, confirming their tumorigenic potential. The process of self-renewal is precisely controlled by critical developmental signaling pathways such as Wnt, Notch, and Hedgehog, which are frequently dysregulated in cancer and represent promising therapeutic targets [7–9].

In addition, CSCs possess differentiation and transdifferentiation capacities, enabling them to generate heterogeneous tumor cell types and even contribute to nontumor lineages. Studies in Severe Combined Immunodeficient (SCID) mouse models show that renal CSCs can give rise to vascular endothelial cells inside neoplastic tissue, highlighting their role in tumor plasticity and progression [10]. CSCs have been shown to differentiate into endothelial cells, contributing to angiogenesis in cancers such as liver cancer and glioblastoma [11, 12]. This differentiation capacity enhances tumor heterogeneity, making treatment difficult as subpopulations within the same tumor may exhibit variable drug responses. A major clinical challenge is the intrinsic chemoresistance of CSCs, which enables them to survive conventional therapies and drive relapse. Resistance mechanisms include enhanced DNA repair, overexpression of drug efflux transporters, evasion of apoptosis, and the capability to remain in a quiescent G0 phase, rendering them less susceptible to therapies targeting proliferating cells [12]. These features allow CSCs to persist after treatment, causing tumor recurrence and progression. Therefore, unraveling the molecular mechanisms underlying CSC self-renewal, differentiation, and therapy resistance is crucial for developing targeted interventions capable of overcoming the limitations of standard chemotherapy.

8.1.2 Role of Metabolic Adaptations in CSC Biology

Metabolic reprogramming is a hallmark of cancer stem cells (CSCs), driving their adaptability, identity, and therapy resistance. Unlike differentiated tumor cells, CSCs can flexibly switch between glycolysis and oxidative phosphorylation (OXPHOS) in response to low oxygen, nutrient scarcity, or treatment, supporting both immediate energy needs and long-term survival (Fig. 8.2) [13].

Glycolysis supports CSC proliferation in low-oxygen regions, while OXPHOS is often linked with quiescence, improved redox balance, and enhanced tumor-initiating capacity. The ability to toggle between these metabolic states, known as the glycolysis-OXPHOS switch, is essential for CSC survival during chemotherapy and radiotherapy. Additionally, other metabolic pathways, including lipid and amino acid utilization, are critical for CSC maintenance. Fatty-acid oxidation (FAO) and lipogenesis supply components for membrane formation, regulate redox equilibrium, and promote metastatic potential, whereas glutamine and one-carbon metabolism provide essential precursors for biosynthesis processes and epigenetic control [14].

Mitochondrial dynamics play a key role in CSC behavior, as biogenesis, fusion/fission, and mito-nuclear signaling control stemness, differentiation, and apoptosis sensitivity. Disrupting mitochondrial function can hinder tumor initiation, making mitochondria a promising therapeutic target. This metabolic flexibility allows CSCs to escape conventional therapies, suggesting that combining metabolic inhibitors with standard treatments could more effectively eliminate CSCs and prevent relapse [15].

CSCs sustain tumor growth through self-renewal and generation of differentiated progeny with limited tumor-initiating potential. Genetic, epigenetic, and microenvironmental interactions drive CSC diversification into subclones with distinct functions. While both CSCs and non-CSCs may acquire migratory traits such as epithelial-mesenchymal transition (EMT), only metastatic CSCs can establish secondary tumors. These circulating CSCs must endure blood circulation, escape immune detection, and colonize distant sites, making metastasis a rare but critical event.

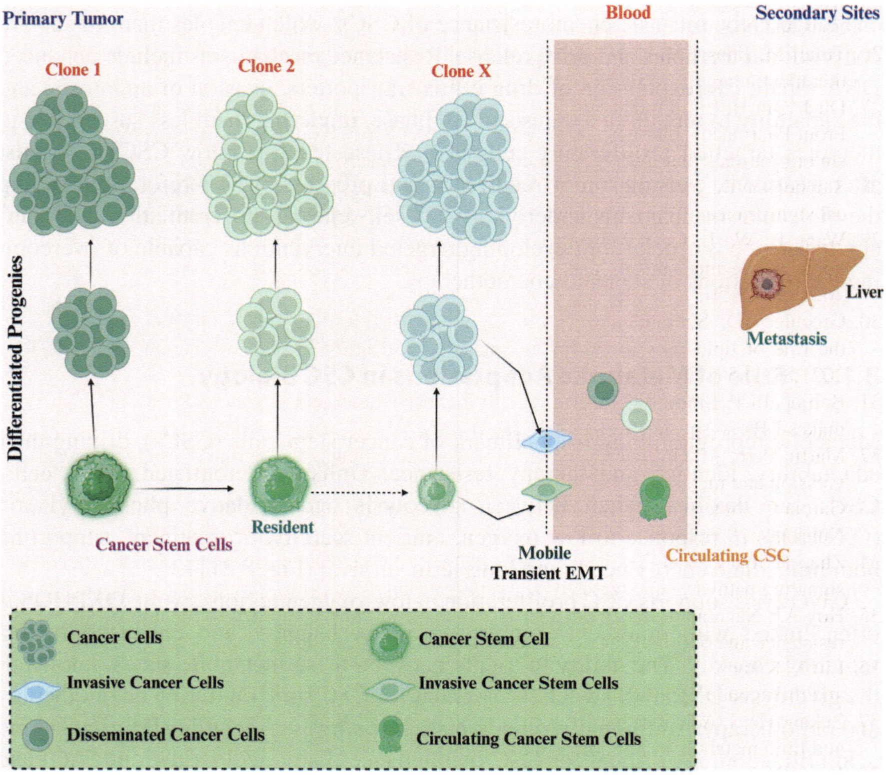

Fig. 8.2 Schematic representation of the cancer stem cell (CSC) model in tumor progression and metastasis. (Figure created using BioRender)

8.1.3 The Role of Tumor Microenvironment in CSC Metabolism

The tumor microenvironment (TME) provides a supportive niche where cancer stem cells (CSCs) adapt their metabolic states and influence neighboring stromal cells. Key components consist of the extracellular matrix, cancer-associated fibroblasts (CAFs), endothelial cells, immune cells, and various soluble signaling molecules [16]. CAFs are major regulators of CSC metabolism. Through signals such as TGF-β, PDGF, hypoxia-inducible factor-1α (HIF-1α), and ROS-driven caveolin-1 suppression, CAFs shift from oxidative phosphorylation (OXPHOS) to aerobic glycolysis [17]. This reprogramming increases production of lactate, glutamine, and ketone bodies, which CSCs import and oxidize to support energy generation and survival, a process termed the reverse Warburg effect [18].

Metabolic symbiosis is reinforced by monocarboxylate transporters: CAFs and differentiated tumor cells predominantly express MCT-4 for lactate export, whereas CSCs express MCT-1 to uptake lactate and channel it into the tricarboxylic acid (TCA) cycle

[19]. This lactate shuttle enhances CSC adaptability in hypoxic and nutrient-limited conditions. Overall, the TME shapes CSC metabolic flexibility, sustaining their tumor-initiating potential, therapeutic resistance, and contribution to disease progression.

8.2 Metabolic Plasticity of CSCs

Cancer stem cells (CSCs) possess remarkable metabolic adaptability, allowing them to reconfigure energy pathways in response to environmental stress or therapy. Unlike differentiated tumor cells with relatively fixed programs, CSCs adapt their metabolism, alternating between glycolysis and OXPHOS based on oxygen, nutrients, and therapeutic stress. This metabolic flexibility enables survival in hypoxic niches through glycolysis and sustains long-term energy needs via OXPHOS in oxygen-rich settings. Such plasticity not only fuels growth and self-renewal but also contributes to resistance against chemotherapy and radiotherapy.

In addition to glucose metabolism, CSCs utilize lipid and amino acid pathways to maintain stemness. Fatty acid oxidation supports energy demands during dormancy, while glutamine metabolism drives biosynthesis and epigenetic regulation. These adaptive strategies provide CSCs with resilience in hostile microenvironments and promote tumor recurrence. Targeting the dynamic metabolic networks of CSCs offers a promising route to weaken their survival mechanisms and improve therapeutic outcomes.

8.2.1 Glycolysis and the Warburg Effect

Glucose serves as the primary energy and biosynthetic source for cell proliferation. It is metabolized through cytoplasmic pathways, glycolysis, the pentose phosphate pathway (PPP), and the serine synthesis pathway (SSP), and mitochondrial oxidative phosphorylation via the TCA cycle. Glycolysis produces pyruvate, which is either converted to lactate for export or transported into mitochondria for the TCA cycle oxidation, while intermediates support the synthesis of nucleotides, amino acids, and lipids.

A defining feature of cancer cell metabolism is its preference for glycolysis, even under oxygen-rich conditions, a phenomenon described by Otto Warburg as the "Warburg effect" or aerobic glycolysis [20]. This metabolic shift is one of the most characteristic hallmarks of cancer and plays a central role in tumor progression. Oncogenic alterations frequently drive it. For example, c-Myc enhances the expression of glycolytic enzymes and activates SSP during nutrient scarcity; Kirsten Rat Sarcoma Viral Oncogene Homolog (KRAS) mutations increase glucose transporter activity and glycolytic flux, while B-Raf proto-oncogene, serine/threonine kinase (BRAF) also contributes to dysregulated glucose metabolism [21]. In hypoxic tumor regions, stabilization of hypoxia-inducible factor-1α (HIF-1α) promotes glycolysis through transcriptional activation of glycolytic enzymes. Importantly, HIF activity is modulated by mitochondrial function, including TCA cycle intermediates, respiratory chain components, biogenesis, apoptosis, and autophagy [22].

The metabolic consequences extend beyond ATP production. Aerobic glycolysis supplies carbon skeletons for macromolecule synthesis, supports rapid proliferation, and results in lactate accumulation. Lactate itself acts as a signaling molecule, shaping the tumor microenvironment by regulating angiogenesis, immune evasion, and inflammatory responses. Clinically, altered glucose metabolism is exploited in diagnostics, with ^18F-fluorodeoxyglucose positron emission tomography (FDG-PET) commonly employed for tumor detection based on elevated glucose uptake in cancer compared to normal tissues. Therapeutically, glucose metabolism is also a target: inhibitors of glycolysis can suppress tumor growth. For instance, the ruthenium-based compound BOLD-100 disrupts glycolysis and sensitizes cancer cells to glucose limitation [23].

8.2.2 Lipid and Fatty Acid Metabolism

Lipids are essential macromolecules that form the architectural framework of biological membranes, act as signaling mediators, and serve as major energy sources. In cancer, lipid metabolism undergoes profound alterations that contribute to tumor initiation and progression [24]. Key enzymes of fatty acid metabolism, such as ATP-citrate lyase (ACLY) and fatty acid synthase (FASN), are frequently upregulated in several cancers, including liver malignancies, and their expression correlates with disease prognosis [25]. Under hypoxic conditions, the synthesis of fatty acids is markedly increased, while enhanced lipid uptake and catabolism further promote tumor growth [26]. For example, fast-proliferating cholangiocarcinoma cells rely heavily on exogenous lipids and lipoproteins to sustain fatty acid breakdown, underscoring the metabolic dependency of certain tumors. These findings have established fatty acid metabolic pathways as a promising therapeutic approach.

Aberrant cholesterol uptake also plays a significant part in tumor development. Disruption of cholesterol homeostasis can promote tumorigenesis and metastasis by conferring resistance to ferroptosis and driving lipid disorders such as hypercholesterolemia [27]. Cholesterol additionally modulates immune responses by influencing the function of tumor-infiltrating immune cells. For instance, regulatory T cells (Tregs), which are central to tumor-induced immunosuppression, depend on lipid synthesis and signaling mediated by sterol regulatory element-binding proteins (SREBPs). Recent evidence shows that SREBP activity is elevated in Tregs within tumors, requiring SREBP cleavage-activating protein (SCAP) for full function. Notably, SCAP deficiency impairs Treg-mediated suppression, reduces tumor growth, and improves the effectiveness of immune checkpoint inhibition (e.g., PD-1 inhibition). Thus, targeting lipid signaling not only interferes with tumor metabolism but also improves antitumor immunity [28].

8.2.3 Oxidative Phosphorylation and Mitochondrial Dynamics

Oxidative phosphorylation (OXPHOS) is the main mitochondrial pathway for ATP generation. In cancer stem cells (CSCs), OXPHOS supplies energy, maintains redox balance, and supports stemness. In contrast to bulk tumor cells that depend on glycolysis, CSCs can alternate between glycolysis and oxidative phosphorylation (OXPHOS concisely. This flexibility helps them survive stress, remain dormant, and later reinitiate growth. High OXPHOS activity is linked with quiescence, therapy resistance, and tumor initiation.

Mitochondrial dynamics also regulate CSC function. Fusion, controlled by MFN1/2 and OPA1, maintains integrity and efficient respiration. Fission, driven by DRP1, aids redistribution during division and promotes stress adaptation. Mitophagy, regulated by PINK1 and Parkin, removes damaged mitochondria and preserves fitness. These processes influence key pathways such as Wnt/β-catenin, Notch, Hedgehog, and STAT3. OXPHOS also regulates the NAD+/NADH ratio and α-ketoglutarate levels, which affect epigenetic control of stemness.

Targeting mitochondrial metabolism offers therapeutic potential. Complex I inhibitors (metformin, phenformin) disrupt OXPHOS. Regulators of PGC-1α alter biogenesis. DRP1 inhibitors disturb fission and block tumor propagation. Since normal stem cells differ metabolically, CSCs can be selectively targeted. Overall, OXPHOS and mitochondrial dynamics form a metabolic network that sustains CSC adaptability, survival, and resistance. These mechanisms represent promising therapeutic vulnerabilities.

8.2.4 Amino Acid Metabolism

Beyond elevated glycolysis and fatty acid synthesis, cancer cells exhibit increased amino acid demand. Amino acids are essential not only for protein synthesis but also for energy production, nucleotide biosynthesis, and redox balance [29]. Key amino acids such as Glutamine, serine, and glycine are essential for cancer cell metabolism. Serine supplies one-carbon units crucial for tumor growth. Extracellular serine supports epidermal stem cell proliferation by inhibiting differentiation, and restricting serine intake or blocking its synthesis can limit tumor progression.

Glycine, glutamine, and aspartate supply carbon and nitrogen for purine synthesis, whereas serine, glycine, and methionine feed into the methionine-folate cycle. Amino acids also maintain redox homeostasis. High ROS levels in tumors disrupt redox balance, prompting cancer cells to increase Nicotinamide Adenine Dinucleotide Phosphate (NADPH) production via glutamine metabolism, the pentose phosphate pathway, and AMP-activated protein kinase (AMPK) activation. Glutamine-derived malate is shuttled to the cytoplasm and converted to NADPH through malic enzyme 1, supporting antioxidant defenses and survival under oxidative stress [30].

In cancer cells, nucleotide breakdown is also reprogrammed to fulfill the high demands of rapid proliferation. Pathways such as glucose-6-phosphate metabolism and one-carbon metabolism connect nucleotide synthesis with glucose and amino acid metabolism. Overall, this metabolic reprogramming supports the progression of the tumor by enhancing proliferation, growth, invasion, and metastasis.

8.3 Regulatory Pathways Linking Metabolism and Stemness

8.3.1 PI3K/Akt/mTOR Signaling

The PI3K/Akt pathway regulates diverse cellular functions through two main mechanisms. In the short term, Akt modifies protein substrates via phosphorylation, affecting their activity, stability, or localization. Over the long term, Akt shapes cellular behavior by phosphorylating transcription factors and altering their activity [31]. Breast cancer stem-like cells depend on the mTOR pathway, triggering colony formation in vitro and driving cancer development in vivo [32]. Suppressing mTOR may reduce aldehyde dehydrogenase 1 (ALDH1) activity, a key marker of colorectal cancer stem cells. Similarly, inhibiting mTORC2 decreases the expression of the hepatic cancer stem cell marker EpCAM and markedly diminishes tumorigenic potential in hepatocellular cancer stem cells [33]. The tumor suppressor Phosphatase and TENsin homolog (PTEN) terminates PI3K/PIP3 signaling by dephosphorylating PIP3 to PIP2. Serving as a principal inhibitor of the PI3K/AKT/mTOR (PAM) pathway, PTEN controls cell growth and survival, while its loss leads to persistent pathway activation [34]. Cancer cell lines with PTEN mutations show elevated Akt activity and resistance to EGFR inhibitors like gefitinib. Restoring PTEN reverses this resistance, as demonstrated, where combined PTEN reconstitution and EGFR blockade suppressed breast cancer xenograft growth, an effect absent with either treatment alone. Similar findings in NSCLC, prostate, and leukemia cells highlight the link between PTEN loss, Akt activation, and reduced EGFR inhibitor sensitivity [35].

8.3.2 AMPK and Energy Sensing

Elevated glycolytic activity is a characteristic shared by many stem cell populations [36]. Activation of glycolysis or its regulators promotes pluripotency during nuclear reprogramming and helps sustain stemness. Early in iPSC generation, the glycolytic pathway undergoes extensive remodeling, which involves increased expression of genes governing glucose uptake, phosphorylation, and later stages of glycolysis. Cancer cells, however, predominantly channel glucose into lactate production even when there is availability of oxygen, a process termed aerobic glycolysis, first identified by Warburg [37]. Cancer cells retain limited OXPHOS but rely mainly on aerobic glycolysis, which yields ATP quickly though inefficiently at just two molecules per glucose. To compensate, they greatly increase glucose uptake, driven by elevated GLUT1 expression [38]. Additionally, several enzymes that drive the Warburg effect, including monocarboxylate transporters 1 and 4 [39], hexokinase 2 (HK2), lactate dehydrogenase A (LDHA), and pyruvate dehydrogenase kinase 1 (PDK1), have been reported to show elevated expression across various cancer types.

8.3.3 HIF-1α and Hypoxic Adaptation

Studies indicate that genetic and epigenetic alterations in adult stem or progenitor cells can transform them into cancer stem or progenitor cells, initiating many human cancers [40]. Supporting this idea, cells with stem-like markers, strong self-renewal capacity, and abnormal differentiation have been isolated from primary tumors, blood, and metastatic tissues [41]. Hypoxia-inducible factor (HIF) plays a central role in maintaining oxygen homeostasis by regulating a wide array of hypoxia-responsive genes. HIF is composed of two subunits: HIF-α and HIF-β [42]. HIF-β is constitutively expressed, whereas HIF-1α, the key regulator of hypoxia, is primarily controlled via post-translational mechanisms [43]. HIF-1α and HIF-2α are the most studied and structurally alike, while HIF-3α (IPAS) has multiple splice variants that can inhibit HIF-1α and HIF-2α activity [44]. HIF-1α is broadly expressed across tissues, whereas HIF-2α and HIF-3α are expressed selectively in certain cell types, including vascular endothelial cells, type II pneumocytes, liver parenchymal cells, renal interstitial cells, and cells of the myeloid lineage [45]. In renewable tissues, mitotic cells respond to damage by either entering senescence or activating apoptosis, though the factors determining this choice remain unclear. Stem cells in hypoxic niches resist oxidative stress, avoiding senescence to preserve tissue regeneration. Nevertheless, adult stem cells accumulate damage over time, contributing to the age-related decline in organ function [46].

8.3.4 Cross Talk with Wnt, Notch, and Hedgehog Pathways

Cancer-associated Wnt pathway deregulation occurs at multiple points in the signaling cascade. R-spondin ligands enhance Wnt signaling in Lgr5+ cells, while the E3 ubiquitin ligases ZNRF3 and RNF43 function as negative feedback regulators by promoting Frizzled (Fz) receptor degradation when R-spondin is absent [47]. Both ZNRF3 and RNF43 require Dishevelled (Dsh), a positive Wnt signaling mediator, for their activity [48]. Key Wnt pathway components, including GSK-3β, also influence Hedgehog signaling. Oncogenic Hedgehog-driven pathological responses have been shown to rely on canonical Wnt/β-catenin signaling [49]. Wnt signaling can inhibit the Hedgehog pathway through various mechanisms, thereby effectively reducing SHH-driven tumorigenesis [50]. Gene network analysis revealed a connection between Wnt and SHH signaling through the Gli2 transcription factor. It highlighted the shared roles of GSK-3β and CK1α1 in both pathways, as they are key regulators of downstream signal inactivation [51]. Under conditions of deregulated Notch signaling, hyperactivation of the Hedgehog-dependent Wnt signaling pathway has been associated with the development of chronic myeloid leukemia, despite the absence of a previously established direct connection between the two pathways [52]. The Notch receptor ligand Jagged1 is activated by β-catenin–mediated transcription, serving as a molecular connection between the Wnt and Notch pathways in cancer [53].

8.4 Metabolic Reprogramming and Therapy Resistance

Metabolic remodeling in cancer, particularly in cancer stem cells (CSCs), contributes significantly to therapy resistance. By altering energy production and biosynthetic pathways, CSCs can survive chemotherapeutic and radiotherapeutic stress. Flexible switching between glycolysis and OXPHOS allows them to adapt to nutrient scarcity or hypoxic conditions, maintaining ATP supply and supporting survival.

This metabolic adaptability also preserves redox balance under oxidative stress, helping CSCs resist apoptosis triggered by therapy. Furthermore, reprogrammed metabolism supports the synthesis of macromolecules required for repair and proliferation, allowing tumor cells to recover rapidly after treatment. Collectively, these metabolic changes give cancer cells a survival edge, reduce therapeutic efficacy, and promote disease recurrence.

8.4.1 Drug Efflux and Redox Balance

Multidrug resistance (MDR) can result from reduced drug entry into target cells. Many drugs enter cells through endocytosis, passive diffusion, or facilitated transport mechanisms [54]. Importantly, the solute carrier (SLC) superfamily, which includes 43 families and 298 transporters, plays a key role in the cellular uptake of many anticancer drugs [55]. Reduced expression or mutations in these transporters can lead to drug resistance. For instance, methotrexate relies on the reduced folate carrier for cellular uptake, and its mutation causes antifolate resistance [56]. Excessive ROS can cause oxidative stress capable of damaging or killing cancer cells. To counter this, cancer cells activate antioxidant defenses, primarily via NRF2, a key transcription factor. Under normal conditions, NRF2 binds KEAP1, undergoes ubiquitination, and is degraded [57]. At low concentrations and within specific cellular compartments, reactive oxygen species (ROS) act as signaling molecules that promote cancer progression [58].

Targeting ROS in cancer cells was proposed to block ROS-driven growth signals. However, because tumors often have elevated antioxidant defences, antioxidant supplementation is ineffective and potentially harmful as a cancer therapy [59]. Epithelial-to-mesenchymal transition (EMT) is crucial for driving tumor metastasis and enhancing therapeutic resistance [60]. In EMT, epithelial cells lose their adhesion and polarity while gaining enhanced motility, migratory capacity, and invasive properties [61]. Cancer stem cells (CSCs) play a major role in the growth of tumors, their survival, and metastasis. Their ability for self-renewal and unlimited proliferation contributes to drug resistance and recurrence. EMT-activated signaling pathways, including Wnt, Hedgehog, and Notch, overlap with those regulating CSCs, linking EMT to stem cell traits in normal and tumor epithelial tissues [62].

8.4.2 Immune Evasion and Tumor Microenvironment Adaptation

During EMT, epithelial cells lose adhesion and polarity while acquiring increased motility, migratory potential, and invasive properties [63]. The tumor microenvironment (TME) exhibits metabolic diversity among tumors due to their heterogeneity and varying proliferation and metastatic demands. Enhancing tumor immunotherapy depends on understanding the TME. Cancer cells rely on high nutrient uptake for growth, while immune cells adapt through multiple metabolic pathways. Recent studies focus on targeting cancer metabolism by modulating immune cell signaling, as cancer cells can impair T-cell function by depleting glucose and altering their activation and proliferation [64]. Recent research in cancer immunotherapy focuses on harnessing the immune system, particularly through immune checkpoint inhibitors. Clinical studies have explored combining these inhibitors with other anticancer drugs to extend patient survival and sustain treatment. Emerging strategies target the tumor microenvironment (TME) to enhance immune responses, as the TME can influence the efficacy of checkpoint inhibitors. Consequently, combination therapies involving TME modulators and immune checkpoint inhibitors are being investigated to improve anticancer outcomes [65].

8.4.3 Plasticity in Response to Metabolic Stress

As tumors grow, cancer cells encounter changing microenvironments with varying nutrients, metabolites, and cell types. Uneven vascularization creates gradients of oxygen and nutrients, leading to metabolic heterogeneity. For example, in human lung tumors, cells in poorly perfused regions rely on glucose, while those in well-perfused areas utilize alternative fuels like lactate [66]. Tumor metabolic flexibility drives resistance to many anticancer therapies, largely due to genetic heterogeneity. Resistance arises through clonal selection of pathways enabling metabolic rewiring to withstand drug-induced stress. This compensatory reprogramming supports cancer cell survival and growth, as seen in chemo-resistance linked to glucose metabolism. For instance, cisplatin treatment in cervical cancer induces key glycolytic enzymes (HK2, PFK, and PKM2) and GLUT-1 via AMPK activation. Enhanced glycolysis produces abundant intermediates for pathways like the PPP, supporting nucleotide synthesis and redox balance. Elevated lactate secretion creates a hypoxic microenvironment that hinders drug uptake. Additionally, increased glucose uptake triggers stress responses under glucose deprivation, promoting autophagy and helping cells evade apoptosis [67].

8.5 Therapeutic Strategies Targeting CSC Metabolism

Targeting metabolic pathways in cancer stem cells (CSCs) offers a promising approach to overcome therapy resistance and prevent tumor relapse. Inhibitors of glycolysis and mitochondrial function can disrupt energy production, impair stemness, and sensitize CSCs to chemotherapy and radiotherapy. Blocking lipid metabolism, including fatty acid synthesis and oxidation, interferes with membrane biogenesis, energy storage, and redox balance, reducing CSC survival.

Modulating amino acid metabolism, such as restricting glutamine, serine, or glycine availability, limits nucleotide synthesis, redox maintenance, and biosynthetic capacity, impairing CSC proliferation. Combining metabolic inhibitors with standard therapies targets both active and quiescent CSCs, exploiting their metabolic vulnerabilities to improve treatment effectiveness.

8.5.1 Glycolysis and Mitochondrial Inhibitors

CSCs are a small subset of tumor cells with stem-like traits, driving tumor growth, therapy resistance, residual disease, and metastasis [68]. While conventional therapies target rapidly dividing, glycolysis-dependent bulk tumor cells, they often spare quiescent CSCs that rely on OXPHOS. Targeting the glycolysis–OXPHOS switch in CSCs could prevent relapse and overcome therapy resistance. Understanding the regulation of this metabolic shift may reveal new therapeutic strategies [69]. In cancer stem cells (CSCs), the shift toward glycolysis is a driver of stemness rather than a result of pluripotency. Research has shown that promoting the metabolic switch from oxidative phosphorylation (OXPHOS) to glycolysis enhances the CSC-like characteristics of CD44 cells in basal-like breast cancer. Notably, HIF-1 was recognized as a key regulator initiating the metabolic reprogramming of CSCs from OXPHOS to glycolysis [70].

8.5.2 Lipid Metabolism Blockers

In cancer cells, the well-known Warburg effect describes a shift to glycolysis, but altered lipid metabolism is also a key adaptation. Rapidly proliferating cancer cells rely on enhanced lipogenesis for membrane synthesis. When glycolysis is inhibited by therapy, lipid droplets are broken down, releasing free fatty acids that fuel mitochondrial energy production via β-oxidation [71]. CSCs leverage metabolic flexibility by activating β-oxidation under glucose-limited conditions. In their hypoxic niches, they show increased fatty acid uptake and lipid droplet accumulation. HIF-α and pyruvate dehydrogenase restrict pyruvate access into the TCA cycle, blocking glucose-driven fatty acid synthesis. Consequently, alternative carbon sources like glutamine are used, undergoing reductive metabolism to produce α-ketoglutarate, isocitrate, and citrate for fatty acid synthesis [72].

8.5.3 Amino Acid Metabolism Modulators

The 20 standard amino acids support key processes for cell proliferation, including protein, nucleotide, lipid, glutathione, glucosamine, and polyamine synthesis, as well as TCA cycle anaplerosis. Amino acid metabolism is highly adaptable, varying by tissue, cancer type, microenvironment, and oncogenic mutations. Common features in cancer include increased nitrogen demand, higher amino acid uptake with transporter upregulation, reliance on certain nonessential amino acids, and altered levels of enzymes for amino acid synthesis or degradation. Redundancy is also observed, as multiple enzymes can catalyze the same reaction; for example, mitochondrial GLS and GLS2 both convert glutamine to glutamate [73]. Several pharmacological inhibitors have been studied to target key enzymes in amino acid metabolism, aiming to hinder cancer progression. Among these enzymes, branched-chain amino acid transaminase (BCAT) is pivotal in promoting the growth and progression of several cancer types [74]. BCAT gene knockdown reduces cancer cell proliferation in vitro and in vivo. Gabapentin, initially developed as a GABA-mimetic, provides anticonvulsant and analgesic effects through blockade of voltage-gated calcium channels in dorsal root ganglion neurons, though its full mechanism remains unclear [75].

8.5.4 Combination Approaches with Conventional Therapies

Cancer immunotherapy has transformed treatment, showing significant success across multiple malignancies [76]. Immunotherapy strategies, such as checkpoint inhibitors, adoptive cell transfer, cancer vaccines, and cytokine therapies, aim to target and modulate specific immune system components [77]. Although multiple immunotherapies have been approved by the FDA, only a small proportion of patients with progressive cancers show a meaningful response to immune checkpoint inhibitors or other single-agent immunomodulatory treatments. Evidence suggests that individuals with strongly immunogenic or detected at an early stage tend to achieve better outcomes with these therapies [78]. Surgery continues to be the primary treatment for solid tumors, but it may be inadequate for aggressive or metastatic cancers. Recently, combining surgical resection with immunotherapy has gained traction, offering improved clinical outcomes. Neoadjuvant therapy followed by surgery is a key multidisciplinary approach for controlling both local and metastatic disease in resectable non-small cell lung cancer. Phase II studies indicate that preoperative PD-1/PD-L1 inhibitors, alone or with chemotherapy, can improve survival. Combining surgery with immunotherapy helps remove tumors while boosting immune responses against residual cells, reducing recurrence and progression [79].

8.6 Challenges in Clinical Transition

Cancer stem cells (CSCs) drive chemotherapy resistance and promote tumor recurrence, making their eradication essential for effective cancer therapy. However, similarities with normal stem cells, such as shared surface markers (CD44) and signaling pathways (Wnt, Notch), pose challenges for selective targeting. Since 2010, metabolic alterations have been identified as a key hallmark of cancer, with evidence supporting the "metabostemness" concept, where metabolic reprogramming enhances EMT and stemness, worsening patient outcomes. CSCs display tissue-specific metabolic heterogeneity and adaptability, complicating therapy development. Nonetheless, vulnerabilities such as glutamine dependence and reliance on autophagy present promising therapeutic targets. Several metabolism-focused drugs, including autophagy modulators like metformin and alisertib, are now under clinical evaluation for their potential relevance to CSCs [80]. Although progress has been made in understanding CSCs, their heterogeneity, plasticity, absence of reliable biomarkers, and intricate interactions with the tumor microenvironment continue to limit clinical translation. Emerging technologies such as single-cell sequencing, multiomics approaches, CRISPR/Cas9 screening, and 3D organoid models hold promise for addressing these challenges. A key obstacle in CSC-targeted therapy is their high metabolic flexibility, which enables them to withstand treatment-induced stress. Unlike differentiated cancer cells with fixed metabolic profiles, CSCs adapt their metabolism by switching between glycolysis and oxidative phosphorylation (OXPHOS) depending on environmental conditions and treatment stress. This adaptability supports survival, resistance to metabolic inhibitors, and escape from therapy-induced death, with ATP production being reprogrammed as needed [81].

8.7 Future Directions

Recent reviews have highlighted CSC plasticity and therapy resistance. Enzymes driving metabolic reprogramming, such as IDH, FASN, and GLS1, are being investigated as biomarkers and therapeutic targets in different cancers. Similarly, regulators of EMT, including transcriptional and epigenetic factors, offer potential intervention points. Given the role of CSCs in resistance and relapse, this review discusses EMT in relation to metabolism and epigenetic regulation, emphasizing their implications for both cancer treatment and regenerative medicine. Understanding how epithelial and metabolic states shift during metastasis is crucial for designing effective therapies. While many drugs now target cancer metabolism, challenges remain, including the need for reliable biomarkers and better insight into the link between metabolism and EMT to avoid treatment-related adverse effects. Addressing these gaps is key to improving strategies against metastatic cancers. Key questions remain about how metabolism shapes cell fate. The mechanisms linking metabolic states to gene expression, the balance between bioenergetic needs and cell identity–driven metabolic choices, and the impact of nutrient availability on cancer progression or development are still unclear. Advancing sensitive methods to study rare cell populations in vivo will help clarify whether metabolic traits drive or follow cellular changes, offering new opportunities for targeted therapies and regenerative medicine.

8.8 Emerging Technologies in CSCs and Precision Oncology

Recent advances in technology are transforming our understanding of cancer stem cells (CSCs) and enabling precision oncology approaches. Single-cell sequencing allows the detailed profiling of CSC heterogeneity, revealing unique metabolic states and therapy-resistant subpopulations. Metabolomics and flux analysis provide insights into real-time nutrient utilization and pathway dependencies, helping identify metabolic vulnerabilities.

Organoid and patient-derived xenograft (PDX) models recreate tumor microenvironments, enabling functional testing of metabolic inhibitors in CSC-rich populations. Coupled with high-throughput screening, these models facilitate the discovery of compounds targeting CSC-specific metabolic pathways. Furthermore, precision oncology integrates molecular and metabolic profiling with computational modeling to predict therapy response, guide combinatorial strategies, and minimize relapse. By combining these technologies with targeted metabolic interventions, it is possible to selectively disrupt CSC survival mechanisms, offering opportunities for more durable and personalized cancer treatments.

Acknowledgments The authors sincerely acknowledge the unwavering support, research facilities, and encouragement extended by their respective institutions, which were instrumental in the successful completion of this study. Mr. Gaurav Ranjan gratefully acknowledges the financial support received from the Department of Science and Technology (DST), Government of India (DST/INSPIRE Fellowship/2020/IF200148).

References

1. Hanahan D, Weinberg RA. Hallmarks of cancer: the next generation. Cell. 2011;144(5):646–74.
2. Beck B, Blanpain C. Unravelling cancer stem cell potential. Nat Rev Cancer. 2013;13(10):727–38.
3. Sell S. On the stem cell origin of cancer. Am J Pathol. 2010;176(6):2584–94.
4. Ye J, Wu D, Wu P, Chen Z, Huang J. The cancer stem cell niche: cross talk between cancer stem cells and their microenvironment. Tumour Biol. 2014;35(5):3945–51.
5. Hatina J. The dynamics of cancer stem cells. Neoplasma. 2012;59(6):700.
6. Yoo YD, Kwon YT. Molecular mechanisms controlling asymmetric and symmetric self-renewal of cancer stem cells. J Anal Sci Technol. 2015;6(1):28.
7. Kanwar SS, Yu Y, Nautiyal J, Patel BB, Majumdar APN. The Wnt/β-catenin pathway regulates growth and maintenance of colonospheres. Mol Cancer. 2010;9(1):212.
8. Wang J, et al. Notch promotes radioresistance of glioma stem cells. Stem Cells. 2010;28(1):17–28.
9. Cochrane CR, Szczepny A, Watkins DN, Cain JE. Hedgehog signaling in the maintenance of cancer stem cells. Cancers (Basel). 2015;7(3):1554–85.

10. Huang Z, Wu T, Liu AY, Ouyang G. Differentiation and transdifferentiation potentials of cancer stem cells. Oncotarget. 2015;6(37):39550.
11. Xiong Y-Q, et al. Human hepatocellular carcinoma tumor–derived endothelial cells manifest increased angiogenesis capability and drug resistance compared with normal endothelial cells. Clin Cancer Res. 2009;15(15):4838–46.
12. Ricci-Vitiani L, et al. Tumour vascularization via endothelial differentiation of glioblastoma stem-like cells. Nature. 2010;468(7325):824–8.
13. Papadaki S, Magklara A. Regulation of metabolic plasticity in cancer stem cells and implications in cancer therapy. Cancers (Basel). 2022;14(23):5912.
14. Xie Y, Ma S, Tong M. Metabolic plasticity of cancer stem cells in response to microenvironmental cues. Cancers (Basel). 2022;14(21):5345.
15. Chu X, et al. Cancer stem cells: advances in knowledge and implications for cancer therapy. Signal Transduct Target Ther. 2024;9(1):170.
16. Li Y, et al. PKM2, a potential target for regulating cancer. Gene. 2018;668:48–53.
17. Schito L, Semenza GL. Hypoxia-inducible factors: master regulators of cancer progression. Trends Cancer. 2016;2(12):758–70.
18. Martinez-Outschoorn UE, Peiris-Pagés M, Pestell RG, Sotgia F, Lisanti MP. Cancer metabolism: a therapeutic perspective. Nat Rev Clin Oncol. 2017;14(1):11–31.
19. Fan Q, et al. Autophagy promotes metastasis and glycolysis by upregulating MCT1 expression and Wnt/β-catenin signaling pathway activation in hepatocellular carcinoma cells. J Exp Clin Cancer Res. 2018;37(1):9.
20. Warburg O. On the origin of cancer cells. Science (80-.). 1956;123(3191):309–14.
21. Sun L, et al. cMyc-mediated activation of serine biosynthesis pathway is critical for cancer progression under nutrient deprivation conditions. Cell Res. 2015;25(4):429–44.
22. Kierans SJ, Taylor CT. Regulation of glycolysis by the hypoxia-inducible factor (HIF): implications for cellular physiology. J Physiol. 2021;599(1):23–37.
23. Baier D, et al. The anticancer ruthenium compound BOLD-100 targets glycolysis and generates a metabolic vulnerability towards glucose deprivation. Pharmaceutics. 2022;14(2):238.
24. Snaebjornsson MT, Janaki-Raman S, Schulze A. Greasing the wheels of the cancer machine: the role of lipid metabolism in cancer. Cell Metab. 2020;31(1):62–76.
25. Gu L, et al. The IKKβ-USP30-ACLY axis controls lipogenesis and tumorigenesis. Hepatology. 2021;73(1):160–74.
26. Munir R, Lisec J, Swinnen JV, Zaidi N. Too complex to fail? Targeting fatty acid metabolism for cancer therapy. Prog Lipid Res. 2022;85:101143.
27. Liu W, Chakraborty B, Safi R, Kazmin D, Chang C, McDonnell DP. Dysregulated cholesterol homeostasis results in resistance to ferroptosis increasing tumorigenicity and metastasis in cancer. Nat Commun. 2021;12(1):5103.
28. Lim SA, et al. Lipid signalling enforces functional specialization of Treg cells in tumours. Nature. 2021;591(7849):306–11.
29. Lieu EL, Nguyen T, Rhyne S, Kim J. Amino acids in cancer. Exp Mol Med. 2020;52(1):15–30.
30. Hayes JD, Dinkova-Kostova AT, Tew KD. Oxidative stress in cancer. Cancer Cell. 2020;38(2):167–97.
31. Lien EC, Lyssiotis CA, Cantley LC. Metabolic reprogramming by the PI3K-Akt-mTOR pathway in cancer. Metab Cancer. 2016;207:39–72.
32. Zhou J, et al. Activation of the PTEN/mTOR/STAT3 pathway in breast cancer stem-like cells is required for viability and maintenance. Proc Natl Acad Sci. 2007;104(41):16158–63.
33. Xia P, Xu X-Y. PI3K/Akt/mTOR signaling pathway in cancer stem cells: from basic research to clinical application. Am J Cancer Res. 2015;5(5):1602.
34. Chow LML, Baker SJ. PTEN function in normal and neoplastic growth. Cancer Lett. 2006;241(2):184–96.
35. Festuccia C, et al. Molecular aspects of gefitinib antiproliferative and pro-apoptotic effects in PTEN-positive and PTEN-negative prostate cancer cell lines. Endocr Relat Cancer. 2005;12(4):983–98.

36. Folmes CDL, et al. Somatic oxidative bioenergetics transitions into pluripotency-dependent glycolysis to facilitate nuclear reprogramming. Cell Metab. 2011;14(2):264–71.
37. Vander Heiden MG, Cantley LC, Thompson CB. Understanding the Warburg effect: the metabolic requirements of cell proliferation. Science (80-). 2009;324(5930):1029–33.
38. Ancey P, Contat C, Meylan E. Glucose transporters in cancer–from tumor cells to the tumor microenvironment. FEBS J. 2018;285(16):2926–43.
39. Jiang B. Aerobic glycolysis and high level of lactate in cancer metabolism and microenvironment. Genes Dis. 2017;4(1):25–7.
40. Mimeault M, Hauke R, Mehta PP, Batra SK. Recent advances in cancer stem/progenitor cell research: therapeutic implications for overcoming resistance to the most aggressive cancers. J Cell Mol Med. 2007;11(5):981–1011.
41. Mukherjee A, Kenny HA, Lengyel E. Unsaturated fatty acids maintain cancer cell stemness. Cell Stem Cell. 2017;20(3):291–2.
42. Muz B, Khan MN, Kiriakidis S, Paleolog EM. Hypoxia. The role of hypoxia and HIF-dependent signalling events in rheumatoid arthritis. Arthritis Res Ther. 2009;11(1):201.
43. Khan WS, Adesida AB, Hardingham TE. Hypoxic conditions increase hypoxia-inducible transcription factor 2$α$ and enhance chondrogenesis in stem cells from the infrapatellar fat pad of osteoarthritis patients. Arthritis Res Ther. 2007;9(3):R55.
44. Kaelin WG, Ratcliffe PJ. Oxygen sensing by metazoans: the central role of the HIF hydroxylase pathway. Mol Cell. 2008;30(4):393–402.
45. Bertout JA, Patel SA, Simon MC. The impact of O_2 availability on human cancer. Nat Rev Cancer. 2008;8(12):967–75.
46. Schultz MB, Sinclair DA. When stem cells grow old: phenotypes and mechanisms of stem cell aging. Development. 2016;143(1):3–14.
47. De Lau W, Peng WC, Gros P, Clevers H. The R-spondin/Lgr5/Rnf43 module: regulator of Wnt signal strength. Genes Dev. 2014;28(4):305–16.
48. Jiang X, Charlat O, Zamponi R, Yang Y, Cong F. Dishevelled promotes Wnt receptor degradation through recruitment of ZNRF3/RNF43 E3 ubiquitin ligases. Mol Cell. 2015;58(3):522–33.
49. Yang SH, et al. Pathological responses to oncogenic Hedgehog signaling in skin are dependent on canonical Wnt/$β$-catenin signaling. Nat Genet. 2008;40(9):1130.
50. Pöschl J, et al. Wnt/$β$-catenin signaling inhibits the Shh pathway and impairs tumor growth in Shh-dependent medulloblastoma. Acta Neuropathol. 2014;127(4):605–7.
51. Mishra S. CSNK1A1 and Gli2 as Novel Targets Identified through an Integrative Analysis of Gene Expression Data, Protein–Protein Interaction and Pathways Networks in Glioblastoma Tumors: can these Two be Antagonistic Proteins? Cancer Inform. 2014;13:CIN–S18377.
52. Sengupta A, et al. Deregulation and cross talk among Sonic hedgehog, Wnt, Hox and Notch signaling in chronic myeloid leukemia progression. Leukemia. 2007;21(5):949–55.
53. Estrach S, Ambler CA, Lo Lo Celso C, Hozumi K, Watt FM. Jagged 1 is a β-catenin target gene required for ectopic hair follicle formation in adult epidermis. Development. 2006;133(22):4427–38.
54. Dobson PD, Kell DB. Carrier-mediated cellular uptake of pharmaceutical drugs: an exception or the rule? Nat Rev Drug Discov. 2008;7(3):205–20.
55. Hediger MA, Romero MF, Peng J-B, Rolfs A, Takanaga H, Bruford EA. The ABCs of solute carriers: physiological, pathological and therapeutic implications of human membrane transport proteins: introduction. Pflügers Arch. 2004;447(5):465–8.
56. Assaraf YG. Molecular basis of antifolate resistance. Cancer Metastasis Rev. 2007;26(1):153–81.
57. Jaramillo MC, Zhang DD. The emerging role of the Nrf2–Keap1 signaling pathway in cancer. Genes Dev. 2013;27(20):2179–91.
58. Schieber M, Chandel NS. ROS function in redox signaling and oxidative stress. Curr Biol. 2014;24(10):R453–62.
59. Chandel NS, Tuveson DA. The promise and perils of antioxidants for cancer patients. N Engl J Med. 2014;371(2):177–8.
60. Chang JC. Cancer stem cells: role in tumor growth, recurrence, metastasis, and treatment resistance. Medicine (Baltimore). 2016;95(1S):S20–5.

61. Brabletz T, Kalluri R, Nieto MA, Weinberg RA. EMT in cancer. Nat Rev Cancer. 2018;18(2):128–34.
62. Du B, Shim JS. Targeting epithelial–mesenchymal transition (EMT) to overcome drug resistance in cancer. Molecules. 2016;21(7):965.
63. Andrejeva G, Rathmell JC. Similarities and distinctions of cancer and immune metabolism in inflammation and tumors. Cell Metab. 2017;26(1):49–70.
64. Munn DH, et al. Prevention of allogeneic fetal rejection by tryptophan catabolism. Science (80-.). 1998;281(5380):1191–3.
65. Ciciola P, Cascetta P, Bianco C, Formisano L, Bianco R. Combining immune checkpoint inhibitors with anti-angiogenic agents. J Clin Med. 2020;9(3):675.
66. Hensley CT, et al. Metabolic heterogeneity in human lung tumors. Cell. 2016;164(4):681–94.
67. Ma L, Zong X. Metabolic symbiosis in chemoresistance: refocusing the role of aerobic glycolysis. Front Oncol. 2020;10:5.
68. Aguilar-Gallardo C, Simón C. Cells, stem cells, and cancer stem cells. In: Seminars in reproductive medicine. Thieme Medical Publishers; 2013. p. 5–13.
69. Fiorillo M, Sotgia F, Lisanti MP. 'Energetic' cancer stem cells (e-CSCs): a new hyper-metabolic and proliferative tumor cell phenotype, driven by mitochondrial energy. Front Oncol. 2019;8:677.
70. Yuen CA, Asuthkar S, Guda MR, Tsung AJ, Velpula KK. Cancer stem cell molecular reprogramming of the Warburg effect in glioblastomas: a new target gleaned from an old concept. CNS Oncol. 2016;5(2):101–8.
71. Baenke F, Peck B, Miess H, Schulze A. Hooked on fat: the role of lipid synthesis in cancer metabolism and tumour development. Dis Model Mech. 2013;6(6):1353–63.
72. Metallo CM, et al. Reductive glutamine metabolism by IDH1 mediates lipogenesis under hypoxia. Nature. 2012;481(7381):380–4.
73. Altman BJ, Stine ZE, Dang CV. From Krebs to clinic: glutamine metabolism to cancer therapy. Nat Rev Cancer. 2016;16(10):619–34.
74. Hattori A, et al. Cancer progression by reprogrammed BCAA metabolism in myeloid leukaemia. Nature. 2017;545(7655):500–4.
75. Kaps L, et al. Liver cell type-specific targeting by Nanoformulations for therapeutic applications. Int J Mol Sci. 2023;24(14):11869. https://doi.org/10.3390/ijms241411869.
76. Seledtsov VI, von Delwig A. Clinically feasible and prospective immunotherapeutic interventions in multidirectional comprehensive treatment of cancer. Expert Opin Biol Ther. 2021;21(3):323–42.
77. Cole K, Al-Kadhimi Z, Talmadge JE. Highlights into historical and current immune interventions for cancer. Int Immunopharmacol. 2023;117:109882.
78. Tan S, Li D, Zhu X. Cancer immunotherapy: pros, cons and beyond. Biomed Pharmacother. 2020;124:109821.
79. Zhong L, et al. Small molecules in targeted cancer therapy: advances, challenges, and future perspectives. Signal Transduct Target Ther. 2021;6(1):201.
80. Ding Y-H, et al. Alisertib, an Aurora kinase A inhibitor, induces apoptosis and autophagy but inhibits epithelial to mesenchymal transition in human epithelial ovarian cancer cells. Drug Des Devel Ther. 2015;9:425–64.
81. Lee H, et al. Cancer stem cells: landscape, challenges and emerging therapeutic innovations. Signal Transduct Target Ther. 2025;10(1):248.

Targeting Metabolism in Cancer Therapy: Inhibitors and Approaches

9

Bhabani Shankar Nayak, Bangmayee Dash, Sisir Nandi, Nebojša Pavlović, and Mohamed Dkhi

9.1 Introduction

Cancer, one of the most complex disorders, has been associated with abnormal mutations in somatic cells and major genes that lead to cell proliferation, inactivating tumor suppressor genes, and forming oncogenes. The cancer cells are characterized by abnormal growth, unlimited cell division, avoidance of apoptosis, invasive nature, reduction of angiogenesis, and metastases. Scientists have conducted various experiments based on the properties, but apart from this, it also involves genetic and biochemical pathways. Based on their alteration in different biochemical pathways associated with the transformation of a normal cell into a cancerous cell. These unhealthy cells enhance continuous cell division and alter the metabolic signaling pathways. Healthy cells depend on the oxidative phosphorylation process of the mitochondria, the powerhouse of the cell, for their growth and development. At the same time, the cancer cells depend on "the Warburg effect". Based on Otto Warburg's research work, Cancer cells never use OXPHOS due to their damaged

B. S. Nayak
KIIT School of Pharmacy, KIMS, KIIT DEEMED to be University, Bhubaneswar, Odisha, India

B. Dash
School of Allied and Health Care Sciences, DRIEMS University, Cuttack, Odisha, India

S. Nandi (✉)
Global Institute of Pharmaceutical Education & Research (GIPER), Kashipur, Uttarakhand, India

N. Pavlović
Department of Pharmacy, Faculty of Medicine, University of Novi Sad, Novi Sad, Serbia

M. Dkhi
Department of Zoology and Entomology, Faculty of Science, Helwan University, Helwan, Egypt

S. Ashique et al. (eds.), *Cancer Metabolism*, Cancer Treatment and Research 195, https://doi.org/10.1007/978-3-032-21861-2_9

mitochondria. However, there has been increasing proof that tumor cells exhibit pliability by utilizing two biochemical pathways, such as glycolysis and respiration. Another hallmark of cancer cells is a high reliance on glutamine [1].

9.2 Altered Metabolism in Cancer

Cancer cells show different biochemical metabolic alterations, which are associated with their rapid development and abnormal cell cycle under stressful conditions. Their cell proliferation depends particularly on the glycolysis cycle due to the conversion of glucose to lactate. This is a major step, which involves the formation of various syntheses of nucleotides, amino acids, and fatty acids, and enables the synthesis of biosynthetic precursors. Glutaminolysis is one of the major biochemical processes involved in the enhancement of cancer cases nowadays. In this process, glutamine is involved in the precursor of carbon and nitrogen, with active involvement in the Krebs cycle, and helps in the synthesis of macromolecules. It is the primary step of the formation of NADPH and maintaining the oxido–redox balance [2]. Mitochondrial metabolism is involved in the reprogramming of mitochondrial metabolism. Based on former research work, Reactive oxygen species, which are produced by the cells of mitochondria, are responsible for the progression of tumor cells by producing signaling molecules. Cancer cells also increased their properties by using the pentose phosphate pathway to form carbohydrates containing ribose sugar and NADPH to initiate a reductive mechanism, and various antioxidant defenses. Fat metabolism is also changed in various cancers. This could be possible due to the enhancement of de novo lipogenesis to form fatty acids to synthesize novel plasma membrane to form fat signaling molecules. On the other hand, fatty acid oxidation is the key pathway to supply energy in the case of nutrient-poor conditions. To live in nutrient–deficient and hypoxic cancer environments, these invasive cells also depend on autophagy and macrophage drinking, i.e., pinocytosis. These are the essential processes to recycle biomolecules and other components to obtain their energy for metabolic reactions. These adaptations enable cancer cells to be remarkably resilient under various conditions, particularly during treatment-induced stress or tumor progression. These metabolic modifications are driven by epigenetic alterations and genetic mutations. Major oncogenes that are involved in various pathways, such as glycolysis and glutaminolysis, are MYC and RAS genes, and p53. On the other hand, transcription factor HIF-1α (hypoxia-inducible factor-1 alpha) is activated in low oxygen conditions [3].

9.2.1 Targeting Metabolism to Inhibit Cancer

The biochemical metabolism has been taken as a promising target to inhibit cancer growth and formation because cancer cells depend on modified pathways for required energy and biosynthesis, and disrupting these major biochemical cycles has an impact on tumor cells. Along with the Warburg effect, drugs inhibit key enzymes that are involved in glycolysis, such as hexokinase 2 and lactate dehydrogenase A, that are being formed to stop these pathways and decrease energy formation in the tumor. Apart from this, the metabolism of glucose is also associated with the growth of cancer cells, such as the presence of glutamine; it is the primary source for carbon and nitrogen-containing elements. Essential biocatalyst that is used to inhibit glutaminase can convert glutamine to glutamate. The fatty acid synthesis pathway is used to synthesize membranes for cancer cells and cell communication. We have to inhibit the enzymes, such as fatty acid synthase, to break down tumor growth and metastasis. Apart from this alteration in the molecular composition of enzymes, isocitrate dehydrogenase 1 and 2 (IDH1/2) are responsible for the formation of oncometabolites, which enhance the tumorigenesis. These enzymes are currently used in clinical trials [4].

Furthermore, it explains therapeutic targets in cancer biochemical metabolism, including glycolysis inhibitors, oxidative phosphorylation, glutaminase, and lipid metabolism. Finally, it addresses challenges and future directions in overcoming metabolic plasticity, developing a combination treatment process, analyzing biomarkers for metabolic targeting, and conducting advanced research for novel therapeutic approaches. Various mechanisms associated with cancer are shown below (Fig. 9.1) [5].

9.3 Overview of Cancer Metabolism

Metabolism of cancer refers to the various ways associated with alterations in energy production and the management of nutrition that support abnormal growth. As compared with normal cells, which mainly depend on mitochondrial oxidative phosphorylation to gain energy (aerobic glycolysis), this phenomenon is known as the Warburg effect. Nucleotides, amino acids, and fatty acids are the major supporting biomolecules for their formation. The metabolic reprogramming promotes cancer cells to oppose cell death by balancing the redox reaction and enhancing their survival under various stressful conditions.

Clinically, these alterations are exploited in diagnostic imaging (e.g., PET scans using radiolabeled glucose) and are being prepared for cancer therapy through metabolic inhibitors that destroy key enzymes involved in glycolysis, glutaminolysis, and lipid synthesis. In summary, altered metabolism is a hallmark of cancer that supports tumor progression and offers promising factors for diagnosis and treatment [5].

9.4 Biochemical Mechanism

The biochemical mechanism of cancer includes a complex series of biomolecular and cellular modifications that convert normal cells into malignant ones. At the core of cancer formation is mutation at the gene level—in oncogenes, tumor suppressor genes, and DNA repair genes—which are responsible for uncontrolled cell division

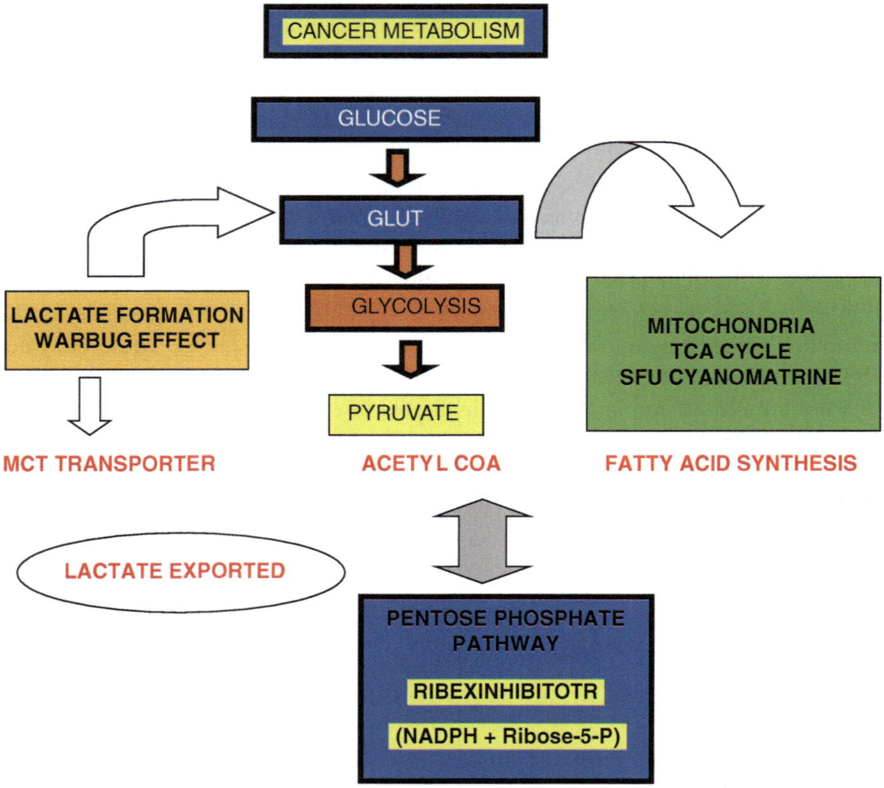

Fig. 9.1 Diagrammatic illustration of the biochemical mechanism associated with the target cancer [5]

and resistance to programmed cell death (apoptosis). Cancer genes such as RAS and MYC in their active form enhance cell proliferation, while the tumor suppressor genes are TP53 and RB. These particular genes remove brakes on the growth of healthy cells. These major genetic alterations modify various biochemical signaling pathways, such as PI3K/AKT/mTOR and MAPK pathways and GPCR pathways. Eventually, these are connected with major metabolism and growth. Furthermore, with the help of pro- and anti-apoptotic proteins (e.g., overexpression of BCL-2) helps the growth of damaged cells to survive. These cells also support angiogenesis by forming factors like VEGF and providing oxygen and other essential nutrients. Biochemical alterations enable cancer cells to invade surrounding tissues and metastasize to distant organs, often including matrix metalloproteinases (MMPs) and epithelial-to-mesenchymal transition (EMT). Another influencing factor is genomic instability due to the formation of BRCA mutations. Eventually, these interconnected biochemical modifications drive the initiation, progression, and aggressiveness of various cancers, making them key targets for modern therapeutic approaches [6–9].

9.5 Targeting Glycolysis Pathways

The glycolysis pathway is the major biochemical metabolism of glucose to pyruvate in the cytoplasm of the cells. Targeting these pathways in cancer is one of the important areas of attention in cancer therapy due to the dependency of many tumor cells on aerobic respiration. Whereas normal healthy cells rely on oxidative phosphorylation of mitochondria. On the other hand, various cancer cells often rely on the glycolysis pathway for the production of multiple ATP and their biosynthesis. This metabolic shift enhances the high-energy and anabolic demands of abnormal proliferation. As a result, glycolytic enzymes and transporters become promising therapeutic targets [10].

9.5.1 Glycolytic Inhibitors

Glycolytic inhibitors are biomolecules that destroy the glycolytic signaling biochemical pathways at different steps, thereby starving the cancerous cell and other precursors of other biosynthetic pathways. Various types of inhibitors and their role are explained below.

Hexokinase Inhibitors (HK Inhibitors)

- *Target Biocatalyst*: Hexokinase (HK), particularly HK2, which is overexpressed in various cancer cells.
- *Example Inhibitor*: *2-Deoxy-D-glucose (2-DG).*

Mode of Biochemical Action

- Glucose transporters are actively involved in taking2-DG. By using the hexokinase enzyme, with the help of the phosphorylation reaction, it converts into 2-DG-6-phosphate, but cannot proceed further in the glycolysis biochemical reaction.
- Formation of 2-DG-6-phosphate is responsible for blocking glycolytic pathways, which are associated with a decrease in the number of ATP synthesized and enhancing the cell death of cancer cells [11].

Phosphofructokinase-1 (PFK-1) Inhibitors

- *Target Biocatalyst*: Phosphofructokinase-1 (PFK-1) is one of the major enzymes of glycolysis pathways, which is responsible for a key rate-limiting enzyme.
- *Example Inhibitor*: 3-(3-Pyridinyl)-1-(4-pyridinyl)-2-propen-1-one (3PO).

Mode of Biochemical Action

- PFKFB3 inhibits 3PO. It is a regulatory isoform in various cancer cells, reducing levels of fructose-2,6-bisphosphate (a potent activator of PFK-1).
- This suppresses glycolytic flux, decreases ATP and lactate formation, and impairs tumor cell proliferation.

Pyruvate Kinase M2 (PKM2) Inhibitors

- *Target Enzyme*: Pyruvate kinase isoform M2 (PKM2), particularly expressed in cancer cells.
- *Example Inhibitor*: Shikonin.

Mode of Action

- Shikonin inhibits Pyruvate kinase isoform M2(PKM2), which stops the conversion of phosphoenolpyruvate (PEP) to pyruvate.
- Inhibition helps to accumulate upstream glycolytic intermediates and suppresses ATP production, enhancing cancer cell apoptosis.

Lactate Dehydrogenase (LDH) Inhibitors

- *Target Enzyme*: Lactate dehydrogenase A (LDH-A), overexpressed in cancer cells for converting pyruvate to lactate.
- *Example Inhibitor*: *FX11* [12].

Mode of Action

- FX11 selectively inhibits Lactate dehydrogenase A (LDH-A), inhibiting the conversion of pyruvate to lactate.
- This causes a buildup of pyruvate and reduces NAD^+ regeneration, which is responsible for the death of cancer cells.
- *Target Protein*: Glucose transporters (GLUT1 especially).
- *Example Inhibitor*: *WZB117*.

Mode of Action

- WZB117 binds to and inhibits GLUT1, decreasing glucose uptake by cancer cells.
- This is responsible for glucose starvation, reduced ATP levels, impaired biosynthesis, and eventually apoptosis of cancer cells.

Significance of Targeting Glycolysis in Cancer

- Cancer cells rely more on glycolysis compared to normal cells, making them selectively vulnerable.
- Glycolytic inhibition decreases tumor growth, angiogenesis, and metastasis.
- May sensitize cancer cells or tumor cells to radiotherapy and chemotherapy.

Challenges and Limitations

- Some normal cells (e.g., immune cells, brain cells) also depend on glycolysis, which can cause off-target toxicity.
- Tumor heterogeneity: Not all cancer types rely equally on glycolysis.
- Adaptive resistance mechanisms: Cancer cells may switch to oxidative phosphorylation or alternative metabolic pathways.

In summary, cancer cells have a unique way of producing energy, where they rely heavily on glycolysis to break down glucose into energy, even when oxygen is available. This abnormal process, known as the Warburg effect, makes cancer cells especially dependent on glycolysis, which provides a potential target for treatment [13–17].

9.6 Glutaminolysis in Cancer Cells

Glutaminolysis is a major metabolic biochemical process in which the breakdown of glutamine occurs to give energy for the growth and development of cells. In the case of cancer, glutamine is essentially required for rapid growth and survival, for which it is important for research in cancer biology. The biochemical reaction starts with the uptake of the amino acid by the cells from the outside environment. In the first step, by using the enzyme glutaminase (GLS), glutamate is produced from glutamine. In the next step, α-ketoglutarate (α-KG) is formed, which is one of the major intermediate products of the Krebs cycle. It is one of the major sources of energy for the formation of ATP. Apart from this, it is very essential for the synthesis of nucleotides, amino acids, and fatty acids. These are also intermediate for the survival of cancer cells, which requires a maximum amount of energy for their abnormal cell division. In normal cells, glutamine plays the role of a non-essential amino acid primarily used in nitrogen transport, protein synthesis, and regulating cellular redox balance, but in the case of cancer cells, it takes a much more essential role by stimulating high-energy requirements and cell proliferation [18].

Impact of Glutaminolysis in Cancer Cells

Altered metabolism is often exhibited by the cancerous cells, which acts as a metabolic reprogramming. However, glutamine addiction can be defined as the process in which cancer cells depend on glutamine not only for energy requirements but also for building blocks. Specific transporters are used to take up glutamine, which is directly involved in the tricarboxylic acid (TCA) cycle (Krebs cycle).

Relationship of Glutaminolysis with Cancer Cells

Glutaminolysis plays various important roles in promoting cancer progression:

1. *Energy Formation*: By utilizing α-KG in the TCA cycle, it allows cancer cells to synthesize ATP molecules in the absence of glucose molecules, even under nutrient-limited conditions.
2. *Biosynthesis of Biomolecules*: Various intermediates from the TCA cycle help in the synthesis of nucleotides such as DNA and RNA, other fat molecules, which are associated with the formation of cell membranes, and the production of proteins, which are essential for the rapid division of cells.
3. *Redox Balance and Survival*: Glutaminolysis helps in the formation of NADPH and *glutathione (GSH)*, which are essential for the cancer cells to regulate oxidative stress and manage redox homeostasis. This decreases cell damage and enhances survival under stressful tumor microenvironment conditions [19–21].

Targeting Glutaminolysis in Cancer Therapy

Inhibiting the major enzymes of glutaminolysis is a promising therapeutic strategy for cancer treatment. Glutaminase is one of the major enzymes involved, which is responsible for converting glutamine into glutamate.

Major Examples Are

- *CB-839 (Telaglenastat)*: The properties of GLS were inhibited by using this drug. It is used to block the synthesis of glutamate and subsequent α-KG production. It is essential to reduce the growth of cancer cells.
- *Biochemical Reaction*
- Glutamine → (GLS) → Glutamate → α-Ketoglutarate (α-KG) → Enters TCA cycle → ATP & biomolecules produced.
- *Mode of Action of GLS Inhibitors (e.g., CB-839)*:
- GLS inhibitors inhibit the enzymatic activity of glutaminase, inhibiting glutamine from being converted into glutamate.

  As a result:

- The supply of α-KG to the TCA cycle is decreased.

- ATP production is reduced, decreasing the energy-dependent processes in cancer cells.
- Biosynthesis of nucleotides, amino acids, and lipids is reduced.

Disruption of Redox Homeostasis

- *Action of Inhibitors*:

By inhibiting glutaminolysis, molecules decrease the synthesis of NADPH and GSH. This is responsible for the accumulation of Reactive oxygen Species in cancer cells. Increased ROS causes damage to DNA, proteins, and lipids, triggering apoptosis or senescence.

Inhibition of Biosynthetic Precursor Supply
Cancer cells need major biosynthesis of nucleotides such as DNA and RNA, lipids, and other amino acids.

Effect of Inhibitors
Blocking glutaminase leads to a reduction of α-KG and other intermediates. Due to a lack of nutrients, cancer cells cannot sustain rapid proliferation and are forced into metabolic arrest or death.

9.7 Decrease of Autophagy and Apoptosis

When cancer cells are deprived of energy and essential metabolites due to glutaminolysis inhibition, they activate stress-response mechanisms.

- *Autophagy*:
- Initially, cells start to survive by breaking down their own organelles to recycle various nutrients.
- However, prolonged glutaminolysis inhibition overwhelms this process, causing cell death.
- *Apoptosis*:
- Lack of energy and accumulated ROS activate pro-apoptotic signaling pathways (e.g., activation of caspases), leading to programmed cancer cell death.

Impact on Cancer Cell Adaptation
Some cancer cells may try to compensate for decreased glutaminolysis by regulating other metabolic pathways, such as glycolysis or fatty acid oxidation, but

combining glutaminolysis inhibitors with other metabolic inhibitors (dual-targeting strategies) can prevent this adaptation and enhance treatment efficacy.

Glutaminolysis inhibitors majorly work by inhibiting the glutaminase, cutting off the supply of critical biomolecules required for energy production, biosynthesis, and redox balance in cancer cells. This results in metabolic stress, which leads to impaired proliferation, oxidative damage, and ultimately cancer cell death. These inhibitors are responsible for a targeted approach to cancer therapy, especially for tumors heavily dependent on glutamine metabolism, although overcoming resistance and minimizing toxicity remain important research challenges [22, 23].

Cancer cells somehow exhibit abnormal metabolism, depending heavily on glutaminolysis to meet their high-energy demands and to provide building blocks needed for rapid growth and division. Because of this dependency nature, targeting the glutaminolysis pathway has emerged as a promising therapeutic approach in cancer treatment.

9.8 Mitochondria Pathway Inhibitors

Mitochondrial pathways play a significant role in cancer by synthesizing energy, inducing cell death, and metabolic reprogramming. In cancer cells, mitochondria are utilized to support rapid proliferation and survival under various stress conditions. Instead of depending solely on oxidative phosphorylation, various cancer cells show enhanced glycolysis and modified tricarboxylic acid (TCA) cycle properties, known as the Warburg effect, even in the presence of oxygen. Moreover, mitochondrial dysfunction relates to apoptosis by regulating the intrinsic apoptosis metabolism, producing proteins like Bcl-2 and cytochrome c. Mitochondria synthesize reactive oxygen species (ROS), which can enhance DNA mutations and form oncogenic signaling pathways. Additionally, changed mitochondrial metabolism enhances biosynthesis of various nucleotides, lipids, and amino acids required for cancer cell growth, making these pathways key targets for cancer treatment.

Mitochondrial pathways are key to cancer formation and progression, as they are associated with both energy metabolism and cell survival. In normal cells, mitochondria create energy mainly through oxidative phosphorylation (OXPHOS), where nutrients like glucose and fatty acids are metabolized in the tricarboxylic acid (TCA) cycle, forming ATP. However, in various cancer cells, this pathway is altered to support rapid growth and proliferation. Instead of primarily using OXPHOS, cancer cells depend on aerobic glycolysis, helping them to synthesize metabolic intermediates needed for nucleotide, amino acid, and lipid formation. Mitochondrial dysfunction in cancer also helps in reducing apoptosis and increasing reactive oxygen species (ROS) generation, which helps further DNA mutations and oncogenic signaling pathways [24–26].

Major enzymes in mitochondrial pathways play a significant role in cancer cell survival and proliferation. One major enzyme is isocitrate dehydrogenase (IDH), particularly its mutated forms (IDH1 and IDH2), which are commonly found in certain cancers like gliomas and acute myeloid leukemia (AML). Normally, IDH is used to convert isocitrate to α-ketoglutarate (α-KG) in the TCA cycle, forming NADPH in the process. Apart from this, when altered, IDH shows a neomorphic property that converts α-KG into 2-hydroxyglutarate (2-HG), an oncometabolite. Formation of 2-HG interferes with DNA and histone demethylation processes, which are responsible for epigenetic alterations that promote tumorigenesis by inhibiting cell differentiation and promoting proliferation.

Another major mitochondrial enzyme used in cancer is pyruvate dehydrogenase kinase (PDK), which modifies the properties of the pyruvate dehydrogenase complex (PDC). In cancer cells, PDK is majorly upregulated, showing in the inhibition of PDC and opposing pyruvate from initiating the TCA cycle as acetyl-CoA. This action is related to various cellular metabolism toward glycolysis even in the presence of oxygen, thus supporting the Warburg effect. This metabolic reprogramming enhances cancer cells to rapidly produce ATP and biosynthetic precursors while decreasing ROS generation from mitochondrial respiration, which could enhance apoptosis. Targeting PDK with various inhibitors like dichloroacetate (DCA) reactivates PDC, helping cancer cells back into oxidative metabolism and enhancing ROS production, indirectly promoting cancer cell death and decreasing the growth of the tumor [27–29].

Cancer therapy targeting mitochondrial enzymes has emerged as a promising strategy to destroy the modified metabolism of cancer cells and enhance cell death. Since many cancer cells depend on metabolic reprogramming and mitochondrial dysfunction for rapid proliferation, inhibiting key mitochondrial enzymes relates to these survival mechanisms. For example, inhibitors of mutant isocitrate dehydrogenase (IDH1/IDH2), such as ivosidenib and enasidenib, stop the production of the oncometabolite 2-hydroxyglutarate (2-HG), restoring the normal epigenetic regulation and enhancing cancer cell differentiation and apoptosis. Somehow, inhibitors of pyruvate dehydrogenase kinase (PDK), like dichloroacetate (DCA), are utilized to shift metabolism back toward oxidative phosphorylation, enhancing reactive oxygen species (ROS) levels and increasing apoptosis in cancer cells. These targeted treatments help to reduce tumor growth and overcome the limitations of conventional treatments.

Moreover, mitochondrial-targeted anticancer therapies rely on degrading mitochondrial membrane potential and are related to the apoptotic signaling pathways. Drugs such as *mitocans* (e.g., elesclomol and alpha-tocopheryl succinate) particularly reduce mitochondrial oxidative stress or reduce major enzymes used in mitochondrial energy metabolism, responsible for mitochondrial dysfunction and enhancing cancer cell death [30–32].

Inhibition of enzymes like glutaminase (GLS) is another major method, as various cancer cells rely particularly on glutaminolysis for their growth, development, and energy. GLS inhibitors, such as CB-839, stop the conversion of glutamine to glutamate, reducing cancer cells' essential metabolites. These major therapeutic strategies are recently being used in clinical trials, creating new hope for more efficacious and selective cancer therapy by specifically inhibiting the unique mitochondrial vulnerabilities of cancer cells [33].

9.9 Pentose Phosphate Pathway

The Pentose Phosphate Pathway (PPP) plays an important role in cancer metabolism by forming biomolecules that are required for cancer cells for growth and survival. Compared to glycolysis, which primarily synthesizes ATP, the PPP helps two important functions: synthesizing ribose-5-phosphate for nucleotide and nucleic acid formation, and creating NADPH, an oxidant required for various metabolic reactions and antioxidant defense. Cancer cells often show an enhanced influx through the PPP to meet the high demands for nucleotides and reducing equivalents, helping rapid cell proliferation and protecting against oxidative stress. This metabolic reprogramming helps cancer cells create their abnormal growth while managing increased levels of reactive oxygen species (ROS) [34, 35].

One of the major biocatalysts in the PPP used in cancer progression is glucose-6-phosphate dehydrogenase (G6PD). G6PD catalyzes the first and rate-decreasing step of the PPP, forming glucose-6-phosphate into 6-phosphoglucono-δ-lactone while forming NADPH. In various cancers, G6PD is increased, leading to increased NADPH formation, which creates lipid synthesis, detoxifies ROS, and maintains redox homeostasis. Increased NADPH levels are particularly important in inhibiting oxidative damage and enabling cancer cells to survive under hypoxic or nutrient-deprived conditions. For this reason, G6PD and other PPP enzymes have become attractive therapeutic targets in cancer therapy.

Focusing on the PPP in cancer therapy relates to disturbing the balance between biosynthesis and redox regulation in cancer cells. Inhibitors of G6PD, such as dehydroepiandrosterone (DHEA) and 6-aminonicotinamide, have been observed for their potential to decrease NADPH formation, thereby enhancing oxidative stress and limiting nucleotide synthesis. This aims to impair DNA replication and repair, which can sensitize cancer cells to chemotherapy or radiation therapy. Apart from this, inhibition of downstream enzymes like transketolase (TK) further disrupts the PPP, limiting the formation of ribose sugars necessary for nucleic acid synthesis. Overall, targeting the PPP offers a dual benefit: starving cancer cells of severe biosynthetic precursors while inhibiting their antioxidant defenses, making it a promising strategy for anti-cancer treatments.

The Pentose Phosphate Pathway (PPP) has gained remarkable attention as a therapeutic target in cancer treatment due to its critical role in supporting tumor growth and survival. Cancer cells depend heavily on the PPP to form ribose-5-phosphate for nucleotide formation and NADPH for maintaining redox balance and biosynthetic processes. Targeting major enzymes of the PPP disrupts these essential functions, leading to impaired cancer cell proliferation and enhanced susceptibility to oxidative damage. One of the key enzymes in this pathway is glucose-6-phosphate dehydrogenase (G6PD), which manages the first and rate-limiting step of the PPP. Inhibiting G6PD reduces NADPH production, making cancer cells vulnerable to oxidative stress, and degrades nucleotide biosynthesis, thereby inhibiting DNA replication and repair, which is critical for rapidly dividing cancer cells.

Several biocatalyst inhibitors are currently being explored for their anti-cancer potential by inhibiting the PPP. For example, 6-aminonicotinamide (6-AN) acts as a competitive inhibitor of G6PD and decreases NADPH levels, enhancing ROS accumulation and reducing apoptosis in cancer cells. In addition, inhibitors of transketolase (TK), such as oxythiamine, block the non-oxidative branch of the PPP, inhibiting the synthesis of ribose-5-phosphate and thus limiting nucleotide supply required for DNA and RNA synthesis. By inhibiting both oxidative and non-oxidative arms of the PPP, these inhibitors can effectively starve cancer cells of biosynthetic building blocks and disrupt their redox homeostasis. Combining PPP enzyme inhibitors with conventional chemotherapy or radiation therapy has shown increased anti-cancer effects in preclinical studies, highlighting the potential of this strategy as part of a combined cancer treatment approach [36–39].

9.10 Fatty Acid Synthesis Inhibitors

Fatty acid synthesis (FAS) plays a critical role in cancer cell survival and proliferation. Unlike normal cells that mainly obtain fatty acids from dietary sources, many cancer cells upregulate de novo fatty acid synthesis to meet the enhanced demand for membrane production, energy storage, and signaling molecules. This metabolic reprogramming is important for rapidly dividing cancer cells. Key enzymes used in the FAS pathway, such as Acetyl-CoA carboxylase (ACC) and Fatty Acid Synthase (FASN), are often overexpressed in different cancers, making them attractive targets for therapeutic intervention.

Fatty acid synthesis inhibitors have emerged as promising agents in cancer therapy by decreasing the metabolic processes that tumors depend on. Inhibitors targeting FASN, such as Orlistat, TVB-2640, and C75, act by reducing critical steps in the fatty acid synthesis pathway. By inhibiting FASN, these agents deprive cancer cells of important lipids required for membrane synthesis, energy formation, and oncogenic signaling, leading to cell cycle arrest and apoptosis. Preclinical studies have demonstrated that FAS inhibitors decrease tumor growth in breast, prostate, and ovarian cancer models, enhancing their potential as anti-cancer agents [40].

The therapeutic utilization of fatty acid synthesis inhibitors is often combined with other treatment modalities to increase efficacy and overcome resistance mechanisms. For example, combining FASN inhibitors with chemotherapy or targeted agents can reduce cancer cells to treatment by exploiting their metabolic vulnerabilities. Additionally, ongoing clinical trials are evaluating the safety and effectiveness of FAS inhibitors in various cancer types, aiming to establish their role in personalized cancer treatment. However, challenges remain, such as potential toxicity and the development of compensatory metabolic pathways, which need careful dosing and combination strategies. Overall, targeting fatty acid synthesis offers a promising avenue for disrupting cancer metabolism and enhancing treatment outcomes [41–45].

9.11 Pros and Cons

Targeting metabolism in cancer treatment using metabolic inhibitors offers a promising strategy due to the unique metabolic dependencies of cancer cells, such as enhanced glycolysis, glutaminolysis, and fatty acid synthesis. The primary advantage is the ability to selectively disrupt the energy formation and biosynthetic processes that cancer cells depend on for rapid growth and survival, potentially leading to reduced tumor progression and overcoming drug resistance. Moreover, metabolic inhibitors can be combined with conventional therapies to enhance treatment efficacy. However, there are significant challenges and drawbacks. Many metabolic pathways targeted by inhibitors are also essential in normal cells, leading to potential toxicity and adverse side effects. Cancer cells can also adapt by activating alternative metabolic pathways, decreasing the long-term effectiveness of these inhibitors. Apart from this, the metabolic heterogeneity among different tumor types and patients complicates the identification of universal metabolic targets, requiring personalized approaches for maximum benefit [46].

9.12 Future Prospective

The future of inhibiting metabolism in cancer therapy creates great promise, as current research focuses on uncovering the difficult metabolic rewiring of cancer cells. Advances in technologies such as metabolomics, single-cell analysis, and CRISPR-based screening are creating a deeper understanding of tumor-specific metabolic vulnerabilities. This knowledge utilizes the way for the formation of highly selective metabolic inhibitors with enhanced safety profiles and efficacy. Future approaches are likely to focus on precision medicine, where metabolic inhibitors are tailored based on the particular metabolic phenotype of a patient's tumor, enhancing treatment response and reducing side effects. Apart from this, combination treatments that pair metabolic inhibitors with immunotherapy, targeted agents, or chemotherapy are being used to overcome adaptive resistance and increase therapeutic outcomes. The combination of artificial intelligence and machine learning to analyze metabolic data will further increase the discovery of novel targets and predictive biomarkers, making metabolism-based cancer therapy an increasingly viable and personalized strategy.

9.13 Conclusion

In conclusion, earmarking metabolism in cancer therapy shows an influential and innovative approach that represents the unique metabolic dependencies of cancer cells. By targeting major metabolic pathways such as glycolysis, glutaminolysis, and fatty acid synthesis, these therapies focus on disrupting the energy supply and biosynthesis essential for tumor growth and survival. While metabolic inhibitors represent significant potential, challenges such as toxicity, tumor heterogeneity, and adaptive resistance remain major problems. However, with modern science and technology advancements in molecular profiling, biomarker discovery, and personalized medicine, metabolism-targeted therapies are focused on becoming an integral part of future cancer treatment strategies. Their combination with conventional therapies and immunotherapies shows a promising method to improve therapeutic potential and patient outcomes in the fight against cancer and tumors.

References

1. Wang J, Shay C, Saba NF, et al. Cancer metabolism and carcinogenesis. Exp Hematol Oncol. 2024;13:10.
2. Urbano AM. Otto Warburg: the journey towards the seminal discovery of tumor cell bioenergetic reprogramming. Biochim Biophys Acta Mol Basis Dis. 2021;1867(1):165965.
3. Kocianova E, Piatrikova V, Golias T. Revisiting the Warburg effect with focus on lactate. Cancers (Basel). 2022;14(24):6028.
4. DePeaux K, Delgoffe GM. Metabolic barriers to cancer immunotherapy. Nat Rev Immunol. 2021;21(12):785–97.
5. Tennant D, Durán R, Gottlieb E. Targeting metabolic transformation for cancer therapy. Nat Rev Cancer. 2010;10:267–77.
6. Ahn CS, Metallo CM. Mitochondria as biosynthetic factories for cancer proliferation. Cancer Metab. 2015;3:1.
7. Pietrocola F, Galluzzi L, Bravo-San Pedro JM, Madeo F, Kroemer G. Acetyl coenzyme A: a central metabolite and second messenger. Cell Metab. 2015;21:805–21.
8. Cortes-Cros M, et al. M2 isoform of pyruvate kinase is dispensable for tumor maintenance and growth. Proc Natl Acad Sci USA. 2013;110:489–94.
9. Kim SY. Cancer energy metabolism: shutting power off cancer factory. Biomol Ther. 2018;26(1):39–44.
10. Yu X, White LT, Alpert NM, Lewandowski ED. Subcellular metabolite transport and carbon isotope kinetics in the intramyocardial glutamate pool. Biochemistry. 1996;35(21):6963–8.
11. Hertz L, Chen Y. Integration between glycolysis and glutamate-glutamine cycle flux may explain preferential glycolytic increase during brain activation, requiring glutamate. Front Integr Neurosci. 2017;11:18.
12. Bak LK, Schousboe A, Sonnewald U, Waagepetersen HS. Glucose is necessary to maintain neurotransmitter homeostasis during synaptic activity in cultured glutamatergic neurons. J Cereb Blood Flow Metab. 2006;26:1285–97.
13. Frahm J, Krüger G, Merboldt KD, Kleinschmidt A. Dynamic uncoupling and recoupling of perfusion and oxidative metabolism during focal brain activation in man. Magn Reson Med. 1996;35:143–8.
14. Ikemoto A, Bole DG, Ueda T. Glycolysis and glutamate accumulation into synaptic vesicles: role of glyceraldehyde phosphate dehydrogenase and 3-phosphoglycerate kinase. J Biol Chem. 2003;278:5929–40.
15. Yaku K, Okabe K, Hikosaka K, Nakagawa T. NAD metabolism in cancer therapeutics. Front Oncol. 2018;8:622.
16. Tufail M, Jiang CH, Li N. Altered metabolism in cancer: insights into energy pathways and therapeutic targets. Mol Cancer. 2024;23:203.
17. Hammoudi N, Ahmed KB, Garcia-Prieto C, Huang P. Metabolic alterations in cancer cells and therapeutic implications. Chin J Cancer. 2011;30(8):508–15.
18. Chelakkot C, Chelakkot VS, Shin Y, Song K. Modulating glycolysis to improve cancer therapy. Int J Mol Sci. 2023;24(3):2606.
19. Zheng S, Li H, Li Y, Chen X, Shen J, Chen M, et al. The emerging role of glycolysis and immune evasion in gastric cancer. Cancer Cell Int. 2023;23:317.

20. DeBerardinis RJ, Lum JJ, Hatzivassiliou G, Thompson CB. The biology of cancer: metabolic reprogramming fuels cell growth and proliferation. Cell Metab. 2008;7:11–20.
21. Liberti MV, Locasale JW. The Warburg effect: how does it benefit cancer cells? Trends Biochem Sci. 2016;41:211–8.
22. Roth KG, Mambetsariev I, Kulkarni P, Salgia R. The mitochondrion as an emerging therapeutic target in cancer. Trends Mol Med. 2020;26(1):119–34.
23. Onodera Y, et al. Arf6-driven cell invasion is intrinsically linked to TRAK1-mediated mitochondrial anterograde trafficking to avoid oxidative catastrophe. Nat Commun. 2018;9:2682.
24. Risi B, Imarisio A, Cuconato G, Padovani A, Valente EM, Filosto M. Mitochondrial DNA (mtDNA) as fluid biomarker in neurodegenerative disorders: a systematic review. Eur J Neurol. 2025;32(1):e70014.
25. Shi S, Liang W, Qie Y, Wu R, Zhu Y. Investigation of mitochondrial DNA methylation-related prognostic biomarkers in hepatocellular carcinoma using the Cancer Genome Atlas (TCGA) database. Transl Cancer Res. 2025;14(3):2095.
26. Lin HY, Chu PY. Mitochondrial calcium uniporter as biomarker and therapeutic target for breast cancer: prognostication, immune microenvironment, epigenetic regulation and precision medicine. J Adv Res. 2025;70:445–61.
27. Hekmatshoar Y. Identification of mitochondrial-related genes as potential biomarkers for docetaxel-resistant prostate cancer. Ankara Üniv Tıp FakMecm. 2025;79(2):137–43.
28. Liu W, Tong B, Xiong J, Zhu Y, Lu H, Xu H, et al. Identification of macrophage polarisation and mitochondria-related biomarkers in diabetic retinopathy. J Transl Med. 2025;23:23.
29. Zhou T, Li H, Zhang Q, Cheng S, Zhang Q, Yao Y, et al. Integrating bioinformatics and experimental validation to identify mitochondrial permeability transition-driven necrosis-related lncRNAs that can serve as prognostic biomarkers and therapeutic targets in endometrial carcinoma. Reprod Sci. 2025;32(3):876–94.
30. Marsh NM, MacEwen MJ, Chea J, Kenerson HL, Kwong AA, Locke TM, et al. Mitochondrial calcium signaling regulates branched-chain amino acid catabolism in fibrolamellar carcinoma. Sci Adv. 2025;11(22):eadu9512.
31. Qiao J, Yu Z, Zhou H, Wang W, Wu H, Ye J. The pentose phosphate pathway: from mechanisms to implications for gastrointestinal cancers. Int J Mol Sci. 2025;26(2):610.
32. Zhou Y, Zhang C, He L, Kang Y, Wang D, Wang S, et al. Glucose-1-phosphate promotes compartmentalization of glycogen with the pentose phosphate pathway in CD8+ memory T cells. Mol Cell. 2025;85:2535.
33. Jin X, Lv Y, Bie F, Duan J, Ma C, Dai M, et al. METTL3 confers oxaliplatin resistance through the activation of G6PD-enhanced pentose phosphate pathway in hepatocellular carcinoma. Cell Death Differ. 2025;32(3):466–79.
34. Loopmans S, Rohlenova K, van Brussel T, Stockmans I, Moermans K, Peredo N, et al. The pentose phosphate pathway controls oxidative protein folding and prevents ferroptosis in chondrocytes. Nat Metab. 2025;7(1):182–95.
35. Jiang X, Wang T, Zhao B, Sun H, Dong Y, Ma Y, et al. KRASG12D-driven pentose phosphate pathway remodeling imparts a targetable vulnerability synergizing with MRTX1133 for durable remissions in PDAC. Cell Rep Med. 2025;6(2):101966.
36. Sánchez-Bayuela T, Peral-Rodrigo M, Parra-Izquierdo I, López J, Gómez C, Montero O, et al. Inflammation via JAK-STAT/HIF-1α drives metabolic changes in pentose phosphate pathway and glycolysis that support aortic valve cell calcification. ArteriosclerThrombVasc Biol. 2025;45(7):e232–9.
37. Peng Y, Xu C, Wen J, Zhang Y, Wang M, Liu X, et al. Fatty acid metabolism-related lncRNAs are potential biomarkers for predicting the overall survival of patients with colorectal cancer. Front Oncol. 2021;11:704038.
38. Yang S, Sun B, Li W, Yang H, Li N, Zhang X. Fatty acid metabolism is related to the immune microenvironment changes of gastric cancer and RGS2 is a new tumor biomarker. Front Immunol. 2022;13:1065927.

39. Tan B, Zhang Y, Zhang T, He J, Luo X, Bian X, et al. Identifying potential serum biomarkers of breast cancer through targeted free fatty acid profiles screening based on a GC–MS platform. Biomed Chromatogr. 2020;34(10):e4922.
40. Shen B, Zhang Y, Tie Y. Fatty acid metabolism influences the immune microenvironment in papillary thyroid cancer and identifies SCD as a novel biomarker. Front Endocrinol. 2025;16:1534393.
41. Li Y, Kong X, Zhang G, Jin H, Li XL, Jin T, et al. Non-targeted and chiral amino acid metabolomics of colon cancer: revealing novel chiral biomarkers and metabolic pathways. J Pharm Anal. 2025;16:101429.
42. Yuan F, Jia G, Wen W, Xu S, Gunchick V, Deng K, et al. Blood metabolic biomarkers and colorectal cancer risk: results from large prospective cohort and Mendelian randomisation analyses. Br J Cancer. 2025;133(1):94–10.
43. Monzon JG, Dancey J. Combination agents versus multi-targeted agents: pros and cons. Curr Oncol 2012;19(2):e51–e54.
44. Vander Heiden MG. Targeting cancer metabolism: a therapeutic window opens. Nat Rev Drug Discov. 2011;10(9):671–84.
45. Dang CV, Hamaker M, Sun P, Le A, Gao P. Therapeutic targeting of cancer cell metabolism. J Mol Med. 2011;89(3):205–12.
46. Giordano S, Petrelli A. From single-to multi-target drugs in cancer therapy: when aspecificity becomes an advantage. Curr Med Chem. 2008;15(5):422–32.

Biomarkers of Cancer Metabolism and Therapeutic Response

10

Hamid Tanzadehpanah, Ali Ahmadizad Firouzjaei, Nafiseh Izadi, Mona Mansourian, Amir Hossein Esfandiari, Khatere Mokhtari, Fatemeh Forouzanfar, Hamed Afkhami, Mahdieh Ameri Shah Reza, Mohsen Sheykhhasan, and Hanie Mahaki

10.1 Introduction

Early clinical presentations of cancer are occult, and patients are diagnosed with advanced- or intermediate-stage disease, thereby missing treatment opportunities. The solution to improve the survival of cancer patients is, therefore, early diagnosis and detection of high-risk groups. Biomarkers are molecules that can be used as indicators to identify the status of diseases, including cancer. Metabolic biomarkers

H. Tanzadehpanah · N. Izadi · A. H. Esfandiari
Antimicrobial Resistance Research Center, Basic Science Research Institute, Mashhad University of Medical Sciences, Mashhad, Iran

A. A. Firouzjaei
Bioinformatics Research Center, Basic Sciences Research Institute, Mashhad University of Medical Sciences, Mashhad, Iran

M. Mansourian
Metabolic Syndrome Research Center, Mashhad University of Medical Sciences, Mashhad, Iran

K. Mokhtari
Department of Cell and Molecular Biology and Microbiology, Faculty of Biological Science and Technology, University of Isfahan, Isfahan, Iran

F. Forouzanfar
Neuroscience Research Center, Mashhad University of Medical Sciences, Mashhad, Iran

H. Afkhami · M. A. S. Reza · M. Sheykhhasan (✉)
Cellular and Molecular Research Center, Qom University of Medical Sciences, Qom, Iran
e-mail: msheykhhasan@muq.ac.ir

H. Mahaki (✉)
Vascular and Endovascular Surgery Research Center, Mashhad University of Medical Sciences, Mashhad, Iran

S. Ashique et al. (eds.), *Cancer Metabolism*, Cancer Treatment and Research 195, https://doi.org/10.1007/978-3-032-21861-2_10

are a group of biomarkers that specifically indicate metabolic changes in cells and can be useful in the diagnosis, prognosis, and treatment of cancer (Fig. 10.1) [1].

These molecules tend to change earlier than genes and proteins do, which can reflect fluctuations in the body's status more timely and effectively. The metabolic flux of cancer cells must first be altered to gain a competitive advantage in the tumor microenvironment (TME) and meet their biosynthetic and energy needs. On the other hand, the abnormal accumulation of metabolites in the TME requires metabolic adaptations in cancer cells to protect themselves from damage, so changes in metabolic markers play a major role in cancer cell survival. Therefore, the metabolism of normal cells is different from that of metastatic cells because the latter generate both energy and biomass for rapid proliferation and survival under various stress conditions [2]. Therefore, our knowledge of cancer-induced alterations in metabolites and their metabolic pathways may lead to better and quicker diagnoses of cancer. Doctors must employ these markers as tools to detect and evaluate diseases, particularly cancer, by integrating clinical information with other disciplines. Analytical tools such as chromatography and mass spectrometry enable the identification and quantification of metabolites with precision and the measurement of small changes in the levels of metabolites that can indicate disease. Here, big data

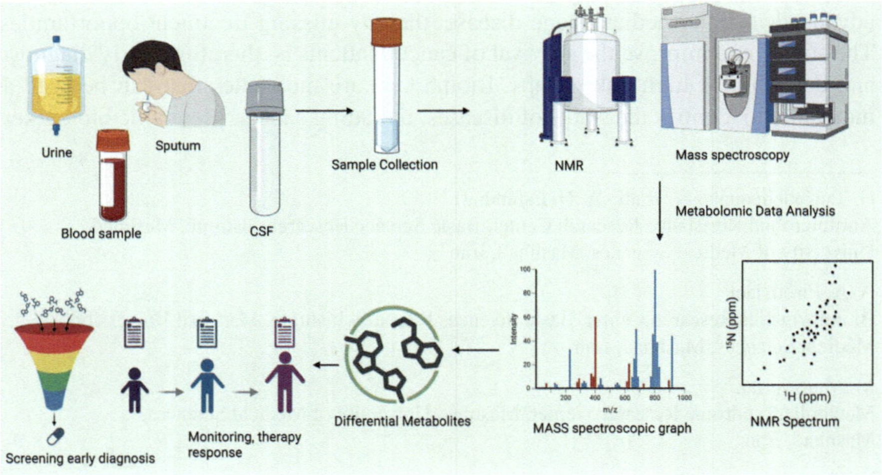

Fig. 10.1 Metabolic biomarker pipeline for identification and use in cancer: The metabolic biomarker pipeline begins with collecting biofluids such as urine, blood, sputum, and CSF, followed by metabolomic analysis using NMR and mass spectrometry. These techniques generate spectral data that are computationally analyzed to identify differential metabolites associated with cancer. The resulting metabolic biomarkers enable early diagnosis, patient stratification, and monitoring of disease progression and therapeutic response in clinical oncology (Concept taken from Wang W et al. [1]). Copyright © 2024 Wang, Zhen, Ping, Wang, and Zhang. This is an open-access article distributed under the terms of the Creative Commons Attribution License (CC BY). The use, distribution, or reproduction in other forums is permitted, provided the original author(s) and the copyright owner(s) are credited and that the original publication in this journal is cited, in accordance with accepted academic practice. No use, distribution, or reproduction is permitted that does not comply with these terms (https://creativecommons.org/licenses/by/4.0/)

Table 10.1 Metabolomic biomarkers for cancer prognosis [4]

Metabolomic Biomarkers of Cancer	Metabolomic Molecules That Change in Cancer
Glucose metabolism	Glucose transporters, including (GLUTs) GLUT1 and GLUT3, pyruvate, lactic acid, myoinositol
Amino acid metabolism	Glutamine and glutamic acid, branched-chain amino acids (BCAAs), amino acids in one-carbon metabolism (serine and glycine), proline, phenylalanine, and tyrosine
Nucleotide metabolism	Inosine, hypoxanthine, and uracil
Lipid metabolism	Palmitic acid, linoleic acid, phosphatidylcholines (PCs) and phosphatidylethanolamines (PEs), sphingomyelins (SMs), ceramides (CERs), glycocholic acid (GCA), estrogens, and estrogen metabolites

collection and processing must be performed, and through statistical means, significant patterns between complex data must be inferred, and associations between metabolites and diseases must be proven. With the help of biomarkers, the patient's response to treatment can be anticipated; hence, doctors can make effective decisions regarding selecting quality treatments. In the long run, with the help of biomarker identification, treatments can be tailored to an individual depending on their metabolic status, which could revolutionize disease diagnosis and treatment as well as enable patients to achieve a good quality of life [3].

In cancer research, this may be the best way to reveal biological phenotypic changes related to function, especially where subtle changes in metabolite concentrations can be monitored. This is why metabolomics is considered one of the fastest-growing research fields in cancer, as are many other aspects of the life sciences. Metabolomic biomarkers for cancer are categorized into distinct groups, including molecules involved in glucose mechanisms, those involved in amino acid metabolism, molecules involved in nucleotide metabolism, and molecules involved in lipid metabolism (Table 10.1). This chapter of the book attempts to explore the factors associated with metabolite biomarkers in more detail.

10.2 Classes of Metabolic Biomarkers

A broad group of molecular markers that define the altered biochemical milieu of cancer cells is termed metabolic biomarkers. They play crucial roles in defining tumor heterogeneity, monitoring the course of the disease, and predicting the outcome of treatment. Three broad categories are amenable to the classification of metabolic biomarkers on the basis of their molecular structure and functional importance: enzymatic proteins, which are representative of cellular activity; metabolite ratios and signatures, which are predictive of pathway flux; and post-translational modifications (PTMs), which dynamically modulate protein function. These categories need to be identified for use in diagnosis, prognosis, and monitoring of therapy [5].

10.2.1 Enzymatic Protein Markers

The quantification of enzymatic protein markers is a mainstay of clinical diagnostics, offering a window into events at the cellular and tissue levels. As catalytically active biomolecules, their presence and quantity in biofluids are valid surrogates for desired states of health. In contrast to structural proteins, increased concentrations of enzymes are frequently directly associated with pathological processes such as necrosis or metabolic dysregulation, as they are released into the circulation after cell injury [6]. These enzymes or enzymatic protein markers are dysregulated and reflect the pathological biochemical pathways of cancer cells. These markers play important roles in the growth, dissemination, and chemoresistance of tumors. Glycolytic enzymes such as pyruvate kinase M2 (PKM2) and hexokinase II (HK2) are often overexpressed in cancer tissues and facilitate increased aerobic glycolysis and glucose consumption [7, 8]. The overexpression of lipid metabolism enzymes such as acetyl-CoA carboxylase (ACC) and fatty acid synthase (FASN) is often associated with increased metastatic potential. They play important roles in the synthesis of membranes and the storage of energy [9, 10]. Glutaminase (GLS) and argininosuccinate synthetase (ASS1) are some of the enzymes responsible for the metabolism of amino acids that facilitate nutritional adjustment and redox homeostasis, particularly in glutamine-addicted tumors [11, 12]. Isocitrate dehydrogenase (IDH1/2) and other mutations of the TCA cycle enzymes yield the oncometabolite 2-hydroxyglutarate, facilitating epigenetic reprogramming and inhibiting cellular differentiation [13]. Methylenetetrahydrofolate dehydrogenase (MTHFD) and other one-carbon-metabolizing enzymes regulate methylation patterns and nucleotide synthesis [14]. In GI cancers, the concentrations of enzymes such as ENO1 greatly increase, which makes them good candidates for early detection markers. In addition to their application in cancer diagnosis and prediction, these enzymatic markers are also therapeutic targets; several inhibitors are being clinically investigated for the disruption of tumor-specific metabolic demand (Table 10.2). Enzymatic biosensors are the technology drivers within this area and take advantage of the well-documented high specificity and catalytic activity of enzymes to convert analyte concentrations to detectable electrochemical or optical signals. This technology is a significant innovation over traditional immunoassays, with a platform that offers ultrarapid, selective, and easy detection, which is essential in modern point-of-care analytical paradigms [15]. The development of enzymatic protein markers as clinical instruments is closely related to continuing technological advances. Future improvements in diagnostic accuracy are more likely to be achieved through the creation of multiplexed assays, which permit the simultaneous measurement of several markers, and by combining biosensor technology with computer science and nanotechnology. However, realization of this potential will depend on surmounting impossible barriers, particularly the absence of standardization across platforms of technology and the imperatives of cost to enable widespread adoption in the clinical environment [16].

Table 10.2 List of the enzymes involved in metabolic pathways and their roles in cancer

Enzyme	Metabolic pathway	Cancer association	Functional role	Refs.
Hexokinase II (HK2)	Glycolysis	Bladder, glioma, breast	Catalyzes glucose phosphorylation; promotes the Warburg effect	[7]
Pyruvate kinase M2 (PKM2)	Glycolysis	Colorectal, glioma, liver	Regulates pyruvate production; supports anabolic growth	[8]
Fatty acid synthase (FASN)	Lipid biosynthesis	Breast, prostate, colorectal	Drives de novo fatty acid synthesis; linked to metastasis	[9]
Acetyl-CoA carboxylase (ACC)	Lipid metabolism	Liver, ovarian, breast	Controls malonyl-CoA production; regulates lipid storage	[10]
Glutaminase (GLS)	Glutamine metabolism	Pancreatic, gastric, ovarian	Converts glutamine to glutamate; supports TCA cycle entry	[11]
Argininosuccinate synthetase (ASS1)	Urea cycle/ arginine metabolism	NSCLC, mesothelioma, sarcoma	Modulates arginine availability; impacts immune response	[12]
Isocitrate dehydrogenase (IDH1/2)	TCA cycle/ epigenetic regulation	Glioma, AML, cholangiocarcinoma	Mutations produce 2-HG; alter DNA/ histone methylation	[13]
MTHFD1/2 (methylenetetrahydrofolate dehydrogenase)	One-carbon metabolism	Breast, colorectal, renal	Regulates folate cycle; supports nucleotide synthesis	[14]

The table provides an overview of major enzymes, associated metabolic pathways, previously reported associations with cancer forms or development, and their biological roles in tumor biology

10.2.2 Metabolite Ratios and Signatures

Contemporary metabolomics has transitioned from the emphasis on quantifying levels of individual metabolites toward the utilization of the diagnostic potential of metabolite ratios and multicomponent metabolic signatures. This transition occurs because relational and multianalyte patterns have been found to provide more stable and physiologically relevant information about physiological states. The pathway-focused approach involves determining ratios between precursors and downstream products within datasets of interest to infer the activity of specific enzymatic pathways. One of the strengths of this method is its inherent capacity to normalize for technical variability in sample processing. In addition, such ratios provide a more direct assessment of metabolic flux—the rate of pathway turnover—than do equilibrium concentration levels per se, which tends to be more dynamic and informative [17]. This strategy is especially valuable for research into complex diseases such as cancer, all of which are characterized by widespread metabolic remodeling. Metabolite ratios such as the lactate/pyruvate ratio, NAD+/NADH ratio, and glutamine/glutamate ratio yield information about pathway dominance (e.g., glycolysis vs. oxidative phosphorylation), redox status, and nutrient dependencies. For example, an increased lactate/pyruvate ratio is an indicator of increased glycolytic flux (Warburg effect), whereas alterations in the NADPH/NADP+ ratio reflect increased antioxidant and biosynthetic demand [18–20]. Together, metabolite ratios and signatures provide a systems-level view of tumor metabolism and are increasingly being integrated into precision oncology pipelines for diagnosis, prognosis, and therapeutic triage. For example, a 2025 pan-cancer study revealed that clustering cell lines by ratios of metabolites (e.g., intermediates of the TCA cycle vs. pyruvate) revealed transparent metabolic subtypes that were not apparent when absolute concentrations were examined [17]. Compared with those with low ratios, cell groups with high TCA cycle ratios presented metabolic features, including increased glutamine cataplerosis and increased susceptibility to drugs related to glutamine metabolism and oxidative phosphorylation. This highlights the way that metabolite ratios may reveal functional metabolic dependencies of immediate therapeutic interest [21]. Similarly, metabolic signatures—multimetabolite panels—have high diagnostic power in that they produce distinctive patterns associated with particular disease states. In the context of neurology studies, a systematic review of drug-resistant epilepsy (DRE) revealed not only individual biomarkers such as glycine and lactate but also repeated derangement of the alanine, aspartate, and glutamate metabolism pathways. This finding suggests that the composite signature across this pathway is a better diagnostic reagent than any one metabolite. Another psychiatric application has utilized metabolomic profiling of dried blood spots to discriminate between major depressive disorder and bipolar disorder by distinctive signature patterns, which provides an avenue for more objective clinical discrimination [22].

10.2.3 Posttranslational Modifications

PTMs are enzymatic alterations to proteins after synthesis, such as phosphorylation, acetylation, ubiquitination, methylation, and O-GlcNAcylation, which are vital in regulating protein function, stability, and localization [23]. PTMs play pivotal roles in cancer metabolism by regulating enzymatic activities and remodulating metabolic pathways to facilitate tumor growth and survival [24]. These alterations can activate or suppress metabolic enzymes, redirect pathway fluxes, and regulate cellular responses to therapy and stress. They can be used as immune evasion, metabolic reprogramming, and drug resistance biomarkers. Their detection by high-technology proteomic approaches allows for dynamic tracking of tumor activity and has potential for targeted interference with PTM-modulating medicines. Aberrant phosphorylation, for example, can drive oncogenic pathways. AMP-activated protein kinase (AMPK) phosphorylation activates energy-stress catabolic processes, whereas the acetylation of glycolytic enzymes can affect their catalytic activity and couple metabolism with epigenetic control [25]. The dbPTM database contains millions of PTM sites and facilitates the mapping of abrogated regulatory networks in cancer. Clinically, proteomics innovations enabled by mass spectrometry allow for large-scale PTM quantitation, which, integrated with other omics data, can identify new drug targets and enable personal treatments by revealing activated oncogenic pathways [19].

10.3 Technologies for Biomarker Discovery

Recent biomarker discovery relies increasingly on sophisticated analytical platforms that provide a systematic, functional interrogation of the mechanisms of disease. This paradigm is driven by advanced methodologies such as metabolomic profiling for signature identification, stable isotope labeling for dynamic pathway mapping, and CRISPR-enabled genomics for deciphering crucial gene function. These advances in molecular phenotyping have enabled the identification of metabolic biomarkers that guide cancer diagnosis, prognosis, and treatment response. Several ancillary technologies are employed to identify these biomarkers, each yielding new insights into metabolic control and functional relevance.

10.3.1 Targeted vs. Untargeted Metabolomics

Metabolomics, the quantitative measurement of small-molecule metabolites, involves two dominant approaches: targeted and untargeted. Untargeted metabolomics is a discovery-oriented approach that broadly profiles all analyzable metabolites, including unknowns, making it possible to identify new biomarkers and determine how a disease works [26]. Its limitations include difficult data analysis, problematic identification of metabolites, and detection bias against more abundant molecules. On the other hand, targeted metabolomics is an analytical strategy designed for the specific quantitation of a preselected set of metabolites. Targeted metabolomics is focused on the quantification of preselected metabolites via high-sensitivity platforms such as LC–MS/MS or NMR. Targeted metabolomics provides precise, reproducible measurements of known metabolic intermediates and is suitable for biomarker candidate validation and monitoring of therapeutic response [20]. Its only drawback is its limited scope. Thus, these approaches are often used together, with untargeted approaches used for discovery and targeted approaches used for validation. Hybridization approaches such as "widely targeted metabolomics" have also been developed to integrate the large scope of untargeted methods with the sensitivity of targeted analysis [27]. Together, these approaches support hypothesis-driven and exploratory biomarker discovery, with untargeted approaches generally guiding targeted assay design.

10.3.2 Stable-Isotope Tracing

Stable-isotope tracing is a versatile tool for metabolic flux mapping in cancer cells. By supplementing nutrients such as glucose, glutamine, or acetate with nonradioactive isotopes (e.g., ^{13}C, ^{15}N, or ^{2}H), researchers can trace their incorporation into downstream metabolites. For example, ^{13}C-glucose tracing discriminates glycolytic versus oxidative metabolism, and ^{13}C-glutamine tracing detects anaplerotic flux into the TCA cycle. Stable-isotope tracing lies at the basis of ascertaining the functional significance of metabolic biomarkers and actionable metabolic vulnerabilities [28]. It rectifies one of the key weaknesses of conventional metabolomics: the inability to quantify pathway activity through the use of isotopically labeled substrates to track nutrient flow through metabolic networks. This provides a dynamic functional readout of metabolic flux, and this is required for quantifying disease-related aspects of metabolic reprogramming, for example, nutrient utilization and biosynthesis. Technologies such as MetTracer have broadened the application of this approach by making global isotope tracing possible. MetTracer employs untargeted mass spectrometry and a targeted data analysis pipeline to precisely quantify isotope incorporation for many metabolites in parallel. When applied to an aging model of Drosophila, this high-coverage approach revealed system-wide dysfunction of metabolic coordination and glucose metabolism rewiring. In addition to mass spectrometry, combining stable-isotope tracing with hyperpolarized MRI provides noninvasive, real-time metabolic imaging in intact organisms, which is one step toward the clinic [29, 30].

10.3.3 CRISPR Screens and Functional Genomics

The long-term goal of functional genomics is to clarify the causal mechanisms underlying the relationships between specific genes and observable phenotypic features. Perturbomics is a core strategy toward this end, where gene function is inferred by systematically monitoring the phenotypes that result from deliberate genetic perturbations. The landscape has been transformed with the arrival of CRISPR–Cas technology, offering a new, unparalleled platform for performing precise, genome-wide screens. These experiments entail the introduction of a library of complex gRNAs into cells to knock out or modify the function of thousands of genes. After exposure to selective pressures, high-throughput gRNA sequencing can identify genes that are required for viability or engaged in particular responses, as revealed through their substantial enrichment or depletion [31]. CRISPR-based genetic screens facilitate the systematic investigation of gene function in cancer cell metabolism. By knocking out or editing genes that participate in metabolism, researchers are able to determine those that are necessary for survival, proliferation, or sensitivity to drugs. The analytical potential and flexibility of CRISPR screens have been further improved by various breakthrough advances. First, the development of CRISPRi and CRISPRa systems has facilitated tunable transcriptional repression or activation, allowing functional studies to be extended to essential genes and noncoding regions. Second, the combination of genetic perturbations with single-cell RNA sequencing (scRNA-seq) creates a multidimensional dataset, recording the transcriptomic effect of every perturbation at single-cell resolution. Third, the utilization of complex disease models, specifically patient-derived organoids, offers a more physiologically relevant screening context, which improves the discovery of therapeutically accessible biomarkers and targets. Together, these new screening paradigms have enabled the discovery of genetic determinants of drug resistance and the discovery of new therapeutic vulnerabilities in cancer [32, 33]. In combination with transcriptomics, proteomics, and metabolomics, CRISPR screens enable the connection of metabolic enzymes and regulators to phenotypic outcomes. Functional genomics also enables biomarker prioritization by revealing context-dependent dependencies, including synthetic lethality or resistance mechanisms. This integrated strategy facilitated the identification of metabolically informative clinical biomarkers and aided in the development of targeted therapies [34, 35].

10.4 Imaging-Based Biomarkers

Imaging-acquired biological markers. These markers can relay helpful information regarding the structure, function, and metabolism of organs and tissues. Some of the common imaging techniques that include imaging-based biomarkers are described below.

10.4.1 PET Tracers

Positron emission tomography (PET) is a noninvasive imaging modality that enables the quantitative visualization of physiological and biochemical processes in vivo [36]. A radioactive tracer, typically labeled with a positron-emitting isotope (such as ^{18}F, ^{11}C, or ^{68}Ga), is injected into the body and is distributed dynamically on the basis of the biological activity of tissues. Once the tracer accumulates in target tissues, the radionuclide undergoes positron emission [37] (Table 10.3). The emitted positron travels a short distance before being annihilated with an electron, resulting in the release of two 511 keV gamma photons in nearly opposite directions (approximately 180° apart). These photons are detected simultaneously (coincidence detection) by the ring of detectors of the PET scanner. With these data, the tomographic images are formulated into three-dimensional pictures of the tracer's distribution, which corresponds to underlying metabolic or molecular activity [2]. Radiotracers, when administered in the body, emit positrons, which, in interaction with other electrons, give off gamma rays. Gamma rays are detected by a PET scanner and lead to maps of metabolism in the body [38]. These maps are able to identify areas of increased metabolism and are employed to quantify tumors, their dimensions, or growth signs.

This technique enables us to predict how tumors metabolize nutrients such as glucose, amino acids, and lipids. Therefore, compared with other imaging

Table 10.3 Classification of Key PET radiotracers and their functional roles in cancer imaging [2, 42]

Metabolic biomarkers	Tracers	Description
Glucose metabolism	[^{18}F] Fluorodeoxyglucose (FDG)	FDG is often upregulated in malignant cells, and the degree of FDG uptake has often been correlated with tumor grade, aggressiveness, and proliferation index.
Amino acid metabolism	[^{11}C]-methionine:	Neoplasms, including high-grade brain gliomas, which have rapid synthesis/proliferation, are associated with high [11C]-methionine uptake.
	[^{18}F]-Fluciclovine	[^{18}F]-Fluciclovine has received FDA approval for imaging in prostate cancer recurrence. It is a synthetic leucine analog taken up by amino acid transporters such as ASCT2 and LAT1, which are frequently upregulated in cancer cells.
	Glutamine-based tracers	Another essential amino acid is glutamine, which sustains cancer cells and their proliferation, including tumors with aberrant glutaminolysis pathways. Some new radiopharmaceuticals.
Hypoxia imaging	[^{18}F]-FMISO (fluoromisonidazole)	[^{18}F]-FMISO, by interacting with macromolecules within the cell, remains in hypoxic regions when oxygen concentrations are low. It has been used to identify hypoxic regions in tumors for radiation therapy, as well as for more challenging cases.
	[^{18}F]-FAZA	A novel hypoxia tracer with enhanced pharmacokinetic properties, leading to higher resolution and more precise measurements of hypoxic regions
Lipid metabolism	Radiolabeled acetate	Lipid metabolism can also be probed using tracers like [^{11}C]-choline and [^{18}F]-fluorocholine, which are taken up by tumors with elevated phospholipid synthesis

techniques that rely on gross anatomical changes, PET scans reflect functional changes or disease progression and can therefore detect tumors earlier and report changes during treatment [39]. Newer developments in PET imaging have gone beyond the conventional applications of this technique. New active molecules are being explored for specific metabolic pathways, which may result in more efficient radiotracers [40]. One of the applications of F-fluorodeoxyglucose (FDG) in cancer diagnosis is related to glucose metabolism. For example, [^{18}F]-FDG is widely used to trace glycolytic metabolism, which is often increased in malignant cells. Its uptake has been correlated with tumor grade, invasiveness, and the proliferation index. Thus, FDG-PET not only aids in diagnosis and staging but also provides semiquantitative insight into the metabolic activity and invasiveness of tumors [41]. One limitation of PET is that it only shows the presence of a radionuclide, not what molecule it is in. A key feature of magnetic resonance spectroscopy (MRS) is chemical shift, where the resonance frequency is a function of the chemical environment; thus, unlike PET, MRS can reveal the molecular origin of the signal [42].

10.4.2 Magnetic Resonance Imaging

Magnetic resonance imaging (MRI) is a noninvasive and safe technique used to analyze soft tissues of the body. MRI plays an important role in the diagnosis of diseases by assessing structural changes. This technique is traditionally used for structural measurements but can also obtain physiological information from other nuclei. MRI probes for cancer metabolism biomarkers are specifically designed to provide more detailed information about the metabolic status of tumors and cancer cells. [1-^{13}C] Pyruvate is widely used as a metabolic tracer in all brain, heart, kidney, liver, and prostate imaging research. Following hyperpolarization, [1-^{13}C] pyruvate is metabolized to [1-^{13}C] lactate and [1-^{13}C] alanine, which can be detected via MRI. This metabolism is a reflection of glycolytic activity and tumor metabolism [43]. Additionally, hyperpolarized (HP) carbon-13 (^{13}C) MRI is a new imaging modality that allows in vivo detection of virtually any HP probe with excellent spatiotemporal resolution. In Kouchkovsky et al. (2024), this technique was used in the diagnosis of cancer of the prostate, and the outcome was that the tumor spread to the right midgland, as identified by HP ^{13}C MRI, which was later confirmed by pathology. Compared with that of adjacent benign prostatic tissue, more LDH-A staining was observed via immunohistochemistry within the tumor [44].

10.4.3 Magnetic Resonance Spectroscopy

MRS measures and identifies metabolites and chemicals within tissues. MRS helps doctors and researchers acquire information about tissue metabolic and biochemical activity [43]. MRS operates on the premise of identifying resonance frequencies of atomic nuclei such as hydrogen-1, carbon-13, and phosphorus-31 when subjected to a strong magnetic field. The resonant frequency is measured and represented in the form of a spectrum reflecting the relative levels of various metabolites within the tissue. The pattern of metabolites observed with MRS may be employed to differentiate among various disease states and to guide the diagnosis and monitoring of treatment. MRS provides functional biochemical data that complement the anatomical data obtained with MRI. Changes in the concentrations of individual metabolites, such as elevated choline or decreased N-acetyl aspartate (NAA), may indicate pathological conditions such as tumors, infection, and demyelination. MRI and the MRS can increase diagnostic accuracy and prognostic value for conditions such as brain tumors through the assessment of structural and metabolic changes [45] (Table 10.4).

The role of MRS in evaluating choline levels in cancer is an important area of research. MRS enables the assessment of metabolite levels within tissues, including those of choline, a component of cell membranes. Elevated choline levels are associated with increased cell proliferation and malignant transformation, making MRS a potential tool for detecting increased choline levels as a biomarker for malignant tumor detection [45]. ^{1}H MRS has been used to detect and grade tumors and monitor their response to treatment, especially for breast, prostate, and brain tumors. In

Table 10.4 Techniques that can be used as tracers in metabolic imaging and to study metabolic processes in cells and tissues

Techniques	Cancers	Description	Refs.
^{1}H magnetic resonance spectroscopy	Gliomas	Mutations in the isocitrate dehydrogenase (IDH) 1 and 2 enzymes are specifically detectable in grade 2 and 3 gliomas through the accumulation of 2-hydroxyglutarate	[47]
	Breast cancer	Decreased citrate and creatine signals and increased tCho signals have been used to detect the presence of cancer. The tCho/creatine signal ratio correlates with tumor grade. In breast cancer, the tCho signal can be used to differentiate between benign and malignant lesions	
13C magnetic resonance spectroscopy	Breast cancer	The detection of ^{13}C labeling increases the sensitivity of the measurement. If tumor metabolism is at steady state, this technique does not provide information about metabolic flux. In the case of lactate metabolism, this technique cannot distinguish between lactate remaining in the inactive metabolic zone and lactate produced from ongoing glycolytic activity	[48]
Hyperpolarized ^{13}C magnetic resonance spectroscopy	Cancers of prostate, breast, brain, and kidney	Metabolic imaging with the introduction of dynamic nuclear polarization (DNP), which can increase the sensitivity of ^{13}C-label detection by more than 10,000-fold. In this method, the electron spins on the radical become completely polarized. One of the first molecules to be polarized was [1-^{13}C] pyruvate. When injected intravenously, there was enough signal to image its location in the body. Clinical studies are now underway in prostate, breast, brain, kidney, and pancreatic cancers. The method can also be used to assess tumor grade and response to early treatment	[42, 49]
^{2}H magnetic resonance spectroscopy	Breast cancer	^{2}H MRSI can image [6,6-$^{2}H_2$] glucose metabolism in the brain (glioblastoma). Oral administration of labeled glucose resulted in the detection of lactate, providing a measure of glycolytic flux, and labeling of glutamate/glutamine (Glx), which provided a surrogate measure of TCA cycle flux. Additionally, in subcutaneous tumor models, rapid imaging after intravenous administration of [6,6-$^{2}H_2$] glucose showed that this flux was significantly reduced after chemotherapy. Deuterium-labeled microarrays can be used to image tumor subtypes, assess grade, and identify response to treatment, similar to those labeled with ^{13}C ^{2}H-fumarate may also be superior in detecting tumor cell death after treatment because it can be administered orally	[50]

the brain, an increase in the total choline signal (tCho) and a decrease in the concentration of N-acetylaspartate (NAA), a neuronal cell marker, is generally considered a diagnostic marker of a brain tumor, whereas an increase in the signal at 1.3 ppm from lipid droplets is associated with a higher grade and poorer survival. The tCho/

NAA signal ratio was shown to distinguish recurrent glioma from necrosis resulting from radiation treatment; however, its ability to discriminate between the two is inferior to that of perfusion imaging [42, 46].

10.5 Liquid Biopsy Approaches

Liquid biopsy is a noninvasive, highly sensitive, and accurate method for tracking cancer and informing treatment decisions [51]. Conventional tissue biopsies are invasive, risky, and do not reflect the dynamic nature of the tumor; thus, liquid biopsies have been developed [52]. Liquid biopsies are used to examine tumor-derived elements, such as cells, DNA, and extracellular vesicles (EVs), in the serum, urine, and cerebrospinal fluid. Liquid biopsies enable real-time tracking of the dynamics of the tumor, such as genetic and metabolic variations, and customized treatment during the progression of the disease [1].

10.5.1 Circulating Metabolites

The study of these small molecules present in circulation within biofluids provides insight into tumor biology, predicts patient prognosis, and directs therapy [1]. Compared with nonneoplastic tissues, tumors exhibit increased aerobic glycolysis and therefore sustained high blood lactate levels (the Warburg effect). Elevated lactate is associated with poor prognosis, enhanced metastatic potential, and immunosuppression [53]. Additionally, glycolytic and TCA cycle metabolites tend to be dysregulated in cancer. Dysregulated amino acid and lipid metabolism, whose metabolites are possible biomarkers for the early detection of cancer and cancer recurrence, is also common in most cancers [54]. It is possible to design treatment more effectively with such analysis and have individualized treatment, ultimately improving patient outcomes. Table 10.5 lists major circulating metabolites observed in different cancers, demonstrating the diversity of pathways involved [1, 54, 55].

10.5.2 Exosomes and Extracellular Vesicles

EVs are small membrane-bound organelles that are released from cells into the extracellular space and have the potential to control the fate of neighboring cells. EVs exist in two important forms: exosomes (50–150 nm in size, which bud from endosomal membranes) and microvesicles (200–800 nm in size, which bud directly from the plasma membrane). They are marked by variability in size, origin, and molecular contents [56]. The vast majority of cell types release exosomes, which are delivered into the extracellular compartment and are found in the blood. Exosomes consist of molecules consisting of lipids, proteins, and RNA, such as microRNAs (miRNAs), that help cells communicate with each other and control biology [56, 57]. Vesicle materials are selectively loaded and reflect the health status

Table 10.5 Circulating metabolites and their metabolic pathway impacts across various cancers

Metabolite class	Specific metabolites	Associated cancers	Reported change	Clinical significance
Carbohydrates	Lactate, pyruvate, glucose, citrate	General solid tumors, colorectal, glioma, breast	↑	Diagnostic, prognostic, reflects Warburg effect
Amino acids	Glutamine, arginine, ornithine, tryptophan	Glioma, pancreatic, colorectal	↓Arginine, ↑Ornithine, Tryptophan	Differentiates tumor grade, immune modulation
Oncometabolites	Succinate, fumarate, 2-hydroxyglutarate	Prostate, colorectal, glioma	↑	Driver of epigenetic changes, diagnostic
Polyamines	N1-acetylspermine, spermidine	Colorectal	↑Acetylated forms in Stage IV	Differentiates metastatic vs. early-stage CRC
Lipids	Phosphatidylcholines (PCs), Sphingomyelins (SMs)	Breast, colorectal, gastric	↑PCs, ↑SMs	High diagnostic accuracy in multimetabolite panels
Other metabolites	Adenosine, hippuric acid, kynurenine	Head and neck, lung, prostate	↑Adenosine, ↑Kynurenine	Immune evasion, prognostic

of the parent cell. EVs can deliver their load to other cells, regulating gene expression and cellular function in healthy and disease states. EVs are involved in organ-to-organ communication, maintaining TME integrity and promoting cancer initiation, drug resistance, and metastasis [57]. Exosomes are potential cancer biomarkers for cancer diagnosis and therapy [58]. Upon analyzing the vesicle contents, we are able to obtain valuable information regarding the metabolic status of tumors. The concentrations of amino acids such as proline and ornithine; fatty acids such as lauric and myristic acids; and oncometabolites such as succinate and fumarate are elevated in EVs derived from tumors [56].

10.5.3 Cell-Free Nucleic Acids

Metabolites and EVs are essential for comprehending the cellular and functional biology of cancer formation, whereas cell-free nucleic acids (cfNAs) constitute an in-the-moment pathway for examining the genomic and transcriptomic structure of tumors. cfNAs include DNA and RNA present within bodily fluids, which are marked by the cellular activity that produces them and reflect the molecular activities occurring in the tumor. Cell-free DNA (cfDNA) consists of 100–200-base fragments of DNA that are released into body fluids as a consequence of cellular processes such as apoptosis, necrosis, or other normal physiological processes (10).

cfDNA is presently an important biomarker in cancer for disease diagnosis and ongoing monitoring. Techniques examining cfDNA, such as mutation profiling, methylation studies, and fragmentomics, provide mixed levels of information on cancer biology and promise much for early detection. Plasma is a particular choice for this use since it is very enriched with cfDNA, allowing for the identification of genomic changes, DNA methylation profiles, and fragmentomic signatures. In the same way, cell-free RNA (cfRNA) includes fragments of RNA shed into biofluids such as blood during apoptosis, necrosis, or excretion. These cfRNA fragments mirror tissue-specific gene expression in tumors and present dynamic insight into gene expression programs, indicating their potential for use in cancer research and clinical applications [59]. Potential biomarkers of cell-free RNA in clinical practice are summarized in Table 10.6.

10.6 Predictive Biomarkers for Targeted and Immunometallic Therapies

Cancer cells reprogram their metabolism to support their growth and accommodate the various tumor microenvironments (TMEs) they encounter during their progression. Metabolites produced by tumors and immune cells can weaken immune responses and promote cancer progression. The TME supports an extensive network of genes, signaling molecules, metabolites, enzymes, and transporters that regulate immune function [60]. Predictive biomarkers are needed to direct targeted and immuno-metabolic therapies by recognizing specific metabolic changes in cancer.

10.6.1 Glycolytic Inhibitors

Glycolytic inhibitors are critical building blocks of immunometabolic therapies, which act on cancer cells by cutting them off from their primary supply of fuel and deranging the immunosuppressive function of the tumor. These inhibitors function by suppressing the key steps of the glycolysis pathway, which augments the metabolism of immune cells fighting tumors and sensitizes cancer cells to other treatments. Among the best-studied inhibitors are 2-deoxy-D-glucose (2-DG), a glucose analog that blocks the enzyme hexokinase (HK). When HK is treated with 2-DG, it accumulates within the cell 2-DG-6-phosphate, which inhibits HK activity and decreases the ATP content of the cell. Other inhibitors affect other parts of the glycolysis process. HK2, for example, is widely overexpressed in cancer cells and is the main target. Lactate dehydrogenase A (LDHA), which facilitates the conversion of pyruvate into lactate, is another important target. Inhibiting LDHA not only inhibits lactate removal but also diminishes the supply of acetyl-CoA for gene regulation via the histone acetylation mechanism. Finally, blocking monocarboxylate transporters (MCTs) will retain lactate inside the cell, lowering the acidic environment of the tumor and providing yet another possible therapeutic avenue [61].

Table 10.6 Candidate biomarkers for clinical practice [59]

Cancer type	Category	Biomarker type	Specimen	Diagnostic/ prognostic value
Lung	miRNAs	miR-23a, miR-96, miR-200 family, miR-181a-5p, miR-574-5p,miR-30a-3p, miR-30e-3p, miR-181-5p, miR-361-5p,miR-10b-5p, miR-15b-5p, and miR-320b	Serum/plasma	Diagnostic/ prognostic
	circRNAs	circSATB2	Serum/plasma	Diagnostic
Breast	miRNAs	miR-1246, miR-155, miR-21-5p, miR-30b/miR-93/miR-23a-3p	Serum/plasma	Diagnostic/ prognostic
Colorectal	miRNAs	miR-15b, miR-16, miR-21, miR-125a-3p, miR-139-3p, miR-23a, miR-126, miR-377-3p, miR-381-3p, miR-940, and miR-1290	Serum/ plasma, stool-derived exosomes	Diagnostic
	circRNAs	circLPAR1, Hsa-circ-0004771	Serum/plasma	Diagnostic/ prognostic
	lncRNAs	CCAT2, LNCV6–38772, LNCV6–84003, LNCV6–98390, LNCV6–98602, LNCV-108266, and LNCV6–116109	Serum/plasma	Prognostic/ treatment-response
Prostate	miRNAs	miR-196a-5p, miR-34a-5p, miR-143-3p, miR-501-3p, miR-92a-1-5p, miR-21, miR-375, miR-125a-5p, miR-141-3p, miR-125a-5p/ miR-141-3p ratio	Serum/ plasma, urine	Diagnostic/ prognostic
	lncRNAs	lncRNA-p21	Urine/ exosome RNA	Diagnostic and monitoring
Kidney	miRNAs	miR-210, miR-1233, miR-92a-1-5p, miR-149-3p, miR-424-3p, miR-30c-5p	Serum/ plasma, urine	Early detection and prognostic information

10.6.2 IDH Mutant Inhibitors

The enzyme isocitrate dehydrogenase (IDH) is an extremely essential enzyme of the TCA cycle, and it is prone to mutation in cancers such as glioma, acute myeloid leukemia (AML), chondrosarcoma, and intrahepatic cholangiocarcinoma. Mutant IDH1 and mutant IDH2 proteins metabolize α-ketoglutarate (α-KG) to 2-hydroxyglutarate (2-HG), and consequently, there are increased levels of 2-HG. This excess 2-HG competes for binding to α-KG-dependent enzymes, interferes with regular cellular differentiation, and potentially has an assisting role with other oncogenes in maintaining carcinogenesis. Mutant IDH is thus a promising potential target for cancer treatment [62].

IDH inhibitors function by decreasing the levels of 2-HG produced from α-KG and reversing the epigenetic effects of the mutation. FDA-certified drugs such as ivosidenib (for IDH1) and enasidenib (for IDH2) specifically bind to the mutant enzyme, changing its structure to reduce its misbehaving activity and reduce 2-HG production [63].

10.6.3 Metabolic Checkpoint Blockade

The use of metabolic checkpoint inhibitors is a new and fascinating method for preventing metabolic activity within the tumor microenvironment to abolish immune suppression and promote antitumor immunity. Some of the major pathways are involved here. One mechanism involves the modulation of the adenosine signaling pathway, where the hypoxia-inducible enzymes CD39 and CD73 convert ATP to form adenosine. This resulting adenosine stimulates A2A and A2B receptors and thus suppresses T-cell and natural killer (NK) cell functions. The other important pathway is tryptophan metabolism, in which enzymes such as indoleamine 2,3-dioxygenase 1 (IDO1) and tryptophan 2,3-dioxygenase (TDO) result in local amino acid deficiencies and support the production of kynurenine, which further increases the level of aryl hydrocarbon receptor (AhR). This mediated activation promotes the differentiation of regulatory T cells (Tregs) and plays a major role in T-cell exhaustion.

Tumor-derived lactate also contributes by inhibiting nuclear factor of activated T cells (NFAT), impairing T-cell and NK-cell function. Finally, tumor cells and myeloid-derived suppressor cells (MDSCs) exploit arginase 1 (Arg1) to deplete arginine, disrupting T-cell receptor (TCR) signaling and further suppressing the immune response [51, 61].

10.7 Integrative Multiomics and Radiomics

10.7.1 Data Fusion Strategies

Integrative multiomics and radiomics strategies seek to harmonize diverse biological and imaging datasets to identify robust biomarkers and predictive signatures related to cancer metabolism and therapeutic response. These approaches can be categorized into at least four key domains: horizontal and vertical integration, radiogenomics, network-based fusion with dimensionality reduction, and feature selection.

Horizontal and Vertical Integration Horizontal integration merges datasets originating from the same omics layer, for example, combining transcriptomic profiles across cohorts or experiments to increase statistical power and reproducibility. Vertical integration fuses information from different omics layers, for example, genomics, proteomics, and metabolomics, enabling the discovery of cross-level interactions, mechanistic links, pathway crosstalk, and multiscale biomarkers that single-layer analyses cannot reveal and improve translational potential in clinical settings [64].

Radiogenomics This approach identifies associations of phenotypic and molecular alterations through the integration of genomic and transcriptome signatures and quantitative imaging features by radiomics. Through the integration of molecular and clinical information and imaging biomarkers, this noninvasive technique can help with individualized treatment planning, biopsy targeting, and the prediction of tumor subtype, prognosis, response to treatment, and geographic heterogeneity [65].

Network-Based Fusion At the systems level, this biomarker prioritization, discovery of mechanisms of relationships, and validation and rapid discovery approach integrate multiomics and radiomics data by applying graph-based models and Bayesian networks. It enables integrated analysis to reveal pathway-level biomarkers, regulatory hubs, and cross-modal interactions [66].

Dimensionality Reduction and Feature Selection involve numerous methods, including principal component analysis (PCA), t-distributed stochastic neighbor embedding (t-SNE), and autoencoder methods. These methods contain concise and informative subsets of features facilitating better downstream modeling tasks, providing rapid and trustworthy interpretations, reducing the noise level, summarizing multimodal data, and emphasizing strong patterns [67].

10.7.2 Machine Learning Algorithms

To better illustrate the complex interactions between radiomics, multiomics features, and clinical endpoints, machine learning should receive prominent focus. These tools can be divided into four broad categories: explainable artificial intelligence (XAI), multimodal deep learning, supervised learning, and unsupervised learning.

Supervised Learning To classify tumor subtypes, make individual and population predictions of drug response, estimate treatment resistance, identify biomarkers, and classify patients by survival risk, supervised learning algorithms use random forests, support vector machines, and deep neural networks. These models are trained on labeled data containing genomic, transcriptomic, imaging, and clinical data. For robustness, repeatability, and clinical relevance, strict cross-validation, selection of features, and interpretation of the model are utilized [68].

Unsupervised Learning approaches enable the discovery of molecular subtypes, reveal hidden structures of multiomics and clinical data, promote biological understanding, serve to inform hypothesis generation, and help downstream analyses. These downstream analyses involve biomarker selection, pathway enrichment, and patient classification for translational research, all of which are aided by unsupervised learning methods using clustering algorithms such as nonnegative matrix factorization and hierarchical clustering [68].

Multimodal Deep Learning Advanced architectures, i.e., transformer-based attention models, multi-input convolutional neural networks, and hybrid encoders, are implemented in the setting of multimodal deep learning to analyze heterogeneous imaging and omics data, enhance predictive power, uncover cross-modal links, and permit model interpretability in the field of translational biomedical research [69].

Explainable AI (XAI) Explainable AI software, e.g., SHAP and LIME, which balances input features, identifies notable biomarkers and bias, provides clinically interpretable explanations, automates biomarker validation workflows, builds confidence, accelerates regulatory approval, and accelerates clinical translation and implementation [70].

Case Study Integrated analysis of a combination of radiomic features and transcriptomic, proteomic, and metabolomic data revealed associated gene signatures of immune metabolism that predict overall survival and distinguished tumor subtypes in distinct microenvironments associated with different treatment responses. Prioritized druggable genes and metabolic networks of 16 cancer types were revealed by investigators through TWAS, PWAS, and Mendelian randomization. Novel targets and therapeutic biomarkers for therapeutic optimization were revealed via integrative analysis. Although radiogenomic models have been developed to noninvasively predict EGFR mutations and PD-L1 expression to inform immunotherapy decisions, multiomics frameworks have enabled the refinement of cancer subtyping and treatment prediction of colorectal, lung, and breast cancers [39].

10.8 Analytical Validation and Regulatory Landscape

10.8.1 Assay Standardization

The first step of integrating biomarker results into clinical practice is assay standardization. The ability to obtain reproducible results on different platforms, in different laboratories, and on different samples while using concise parameters of sensitivity, specificity, accuracy, and precision is a key component of proper analytical validation. The use of standardized reference materials and controls, such as synthetic spike-ins and aggregate patient samples, allows benchmarking and interstudy comparability. To reduce variability and ensure analyte integrity, preanalytical factors must be harmonized and include the methods of collection, transportation, storage, and processing. To ensure the interoperability of multiomics and radiomics outputs, cross-platform harmonization is required to align the sequencing, imaging, and computer workflow technologies. Moreover, external proficiency testing and quality management are essential for the discovery of drift and demonstration of competency. The use and ensurance of clinical guideline application are heightened through the validation of their clinical value by well-crafted prospective studies.

Biomarkers become trustworthy, scalable, and therapeutically viable instruments by means of aligned implementation avenues consisting of technological normalization, regulatory harmonization, and education of clinicians [71].

10.8.2 Companion Diagnostics

Companion diagnostics are tests codeveloped with targeted treatments to aid in clinical decision-making by assessing biomarker status. They are predictive biomarkers that define patients likely to benefit most from given therapeutic agents, exemplified by EGFR mutation testing informing tyrosine kinase inhibitor treatment in non-small cell lung cancer. They enable therapeutic stratification by classifying patients into likely responders and likely nonresponders and thus enable personalized treatment approaches. As approval processes can be accelerated by codevelopment models whereby pharmaceuticals and diagnostics are developed side by side, regulatory authorities encourage these models. Validation of clinical utility and reducing access delay are additional advantages that facilitate approval processes.

To increase sensitivity, track resistance, and widen the patient population for whom targeting would be practical, new modalities are broadening companion diagnostics beyond single-gene tests alone to liquid biopsies, radiogenomic signatures, and multianalyte panels. These modalities also open the door to adaptive trial designs and the formation of real-world evidence, both of which are deployed to enhance predictive ability and shape globally implemented regulatory decisions [72].

10.8.3 FDA/EMA Regulatory Pathways

The clinical use of cancer biomarkers must navigate complex regulations requiring well-defined processes and strong data to guarantee safety, efficacy, and worldwide use. In the United States, premarket approval of high-risk companion diagnostics offers new clinical information, the 510(k) program for assays is substantially equivalent to already approved tests, and breakthrough device programs are regulatory options facilitating the review of new technologies targeting the fulfillment of unreconciled medical needs. In the European Union, the CE marking, which demonstrates the compliance of products and related accessories by ensuring the conformity of the products and accessories to the EU safety and performance requirements, represents evidence of adherence.

The In Vitro Diagnostic Regulation (IVDR) requires stronger clinical evidence, risk classification, and postmarket surveillance. Global harmonization initiatives try to bring standards into line, eliminate duplicative requirements, and enable the wider and earlier application of verified cancer biomarkers within various jurisdictions. These are driven by associations such as the International Medical Device Regulators Forum and mutual collaborations between the FDA and EMA [73].

10.9 Clinical Trial Design and Real-World Evidence

The crucial functions of some metabolic chemicals in a variety of malignancies, such as colorectal and breast cancer, have been investigated in certain trial studies (Table 10.7). These results demonstrate the potential use of these compounds in therapeutic and prognostic approaches. For example, research on genes related to amino acid metabolism (AAMRGs) revealed that the expression of these genes is associated with variations in patient survival outcomes.

AAMRG expression is linked to immune pathways in malignancies according to functional analysis, and patients who have good AAMRG profiles and greater immune infiltration typically have better survival rates. Three genes—AIMP2, IYD, and QARS1—were used to construct a risk model that showed how breast cancer cell proliferation was regulated and that tumor growth was suppressed. These findings suggest that AAMRGs could be useful biomarkers for prognosis and novel therapeutic approaches in breast cancer [74]. To elaborate on the function of amino acids, certain malignancies have decreased levels of arginine and glutamine, which are critical for immunological regulation, cell proliferation, and nitrogen balance. This may result in increased nitrogenous waste and tumor aggression. However, altered glutamine routes can provide energy for cell division and increase anaplerotic flux into the TCA cycle. Tumors are interesting candidates for therapeutic intervention and monitoring because these metabolic pathways reveal how they use amino acids to fuel development and elude immune surveillance [75]. Compared with those from healthy individuals with hematologic malignancies, plasma samples from patients with diffuse large B-cell lymphoma (DLBCL) presented variations in the expression of eight amino acids. Among the amino acids, glycine (Gly), histidine (His), serine (Ser), and tryptophan (Trp) decreased, whereas aspartic acid (Asp), glutamic acid (Glu), phenylalanine (Phe), and threonine (Thr) increased. Tryptophan and glutamine levels have been shown to be strongly correlated with patient prognosis. These amino acids, along with a number of clinical factors, such as age, LDH levels, extranodal involvement, and the IPI score, are used in the SVR prediction model. With an R^2 of 0.89 and a low prediction error, this model demonstrated exceptional performance and could be used to predict progression-free survival (PFS). These findings provide compelling evidence for the use of amino acids as a clinical diagnostic and prognostic tool for DLBCL, indicating that some biomarkers derived from plasma amino acid profiles may facilitate detection and enhance diagnosis and therapy [76].

Two purine metabolites, adenine and hypoxanthine, are essential for the metabolism of cancer cells, particularly MCF-7 breast cancer cells. Adenine and hypoxanthine levels have been shown to fluctuate in certain ways and have been linked to metabolic activity and cell survival. Hypoxanthine levels are relatively low during the lag phase, the initial phase of cell development. Nevertheless, hypoxanthine levels sharply increase as cells enter the logarithmic development phase. The rapid growth of DNA and RNA depends on this rise. These results emphasize nucleotide synthesis as a useful indicator and early biomarker for metabolic activation and cell proliferation in cancer, highlighting the roles of purines and hypoxanthine [77].

Table 10.7 Biomarkers identified in clinical applications

Biomarker type	Cancer type	Key findings	Ref.
Amino acids	Breast cancer	AAMRGs: Immune infiltration and better survival; potential for prognosis and therapy	[74]
	Cholangiocarcinoma	Arginine and glutamine downregulation: Tumor aggressiveness; growth and immune evasion.	[75]
	DLBCL	Asp, Glu, Phe, Thr ↑; Gly, His, Ser, Trp ↓; A model (Trp and Glu) for prediction of progression-free survival	[76]
	Colorectal cancer	Histidine, methionine, tryptophan ↓; glutamic acid, iso-glutamine, proline, putrescine ↑; Contradictory trends across studies in alanine and taurine	[81]
Purines/ nucleotides	Breast cancer (MCF-7)	Hypoxanthine during proliferation↑; Early biomarker for DNA/RNA synthesis and metabolic activation	[77]
	Colorectal cancer	Uracil, hypoxanthine ↑; phenol, urea ↓.	[81]
Lipids and fatty acids	Colorectal cancer	SFA, MUFA, glycoprotein acetyls, 3-hydroxybutyrate, and triglycerides increase, and linoleic acid decreases, the risk of CRC (by inhibiting arachidonic acid synthesis)	[78]
	Colorectal cancer	PC species with arachidonic acid increase, and omega-6 and MUFA PC species decrease the risk of CRC	[79]
	Lung adenocarcinoma	PC and PE: Membrane changes and metabolic reprogramming; potential noninvasive biomarkers for early detection	[80]
	Colorectal cancer	Hydroxybutyrate, choline, succinate, oleic acid, glycochenodeoxycholate ↑; phosphocholine ↑; linked to tumor progression and staging	[81]
Carbohydrates	Colorectal cancer	Glucose, galactose, mannose, arabitol, pyruvate ↓; lactate, glycerol, succinate ↑; Warburg effect and energy metabolism reprogramming	[81]

Colorectal cancer (CRC) has also been linked to lipid metabolism. A comprehensive investigation examined the relationships between the risk of CRC and several blood metabolic indicators. An increased risk of colorectal cancer is associated with increased amounts of triglycerides, 3-hydroxybutyrate, glycoprotein acetyls, monounsaturated fatty acids (MUFAs), and saturated fatty acids (SFAs) in very large VLDL particles. However, by delaying the manufacture of arachidonic acid, a precursor to proinflammatory chemicals, biomarkers such as linoleic acid lower the risk of colorectal cancer by up to 11%. These results imply that lipid metabolism plays an important role in the development of colorectal cancer and might enhance future preventative measures to decrease the incidence of this disease [78]. Furthermore, an increased risk of CRC is associated with increased levels of phosphatidylcholine (PC) molecules, which are precursors to inflammatory mediators and include polyunsaturated fatty acids, arachidonic acid, and docosapentaenoic acid. Other PC species, such as monounsaturated and omega-6 fatty acids, are known to lower the incidence of colorectal cancer [79]. Furthermore, the levels of PC and PE not only cause structural changes in tumor cell membranes but are also involved in the metabolic reprogramming of lung adenocarcinoma in its early stage. These findings demonstrate their potential as noninvasive biomarkers for early detection and pave the way for personalized treatment strategies based on metabolic profiling [80].

10.10 Future Directions and Challenges

As a rapidly emerging subject in oncology, metabolomics has promise for understanding cancer biology, early detection, diagnosis, and individualization. Metabolomic profiling of amino acids, lipids, and nucleosides has been performed in studies on several cancer types to identify certain biochemical alterations. Notwithstanding their promise, several obstacles need to be taken into account, including cross-platform data integration and sample preparation. One of the most promising avenues for future research in cancer metabolomics is the combination of microbiome–metabolome data. Prostate and colorectal cancers have been linked to the impact of the gut microbiota on immune responses and host metabolism. Trimethylamine N-oxide (TMAO), polyamines, bile acids, and short-chain fatty acids are examples of microbial metabolites that are known to contribute to immunological regulation and carcinogenesis. Certain dietary trans-fatty acids, which are thought to be detrimental, have been demonstrated to increase antitumor immunity, indicating the possibility of using nutrition to cure cancer. Combining metabolomic and microbiome analyses may help identify new treatment targets and biomarkers, particularly for improving immunotherapy and early illness diagnosis. Although metabolic pathways in tumors may be identified via traditional approaches, they are not sensitive enough to capture the temporal and spatial variability of the TME. Currently, more sophisticated methods, such as scRNA-seq and CyTOF, shed light on protein-level regulation and metabolic gene expression. These methods have shown that immunosuppression results from cancer cells frequently outcompeting immune cells for essential nutrients such as glucose and glutamine. The interactions between cancer and the immune system are significantly influenced by systemic variables, including the tumor organismal environment (TOE), in addition to the TME. Immunometabolic processes are governed by the microbiome, neuroendocrine signals, physical activity, and nutritional metabolites. However, significant challenges abound. Interplatform, interspecimen type, and interanalytic strategy variability of biomarkers identified arise because of the dissimilarities of methodologies, specimen varieties, and analytic approaches. The insufficient external validation cohort supports the clinical utility of hundreds of investigations. In addition, the integration of metabolomics data with genetic and microbial information has gained increasing ethical prominence. To effectively navigate issues of informed consent, data confidentiality, risks of reidentification, and equitable access to new screening technologies, open mechanisms of governance and participatory processes of investigation are essential. In short, the start of the new cancer research century has been framed by the intersection of metabolomics, microbial investigations, spatial imaging, and sensitivity toward ethical issues. These technologies have the ability to transform screening strategies, improve prognostics, and make therapeutic approaches better suited to the individual needs of patients. To make this happen, however, collaborative endeavors under well-defined protocols, vigorous validation, and sensitivity toward the clinical application of ethical rigor are necessary [82–86].

References

1. Wang W, Zhen S, Ping Y, Wang L, Zhang Y. Metabolomic biomarkers in liquid biopsy: accurate cancer diagnosis and prognosis monitoring. Front Oncol. 2024;14:1331215. https://doi.org/10.3389/fonc.2024.1331215.
2. Garg P, Singhal G, Horne D, Kulkarni P, Salgia R, Singhal SS. Molecular PET imaging: unlocking the secrets of cancer metabolism. Biochem Pharmacol. 2025;242:117202. https://doi.org/10.1016/j.bcp.2025.117202.
3. Qiu S, Cai Y, Yao H, Lin C, Xie Y, Tang S, et al. Small molecule metabolites: discovery of biomarkers and therapeutic targets. Signal Transduct Target Ther. 2023;8(1):132. https://doi.org/10.1038/s41392-023-01399-3.
4. Bamji-Stocke S, van Berkel V, Miller DM, Frieboes HB. A review of metabolism-associated biomarkers in lung cancer diagnosis and treatment. Metabolomics. 2018;14(6):81.
5. Wu F, Li W, Lu H, Li L. Recent advances in mass spectrometry-based studies of post-translational modifications in Alzheimer's disease. Mol Cell Proteomics. 2025;24(7):101003. https://doi.org/10.1016/j.mcpro.2025.101003.
6. Kaur A, Rohilla R, Rana S, Rani S, Prabhakar N. Recent advances in protein biomarkers based enzymatic biosensors for non-communicable diseases. TrAC Trends Anal Chem. 2024;174:117683. https://doi.org/10.1016/j.trac.2024.117683.
7. Afonso J, Gonçalves C, Costa M, Ferreira D, Santos L, Longatto-Filho A, et al. Glucose metabolism reprogramming in bladder cancer: hexokinase 2 (HK2) as prognostic biomarker and target for bladder cancer therapy. Cancers (Basel). 2023;15(3) https://doi.org/10.3390/cancers15030982.
8. Zahra K, Dey T, Ashish MSP, Pandey U. Pyruvate kinase M2 and cancer: the role of PKM2 in promoting tumorigenesis. Front. Oncologia. 2020;10:159. https://doi.org/10.3389/fonc.2020.00159.
9. Andolino C, Cotul EK, Xianyu Z, Li Y, Bhat D, Ayers M, et al. Fatty acid synthase-derived lipid stores support breast cancer metastasis. Cancer Metab. 2025;13(1):35. https://doi.org/10.1186/s40170-025-00404-3.
10. Yu Y, Nie Q, Wang Z, Di Y, Chen X, Ren K. Targeting acetyl-CoA carboxylase 1 for cancer therapy. Front Pharmacol. 2023;14:1129010. https://doi.org/10.3389/fphar.2023.1129010.
11. Yu W, Yang X, Zhang Q, Sun L, Yuan S, Xin Y. Targeting GLS1 to cancer therapy through glutamine metabolism. Clin Transl Oncol. 2021;23(11):2253–68. https://doi.org/10.1007/s12094-021-02645-2.
12. Sun N, Zhao X. Argininosuccinate synthase 1, arginine deprivation therapy and cancer management. Front Pharmacol. 2022;13:935553. https://doi.org/10.3389/fphar.2022.935553.
13. Cairns RA, Mak TW. Oncogenic isocitrate dehydrogenase mutations: mechanisms, models, and clinical opportunities. Cancer Discov. 2013;3(7):730–41. https://doi.org/10.1158/2159-8290.Cd-13-0083.
14. Zhu Z, Leung GKK. More than a metabolic enzyme: MTHFD2 as a novel target for anticancer therapy? Front Oncol. 2020;10:658. https://doi.org/10.3389/fonc.2020.00658.

15. Almohanna T, Auda FM, Ali BM. Early detection of digestive system cancers: insights from enzymatic and non-enzymatic tumour markers. J Med Biochem. 2025;44(3):631–6. https://doi.org/10.5937/jomb0-56390.
16. Kim C, Kang MS, Raja IS, Joung YK, Han DW. Advancements in nanobiosensor technologies for in-vitro diagnostics to point of care testing. Heliyon. 2024;10(22):e40306. https://doi.org/10.1016/j.heliyon.2024.e40306.
17. Santiappillai NT, Cao Y, Hakeem-Sanni MF, Yang J, Quek LE, Hoy AJ. Pathway metabolite ratios reveal distinctive glutamine metabolism in a subset of proliferating cells. Mol Syst Biol. 2025;21(8):983–1003. https://doi.org/10.1038/s44320-025-00099-0.
18. Mortazavi Farsani SS, Verma V. Lactate mediated metabolic crosstalk between cancer and immune cells and its therapeutic implications. Front Oncol. 2023;13:1175532. https://doi.org/10.3389/fonc.2023.1175532.
19. Chung CR, Tang Y, Chiu YP, Li S, Hsieh WK, Yao L, et al. dbPTM 2025 update: comprehensive integration of PTMs and proteomic data for advanced insights into cancer research. Nucleic Acids Res. 2025;53(D1):D377–d86. https://doi.org/10.1093/nar/gkae1005.
20. Wang W, Rong Z, Wang G, Hou Y, Yang F, Qiu M. Cancer metabolites: promising biomarkers for cancer liquid biopsy. Biomark Res. 2023;11(1):66. https://doi.org/10.1186/s40364-023-00507-3.
21. Liu M-X, Jin L, Sun S-J, Liu P, Feng X, Cheng Z-L, et al. Metabolic reprogramming by PCK1 promotes TCA cataplerosis, oxidative stress and apoptosis in liver cancer cells and suppresses hepatocellular carcinoma. Oncogene. 2018;37(12):1637–53.
22. Lim ZD, Abdullah NAS, Lim KS, Ho PC, Arulsamy A, Fong SL, et al. Exploring metabolic biomarkers and pathways in pharmacoresistant epilepsy: a systematic review. Epilepsy Res. 2025;218:107656. https://doi.org/10.1016/j.eplepsyres.2025.107656.
23. Vo DK, Trinh KTL. Emerging biomarkers in metabolomics: advancements in precision health and disease diagnosis. Int J Mol Sci. 2024;25(23) https://doi.org/10.3390/ijms252313190.
24. Hu Y, Xu W, Chen L. Post-translational modifications and the reprogramming of tumor metabolism. Discov Oncol. 2025;16(1):929. https://doi.org/10.1007/s12672-025-02674-1.
25. Feng T, Zhang H, Zhou Y, Zhu Y, Shi S, Li K, et al. Roles of posttranslational modifications in lipid metabolism and cancer progression. Biomark Res. 2024;12(1):141. https://doi.org/10.1186/s40364-024-00681-y.
26. Ribbenstedt A, Ziarrusta H, Benskin JP. Development, characterization and comparisons of targeted and non-targeted metabolomics methods. PLoS One. 2018;13(11):e0207082.
27. Lin C, Tian Q, Guo S, Xie D, Cai Y, Wang Z, et al. Metabolomics for clinical biomarker discovery and therapeutic target identification. Molecules. 2024;29(10) https://doi.org/10.3390/molecules29102198.
28. Hilovsky D, Hartsell J, Young JD, Liu X. Stable isotope tracing analysis in cancer research: advancements and challenges in identifying dysregulated cancer metabolism and treatment strategies. Meta. 2024;14(6) https://doi.org/10.3390/metabo14060318.
29. Wang R, Yin Y, Li J, Wang H, Lv W, Gao Y, et al. Global stable-isotope tracing metabolomics reveals system-wide metabolic alternations in aging drosophila. Nat Commun. 2022;13(1):3518. https://doi.org/10.1038/s41467-022-31268-6.
30. Fan TW, Lorkiewicz PK, Sellers K, Moseley HN, Higashi RM, Lane AN. Stable isotope-resolved metabolomics and applications for drug development. Pharmacol Ther. 2012;133(3):366–91. https://doi.org/10.1016/j.pharmthera.2011.12.007.
31. Park B-S, Lee M, Kim J, Kim T. Perturbomics: CRISPR–Cas screening-based functional genomics approach for drug target discovery. Exp Mol Med. 2025;57(7):1443–54. https://doi.org/10.1038/s12276-025-01487-0.
32. Nguyen LV, Caldas C. Functional genomics approaches to improve pre-clinical drug screening and biomarker discovery. EMBO Mol Med. 2021;13(9):e13189. https://doi.org/10.15252/emmm.202013189.
33. He Y, Tu X, Xue Y, Chen Y, Ye B, Li X, et al. CRISPR screening redefines therapeutic target identification and drug discovery with precision and scalability. J Pharm Analy. 2025:101357. https://doi.org/10.1016/j.jpha.2025.101357.

34. Dubrot J, Du PP, Lane-Reticker SK, Kessler EA, Muscato AJ, Mehta A, et al. In vivo CRISPR screens reveal the landscape of immune evasion pathways across cancer. Nat Immunol. 2022;23(10):1495–506. https://doi.org/10.1038/s41590-022-01315-x.
35. Li YR, Lyu Z, Tian Y, Fang Y, Zhu Y, Chen Y, et al. Advancements in CRISPR screens for the development of cancer immunotherapy strategies. Mol Ther Oncol. 2023;31:100733. https://doi.org/10.1016/j.omto.2023.100733.
36. Sun Y, Cheng Z, Qiu J, Lu W. Performance and application of the total-body PET/CT scanner: a literature review. EJNMMI Res. 2024;14(1):38. https://doi.org/10.1186/s13550-023-01059-1.
37. Trotter J, Pantel AR, Teo B-KK, Escorcia FE, Li T, Pryma DA, et al. Positron emission tomography (PET)/computed tomography (CT) imaging in radiation therapy treatment planning: a review of PET imaging tracers and methods to incorporate PET/CT. Adv Radiat Oncol. 2023;8(5):101212. https://doi.org/10.1016/j.adro.2023.101212.
38. Rong J, Haider A, Jeppesen TE, Josephson L, Liang SH. Radiochemistry for positron emission tomography. Nat Commun. 2023;14(1):3257. https://doi.org/10.1038/s41467-023-36377-4.
39. Yan Q, Yan X, Yang X, Li S, Song J. The use of PET/MRI in radiotherapy. Insights Imaging. 2024;15(1):63. https://doi.org/10.1186/s13244-024-01627-6.
40. Vercellino L, de Jong D, Dercle L, Hosten B, Braumuller B, Das JP, et al. Translating molecules into imaging-the development of new PET tracers for patients with melanoma. Diagnostics (Basel). 2022;12(5) https://doi.org/10.3390/diagnostics12051116.
41. Ali FB, Qmichou Z, Oukabli M, Dakka N, Bakri Y, Eddouks M, et al. Alteration of glucose metabolism and expression of glucose transporters in ovarian cancer. Explor Target Anti-tumor Ther. 2024;5(2):384.
42. Brindle KM. Imaging cancer metabolism using magnetic resonance. Npj Imaging. 2024;2(1):1.
43. Khan AS, Laustsen C. Technologies and strategies for metabolic and molecular imaging with hyperpolarized MRI. J Magn Reson Imaging. 2025;
44. de Kouchkovsky I, Nguyen H, Chen H-Y, Liu X, Qin H, Stohr BA, et al. Dual hyperpolarized [1-13C]pyruvate and [13C]urea magnetic resonance imaging of prostate cancer. J Magnet Reson Open. 2024;21:100165. https://doi.org/10.1016/j.jmro.2024.100165.
45. Kumari A, Mishra G, Parihar P, Dudhe SS, Mishra GV. Role of magnetic resonance spectroscopy in evaluating choline levels in gallbladder carcinoma: a comprehensive review. Cureus. 2024;16(8)
46. Fardanesh R, Marino MA, Avendano D, Leithner D, Pinker K, Thakur SB. Proton MR spectroscopy in the breast: technical innovations and clinical applications. J Magn Reson Imaging. 2019;50(4):1033–46.
47. Choi C, Ganji SK, DeBerardinis RJ, Hatanpaa KJ, Rakheja D, Kovacs Z, et al. 2-hydroxyglutarate detection by magnetic resonance spectroscopy in IDH-mutated patients with gliomas. Nat Med. 2012;18(4):624–9.
48. Rothman D, Howseman A, Graham G, Petroff O, Lantos G, Fayad PB, et al. Localized proton NMR observation of [3-13C] lactate in stroke after [1-13C] glucose infusion. Magn Reson Med. 1991;21(2):302–7.
49. Ardenkjær-Larsen JH, Fridlund B, Gram A, Hansson G, Hansson L, Lerche MH, et al. Increase in signal-to-noise ratio of> 10,000 times in liquid-state NMR. Proc Natl Acad Sci. 2003;100(18):10158–63.
50. Kreis F, Wright AJ, Hesse F, Fala M, Hu D-e, Brindle KM. Measuring tumor glycolytic flux in vivo by using fast deuterium MRI. Radiology. 2020;294(2):289–96.
51. Borea R, Saldanha EF, Maheswaran S, Nicolo E, Singhal S, Pontolillo L, et al. Cancer in a drop: advances in liquid biopsy in 2024. Crit Rev Oncol Hematol. 2025;213:104776. https://doi.org/10.1016/j.critrevonc.2025.104776.
52. Pandey S, Yadav P. Liquid biopsy in cancer management: integrating diagnostics and clinical applications. Pract Lab Med. 2025;43:e00446. https://doi.org/10.1016/j.plabm.2024.e00446.
53. Hammond NG, Cameron RB, Faubert B. Beyond glucose and Warburg: finding the sweet spot in cancer metabolism models. NPJ Metab Health Dis. 2024;2(1):11. https://doi.org/10.1038/s44324-024-00017-2.

54. Suri GS, Kaur G, Carbone GM, Shinde D. Metabolomics in oncology. Cancer Rep (Hoboken). 2023;6(3):e1795. https://doi.org/10.1002/cnr2.1795.
55. Ishizaki T, Sugimoto M, Kuboyama Y, Mazaki J, Kasahara K, Tago T, et al. Stage-specific plasma metabolomic profiles in colorectal cancer. J Clin Med. 2024;13(17) https://doi.org/10.3390/jcm13175202.
56. Harmati M, Bukva M, Boroczky T, Buzas K, Gyukity-Sebestyen E. The role of the metabolite cargo of extracellular vesicles in tumor progression. Cancer Metastasis Rev. 2021;40(4):1203–21. https://doi.org/10.1007/s10555-021-10014-2.
57. Cunha ERK, Ying W, Olefsky JM. Exosome-mediated impact on systemic metabolism. Annu Rev Physiol. 2024;86:225–53. https://doi.org/10.1146/annurev-physiol-042222-024535.
58. Zhang Y, Liang F, Zhang D, Qi S, Liu Y. Metabolites as extracellular vesicle cargo in health, cancer, pleural effusion, and cardiovascular diseases: an emerging field of study to diagnostic and therapeutic purposes. Biomed Pharmacother. 2023;157:114046. https://doi.org/10.1016/j.biopha.2022.114046.
59. Xu Y, Zhu S, Xia C, Yu H, Shi S, Chen K, et al. Liquid biopsy-based multi-cancer early detection: an exploration road from evidence to implementation. Sci Bull (Beijing). 2025;70(17):2852–67. https://doi.org/10.1016/j.scib.2025.06.030.
60. Lv Y, Li Z, Liu S, Zhou Z, Song J, Ba Y, et al. Metabolic checkpoints in immune cell reprogramming: rewiring immunometabolism for cancer therapy. Mol Cancer. 2025;24(1):210. https://doi.org/10.1186/s12943-025-02407-6.
61. Wang H, Zhou F, Qin W, Yang Y, Li X, Liu R. Metabolic regulation of myeloid-derived suppressor cells in tumor immune microenvironment: targets and therapeutic strategies. Theranostics. 2025;15(6):2159–84. https://doi.org/10.7150/thno.105276.
62. Cai Z, Yang H, Yu Z, Su J, Zhang J, Ye Z, et al. Efficacy and safety of IDH inhibitors in IDH-mutated cancers: a systematic review and meta-analysis of 4 randomized controlled trials. World J Surg Oncol. 2024;22(1):295. https://doi.org/10.1186/s12957-024-03579-z.
63. Tufail M, Jiang CH, Li N. Altered metabolism in cancer: insights into energy pathways and therapeutic targets. Mol Cancer. 2024;23(1):203. https://doi.org/10.1186/s12943-024-02119-3.
64. Ulfenborg B. Vertical and horizontal integration of multi-omics data with miodin. BMC Bioinform. 2019;20(1):649. https://doi.org/10.1186/s12859-019-3224-4.
65. He W, Huang W, Zhang L, Wu X, Zhang S, Zhang B. Radiogenomics: bridging the gap between imaging and genomics for precision oncology. MedComm (2020). 2024;5(9):e722. https://doi.org/10.1002/mco2.722.
66. Valous NA, Popp F, Zörnig I, Jäger D, Charoentong P. Graph machine learning for integrated multi-omics analysis. Br J Cancer. 2024;131(2):205–11. https://doi.org/10.1038/s41416-024-02706-7.
67. Chang Y-cI. A Survey: Potential Dimensionality Reduction Methods. arXiv preprint arXiv:250211036. 2025;
68. Sartori F, Codicè F, Caranzano I, Rollo C, Birolo G, Fariselli P, et al. A comprehensive review of deep learning applications with multi-omics data in cancer research. Genes (Basel). 2025;16(6) https://doi.org/10.3390/genes16060648.
69. Ballard JL, Wang Z, Li W, Shen L, Long Q. Deep learning-based approaches for multi-omics data integration and analysis. BioData Min. 2024;17(1):38. https://doi.org/10.1186/s13040-024-00391-z.
70. Vimbi V, Shaffi N, Mahmud M. Interpreting artificial intelligence models: a systematic review on the application of LIME and SHAP in Alzheimer's disease detection. Brain Inform. 2024;11(1):10. https://doi.org/10.1186/s40708-024-00222-1.
71. Chen G, Huang S, Weng W, Su C. Biomarker assay development, qualification, and validation. In: Fang L, Su C, editors. Statistical methods in biomarker and early clinical development. Cham: Springer International Publishing; 2019. p. 87–115.
72. Sato Y. Clinical utility of liquid biopsy-based companion diagnostics in the non-small-cell lung cancer treatment. Explor Target Antitumor Ther. 2022;3(5):630–42. https://doi.org/10.37349/etat.2022.00104.

73. Ibrahim S. Comparing FDA and EMA decisions for market authorization of generic drug applications covering 2017–2020. Office of Generic. Drugs. 2022;
74. Zhou Y, Yu S, Zhu L, Wang Y, Duan C, Li D, et al. Molecular biomarkers for the prognosis of breast cancer: role of amino acid metabolism genes. J Physiol Biochem. 2025;81(2):441–57. https://doi.org/10.1007/s13105-025-01088-5.
75. Prajumwongs P, Titapun A, Thanasukarn V, Jareanrat A, Khuntikeo N, Namwat N, et al. Identification of serum metabolite biomarkers and metabolic reprogramming mechanisms to predict recurrence in cholangiocarcinoma. Sci Rep. 2025;15(1):12782. https://doi.org/10.1038/s41598-025-97641-9.
76. Zhang C, Cai M, Yao W, Hong Q, Han Y, Chen N. Amino acid-based risk stratification model improves prognostic precision in diffuse large B-cell lymphoma. Cancer Cell Int. 2025;25(1):221. https://doi.org/10.1186/s12935-025-03879-8.
77. Zhang S, Qu Y. Spatially isolated dual-active sites enabling selective hydrogenation. Cell reports physical Science. 2024;5(2) https://doi.org/10.1016/j.xcrp.2024.101793.
78. Yuan F, Jia G, Wen W, Xu S, Gunchick V, Deng K, et al. Blood metabolic biomarkers and colorectal cancer risk: results from large prospective cohort and Mendelian randomisation analyses. Br J Cancer. 2025;133(1):94–103. https://doi.org/10.1038/s41416-025-02997-4.
79. Wu H, Gu J, He Y, Ji Y, Cao W, Li R, et al. Exploring the causal relationship between lipid profiles and colorectal cancer through Mendelian randomization: a multidimensional plasma lipid composition perspective. J Cancer. 2025;16(6):1848–59. https://doi.org/10.7150/jca.103247.
80. Wu B, Zheng M, Guo Q, Wang N, Zhu C, Zhao W, et al. Early potential metabolic biomarkers of T1 stage lung adenocarcinoma based on serum metabolomics. Front Mol Biosci. 2025;12:2025. https://doi.org/10.3389/fmolb.2025.1544774.
81. Erben V, Bhardwaj M, Schrotz-King P, Brenner H. Metabolomics biomarkers for detection of colorectal neoplasms: a systematic review. Cancer. 2018;10(8):246.
82. Chen S, Zhang Y, Li X, Zhang Y, Zeng Y. Driving innovations in cancer research through spatial metabolomics: a bibliometric review of trends and hotspot. Front Immunol. 2025;16:2025. https://doi.org/10.3389/fimmu.2025.1589943.
83. Holmes L, LaHurd A, Wasson E, McClarin L, Dabney K. Racial and ethnic heterogeneity in the association between Total cholesterol and pediatric obesity. Int J Environ Res Public Health. 2016;13(1):19.
84. Taunk K, Jajula S, Bhavsar PP, Choudhari M, Bhanuse S, Tamhankar A, et al. The prowess of metabolomics in cancer research: current trends, challenges and future perspectives. Mol Cell Biochem. 2025;480(2):693–720. https://doi.org/10.1007/s11010-024-05041-w.
85. Xiao Y, Li Y, Zhao H. Spatiotemporal metabolomic approaches to the cancer-immunity panorama: a methodological perspective. Mol Cancer. 2024;23(1):202. https://doi.org/10.1186/s12943-024-02113-9.
86. Zhang F, Zhang Y, Zhao W, Deng K, Wang Z, Yang C, et al. Metabolomics for biomarker discovery in the diagnosis, prognosis, survival and recurrence of colorectal cancer: a systematic review. Oncotarget. 2017;8(21):35460.

Cancer and Immune Cells: A Metabolic Battle in the Tumor Microenvironment

11

Sam Pournezhad, Ramyar Azar, and Farzad Taghizadeh-Hesary

11.1 Introduction

The significance of metabolism within the immune system has become increasingly evident over the past three decades [1]. *Immunometabolism* refers to a field of immunology that investigates how the metabolic state of immune cells influences their function, and conversely, how immune activity and interactions with the surrounding microenvironment modulate cellular metabolism [2].

The immune system plays a pivotal role in cancer treatment, either as an independent therapeutic component [3] or in combination with various anti-cancer therapies, such as radiotherapy [4], chemotherapy [5], and immunotherapy [6]. Consequently, immunometabolism holds great importance in oncology, as it determines how immune cells communicate and compete metabolically with cancer cells. Understanding the metabolic dynamics underlying these interactions provides an essential framework for designing more effective therapeutic approaches against cancer.

With this background, the present chapter aims to provide a comprehensive overview of immunometabolism in the context of oncology, serving as a practical guide for oncologists, immunologists, cancer biologists, and researchers interested in the

Authors Sam Pournezhad and Ramyar Azar contributed equally to this chapter.

S. Pournezhad
Marcus Stroke and Neuroscience Center, Grady Memorial Hospital, Atlanta, GA, USA

Department of Clinical Sciences, Touro University California College of Pharmacy, Vallejo, CA, USA

R. Azar
Iran University of Medical Sciences, Tehran, Iran

F. Taghizadeh-Hesary (✉)
Breast Cancer Research Center, Iran University of Medical Sciences, Tehran, Iran

ENT and Head and Neck Research Center and Department, The Five Senses Health Institute, School of Medicine, Iran University of Medical Sciences, Tehran, Iran
e-mail: taghizadeh_hesary.f@iums.ac.ir

S. Ashique et al. (eds.), *Cancer Metabolism*, Cancer Treatment and Research 195, https://doi.org/10.1007/978-3-032-21861-2_11

intricate interplay between cancer and the immune system. In this chapter, we first introduce the main immune components involved in antitumor defense and discuss their characteristic metabolic profiles. We then describe the mechanisms by which cancer cells evade immune surveillance. Section 11.4 outlines current and emerging strategies in cancer immunotherapy, while Sect. 11.5 explores the metabolic crosstalk between immune and cancer cells.

11.2 Immune Cells in Response to Cancer Cells: Two Groups with Two Distinct Features

The immune system is a complex network of cells, tissues, and molecules that work together to protect the host by recognizing and eliminating harmful invaders. Effective and timely identification of these invaders is crucial for maintaining homeostasis and preventing disease progression. In the context of oncology, the "invaders" are cancer cells—aberrant cells that arise from the body's own tissues but acquire the ability to evade normal immune surveillance and destruction.

In the context of cancer, the immune system represents a highly complex network of cellular populations that can broadly be divided into two major categories based on their functional response to tumors. The first group consists of antitumoral immune cells, which aim to recognize and eliminate cancer cells [7]. The second group includes pro-tumorigenic immune cells, which, instead of suppressing tumor growth, facilitate cancer cell survival, proliferation, and metastasis. Notably, many of these pro-tumorigenic immune cells acquire their tumor-promoting characteristics in response to various biomolecules and signaling factors secreted by cancer cells within the tumor microenvironment (TME) [8].

The antitumoral immune cells comprise several key components: (1) $CD8^+$ cytotoxic T lymphocytes (CTLs), which serve as the primary effector cells responsible for directly recognizing and destroying malignant cells; (2) $CD4^+$ T helper 1 (Th1) cells, which support CTL activity by secreting pro-inflammatory cytokines such as IFN-γ and IL-2; (3) natural killer (NK) cells, innate lymphocytes capable of targeting and lysing tumor cells independently of antigen presentation; (4) macrophages of the M1 phenotype, which phagocytose tumor cells, release reactive oxygen species (ROS), and participate in antigen presentation to activate effector T cells; (5) B lymphocytes, which contribute to antitumor immunity through the production of antibodies against tumor-associated antigens and facilitation of antibody-dependent cellular cytotoxicity (ADCC); and (6) dendritic cells (DCs), which act as professional antigen-presenting cells, as well as capture and process tumor antigens to prime adaptive immune responses [7].

In contrast, the pro-tumorigenic immune cells encompass several immunosuppressive or tumor-supportive populations that promote cancer progression through distinct mechanisms. These include regulatory (1) T cells (Tregs), which inhibit effector T-cell function via cytokines such as IL-10, adenosine, and TGF-β; (2) myeloid-derived suppressor cells (MDSCs), which impair T and NK cells activation and dendritic cell maturation; (3) tumor-associated macrophages (TAMs) of the M2 phenotype, which leads immunosuppression by recruiting Tregs to TME; (4)

tumor-associated neutrophils (TANs), which induce programmed cell death ligand 1 (PD-L1) on cancer cells and T cell apoptosis [8]; and mast cells through interaction with Tregs and MDSCs [9]. Among these, eosinophils may have both pro-tumoral and antitumoral effects on TME [10].

Collectively, the dynamic balance between antitumoral and pro-tumorigenic immune cells within the TME determines whether the immune system suppresses or supports tumor development. Understanding these opposing forces is fundamental to designing effective immunotherapies that restore antitumor immunity and counteract immune suppression.

11.3 How Cancer Cells Evade Immune System?

Immune cells are designed to detect and eliminate cancer cells. However, cancer cells are equipped with various abilities that enable them to hide themselves from the antitumor immune system. Collectively, these protective mechanisms are categorized as *immune evasion*. This section outlines the most common mechanisms by which cancer cells evade the immune system.

11.3.1 The Role of Immune Checkpoints in Immune Evasion

Immune checkpoints are regulatory surface molecules expressed on cell membranes that help maintain immune tolerance by signaling to immune cells that a given cell is "self" and should not be targeted. This mechanism is essential for preventing autoimmunity and maintaining immune homeostasis. However, cancer cells exploit immune checkpoints to evade immune surveillance. By overexpressing checkpoint ligands, tumor cells transmit inhibitory signals to activated T cells and NK cells, falsely presenting themselves as normal, non-threatening cells [11].

Several immune checkpoint pathways have been identified in oncology, including cytotoxic T-lymphocyte–associated protein 4 (CTLA-4), programmed death-ligand 1 (PD-L1), T-cell immunoglobulin and mucin-domain containing-3 (TIM-3), lymphocyte activation gene-3 (LAG-3), and V-domain Ig suppressor of T-cell activation (VISTA) [11]. Understanding these pathways has led to the development of immune checkpoint inhibitors—monoclonal antibodies that block checkpoint molecules or their receptors on immune cells. These therapies restore antitumor immunity by preventing inhibitory signaling, thereby allowing immune cells to recognize and eliminate cancer cells.

11.3.2 Reduced Antigen Presentation

Effector immune cells eliminate cancer cells either directly, by recognizing tumor-specific antigens, or indirectly, through interactions with antigen-presenting cells (APCs) such as dendritic cells (DCs) and macrophages. In both mechanisms, recognition of cancer-associated antigens is essential for the activation, proliferation, and cytotoxic function of effector lymphocytes. However, cancer cells have evolved immune evasion strategies to disrupt this process, primarily by impairing antigen presentation. One of the most common mechanisms involves the downregulation of major histocompatibility complex class I (MHC-I) molecules, which are required for antigen presentation to cytotoxic $CD8^+$ T cells [12]. By reducing MHC-I expression or altering antigen-processing machinery components, tumor cells escape immune detection and avoid cytolytic attack.

11.3.3 Immunosuppressive Biomolecules

In addition to immune checkpoint expression and antigen presentation downregulation, cancer cells employ cytokine-mediated suppression to inhibit activated immune responses. Under hypoxic conditions, stabilization of hypoxia-inducible factor 1 (HIF-1) in tumor cells promotes the secretion of immunosuppressive cytokines such as interleukin-10 (IL-10) and transforming growth factor-beta (TGF-β), both of which impair cytotoxic T-cell and NK cell functions [13]. Similarly, activation of the PI3K signaling pathway in tumor cells reduces the production of pro-inflammatory cytokines while further enhancing IL-10 secretion, contributing to an immunosuppressive tumor microenvironment [14]. Moreover, tumor cells can release exosomes enriched with programmed death-ligand 1 (PD-L1), which binds to PD-1 on effector T cells and suppresses their activity, thereby reinforcing immune escape [15].

11.3.4 Interplay Between Immune System and Tumor Microenvironment

The TME plays a central role in enabling cancer immune evasion by recruiting and reprogramming stromal and immune cells into immunosuppressive phenotypes. MDSCs are pivotal contributors to immune suppression; they are recruited by tumor-derived CCR2 ligands and lactate, where they inhibit T-cell and NK cell cytotoxicity, suppress DC antigen presentation, promote Treg recruitment, and induce M2-like macrophage transformation. Similarly, TAMs are reprogrammed from an M1 to an M2 phenotype by tumor-secreted IL-6, M-CSF, and PGE2. These TAMs release IL-10 and TGF-β to suppress effector immune cells and secrete CCL22 to recruit Tregs. Tregs per se accumulate in the TME in response to cancer-derived chemokines, VEGFA, and hypoxia. Tregs inhibit antitumor immunity by blocking APC–T-cell interactions, consuming IL-2 required for effector T-cell survival, and secreting suppressive mediators such as TGF-β, IL-10, and adenosine. TANs further contribute to immune evasion by forming neutrophil extracellular traps (NETs), activating KRAS/MAPK signaling, expressing PD-L1 to inhibit T cells, triggering apoptosis of cytotoxic T cells through TNF-α, and promoting angiogenesis [8].

In addition to immune cells, cancer-associated fibroblasts (CAFs) are major stromal components of the TME involved in immune escape. Activated by tumor-derived TGF-β, FGF, PDGF, IL-6, and SHH signaling, CAFs promote tumor progression by suppressing immune activity. CAFs inhibit NK cell activation, DC maturation, and cytotoxic T-cell recruitment while promoting the recruitment of TAMs, TANs, MDSCs, and Tregs [8]. Collectively, these TME components create a profoundly immunosuppressive niche that undermines antitumor immunity and facilitates tumor survival and progression.

11.3.5 Cancer Cells Improve Their Mitochondrial Content Over Immune Cells

Emerging evidence has revealed a new dimension in the crosstalk between cancer cells and immune cells, highlighting the role of mitochondrial dynamics in tumor immune evasion. In 2022, Saha et al. reported that cancer cells are capable of hijacking functional mitochondria from co-cultured T cells and natural killer (NK) cells. They demonstrated that tumor cells extend tunneling nanotubes toward immune cells, physically extracting their mitochondria to enhance tumor bioenergetics and survival [16]. Building on this discovery, Ikeda et al. (2025) showed that this interaction is bidirectional: in addition to stealing functional mitochondria, cancer cells also transfer their own damaged and metabolically exhausted mitochondria to immune cells. Moreover, tumor cells release mitophagy-inhibitory factors that prevent immune cells from clearing these dysfunctional mitochondria, leading to mitochondrial dysfunction and bioenergetic collapse in immune cells [17]. Through these mechanisms, cancer cells shift the mitochondrial balance in their favor, gaining metabolic dominance within the tumor microenvironment and suppressing antitumor immunity.

The metabolic consequences of mitochondrial hijacking are profound. By depriving immune cells of healthy mitochondria while burdening them with dysfunctional ones, cancer cells induce immune exhaustion and impair cytotoxic effector functions. Energy-depleted T cells and NK cells exhibit reduced production of interferon-γ (IFN-γ) and granzymes, compromising their ability to eliminate tumor cells [18]. Furthermore, mitochondrial stress promotes the upregulation of immune checkpoint molecules such as PD-1, Lag-3, and Tim-3 on immune cells, reinforcing their dysfunctional state [19]. As a result, cancer cells effectively evade immune surveillance while establishing a metabolically immunosuppressive microenvironment. This emerging concept of mitochondrial immune reprogramming provides a compelling new target for cancer immunometabolism-based therapies.

11.4 Immunotherapy: Current Landscape

Understanding the various strategies by which cancer cells evade the immune system has enabled the development of therapeutic approaches collectively known as immunotherapies, which are designed to empower and restore antitumor immunity. This section provides a practical overview of the major immunotherapeutic modalities currently in use or under investigation in clinical and experimental settings.

11.4.1 Immune Checkpoint Inhibitors

Immune checkpoint inhibitors (ICIs) represent one of the most transformative advances in modern oncology. Under physiological conditions, immune checkpoints such as CTLA-4, PD-1, and its ligand PD-L1 are essential for maintaining immune tolerance and preventing autoimmunity. However, cancer cells exploit these regulatory pathways to suppress cytotoxic T-cell activity and evade immune destruction. ICIs are monoclonal antibodies that block these inhibitory signals, thereby restoring T-cell–mediated antitumor immunity. CTLA-4 inhibitors (e.g., ipilimumab) act primarily at the lymph node level by enhancing T-cell priming, while PD-1/PD-L1 inhibitors (e.g., nivolumab, pembrolizumab, atezolizumab) function mainly within the TME to reinvigorate exhausted T cells [20]. ICIs have demonstrated durable clinical responses in melanoma, non-small cell lung cancer, renal cell carcinoma, colorectal cancer with mismatch repair deficiency, and many others. However, only a subset of patients responds, and immune-related adverse events such as colitis, pneumonitis, and dermatitis remain significant limitations [21]. Ongoing research aims to improve response rates through biomarker-based patient selection and combination strategies.

11.4.2 CAR-T Cell Therapy

Chimeric Antigen Receptor T-cell (CAR-T) therapy constitutes a personalized form of adoptive cell transfer that harnesses a patient's own immune system to better target cancer cells. In this approach, T cells are obtained from the patient, genetically engineered to express a synthetic receptor (i.e., CAR) that identifies a specific tumor antigen, expanded ex vivo, and reinfused into the patient. Unlike conventional T cells, CAR-T cells can recognize tumor surface antigens independent of MHC presentation, enabling them to overcome one of the key immune evasion strategies of cancer (see Sect. 11.3.2). CAR-T therapy has achieved remarkable success in hematological malignancies. However, several challenges limit their application in solid tumors, including antigen heterogeneity, T-cell exhaustion, and the immunosuppressive TME [22].

11.4.3 Cancer Vaccines

Cancer vaccines are engineered to induce the immune system activation to recognize and destroy tumor cells by presenting tumor-specific antigens to immune cells. Unlike prophylactic vaccines against viruses such as HPV and HBV, therapeutic cancer vaccines aim to treat established cancers by amplifying antigen-specific T-cell responses. There are several types of cancer vaccines: peptide-based vaccines, virus-based vaccines (virus vector-based and oncolytic virus), nucleic acid vaccines (DNA or mRNA), and cell-based vaccines (tumor cell-based and dendritic cell-based) [23]. Personalized neoantigen vaccines are an emerging approach, exploiting tumor-specific mutations to induce a targeted immune response [24]. However, cancer vaccines face limitations such as weak immunogenicity, antigen escape, and the need for combination therapies with checkpoint inhibitors or adjuvants to improve efficacy. Nevertheless, advances in genomics and mRNA technology are rapidly enhancing their clinical potential [23].

11.4.4 Emerging Approaches

In addition to established immunotherapies, several innovative strategies are advancing toward clinical application. Bispecific antibodies simultaneously bind a tumor antigen and a T cell receptor, such as CD3, physically redirecting cytotoxic T cells to kill tumor cells independent of MHC recognition [25]. TCR-engineered T cells offer another strategy by modifying T cells to express high-affinity T-cell receptors capable of recognizing intracellular antigens presented on MHC molecules, expanding therapeutic targets beyond cell-surface proteins [26]. Adoptive NK cell therapy implements allogeneic or engineered NK cells to overcome tumor immune evasion with minimal adverse effects like graft-versus-host disease (GVHD) and cytokine release syndrome [27]. These emerging therapies aim to overcome resistance to conventional immunotherapies and expand treatment options for solid tumors.

11.5 Immunometabolic Interactions in Cancer

This section describes how cancer cells adapt to the harsh conditions of the TME and how these stresses create opportunities for tumor cells to evade activated immune cells more effectively.

11.5.1 Tumor Microenvironment: A Metabolic Battleground

The TME represents a metabolically harsh ecosystem shaped by hypoxia, nutrient deprivation, and accumulation of lactate, leading to acidosis. These features are due to rapidly proliferating tumor cells, outpacing the development of the vascular network, that results in regions of marked hypoxia, nutrient scarcity, and extracellular acidosis [28]. These conditions provide several benefits for cancer cells, ultimately resulting in tumor progression, metabolic reprogramming, treatment resistance, and immune escape.

Among these factors, hypoxia is a major determinant of metabolic adaptation. Secondary to hypoxia, stabilization of HIFs induces a metabolic shift from OXPHOS to glycolysis, ensuring ATP generation under hypoxic conditions [29]. Hypoxia not only enhances tumor survival but also promotes angiogenesis, epithelial–mesenchymal transition, metastasis, and treatment resistance [30]. In parallel, loss of nutrients, particularly glucose and glutamine, forces cancer cells to adopt alternative energy sources such as fatty acid oxidation (FAO) and to activate catabolic pathways like autophagy [31]. In addition, as stated in Sect. 11.3.5, cancer cells can provide their ATP by hijacking mitochondria from adjacent immune cells [16]. These adaptations enable cancer cells to scavenge nutrients from the extracellular matrix and necrotic cells, maintaining biosynthesis and redox balance despite metabolic stress. Another defining metabolic feature of the TME is acidosis, resulting from increased lactate export due to elevated glycolysis and overexpression of specific proton transporters [32]. Acidosis can promote tumor invasion by degrading the extracellular matrix [33] and enhancing chemoresistance [34]. One remarkable outcome of metabolic heterogeneity in tumors is the emergence of *metabolic symbiosis* between cancer cell subpopulations. In this strategy, hypoxic tumor regions secrete large amounts of lactate due to upregulated glycolysis. This lactate is not only a waste product for cancer cells, but also it is taken up by normoxic tumor cells through specific transporters and used as a carbon source in the tricarboxylic acid (TCA) cycle. This strategy is also called the *lactate shuttle* in the literature [35].

Beyond supporting tumor cell adaptation, hypoxia, nutrient shortage, and acidosis collectively dampen activated immune cells, which require physiologic conditions for their proper actions [36]. In addition, hypoxia induces expression of PD-L1 on cancer cells [37], and drives the recruitment of immunosuppressive MDSCs [38] and Tregs [39], and promotes the polarization of TAMs toward an antiinflammatory M2 phenotype [40]. These effects can further suppress the antitumor immune system (see Sect. 11.3.4).

Collectively, these metabolic constraints create a hostile immune landscape that favors cancer immune evasion. Therefore, the TME is not only a metabolic battleground that shapes tumor evolution but also a central regulator of immune suppression, offering critical opportunities for therapeutic intervention via metabolic reprogramming.

11.5.2 Cancer Cells Metabolic Rewiring

Cancer cells are not static entities; they evolve dynamically throughout tumor progression by acquiring new genetic and phenotypic traits. This gradual evolution, known as *malignant transformation*, results in intratumoral heterogeneity, where tumor masses consist of cancer cells with diverse behaviors, phenotypes, and treatment sensitivities [41].

In 2000, Hanahan and Weinberg described a set of biological capabilities acquired during tumor development, calling them the *Hallmarks of Cancer*. The first six classical hallmarks include: self-sufficiency in growth signals, insensitivity to anti-growth signals, evasion of apoptosis, sustained angiogenesis, limitless replicative potential, and tissue invasion and metastasis [42]. These hallmarks summarize the essential processes cancer cells must acquire to initiate and sustain malignant growth. With advances in cancer research, this framework expanded. In 2011, four emerging hallmarks were added: genome instability, tumor-promoting inflammation, deregulated cellular energetics (altered metabolism), and immune evasion

[43]. In 2022, Douglas Hanahan proposed an updated model, incorporating non-mutational epigenetic reprogramming, phenotypic plasticity, cellular senescence, and the influence of polymorphic microbes, reflecting deeper mechanistic understanding of cancer biology [44].

Figure 11.1 illustrates the main events that happen during malignant transformation. During early malignant transformation, cancer cells reside in a nutrient-rich and oxygenated environment. At this stage, they primarily depend on OXPHOS to generate biosynthetic precursors, including amino acids, fatty acids, and nucleotides, required for rapid proliferation. As tumors grow, the imbalance between cellular demand and nutrient supply leads to hypoxia, acidosis, and metabolic stress within the TME. To survive, cancer cells shift toward aerobic glycolysis (the Warburg effect), allowing continued proliferation despite low oxygen availability. This metabolic switch is driven by HIF-1, which activates gene programs that promote glycolysis, angiogenesis, and survival [41].

As cancer progresses, some tumor cells undergo epithelial–mesenchymal transition (EMT), gaining invasive and migratory ability necessary for metastasis—one of the original six hallmarks of cancer. EMT is controlled by transcription factors such as Snail, Twist, and ZEB, many of which are induced by HIF-1, linking metabolic stress to metastatic potential. EMT also contributes to the emergence of cancer stem cells (CSCs), a subpopulation with enhanced self-renewal and therapy resistance. These CSCs exhibit metabolic plasticity, switching between glycolysis and

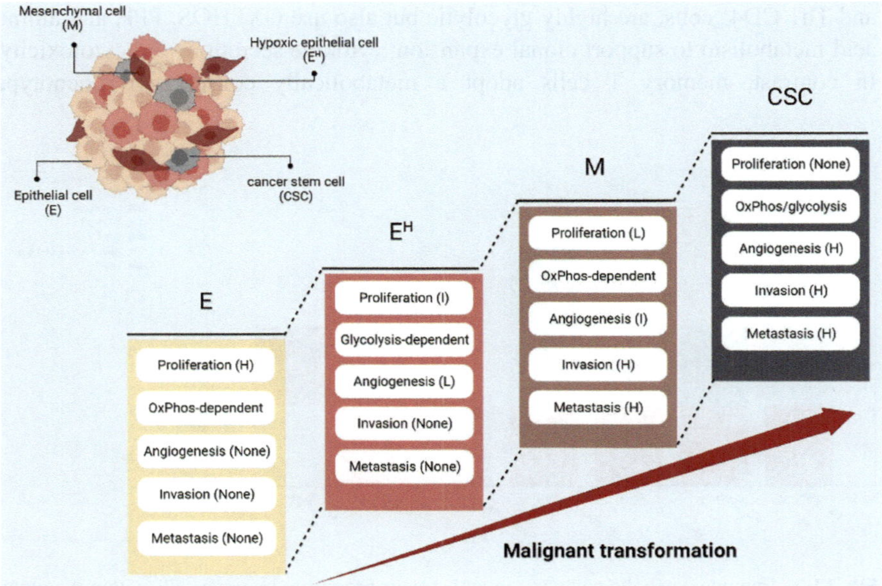

Fig. 11.1 Evolution of cancer metabolism and capabilities during malignant transformation. CSC indicates cancer stem cells, E epithelial cancer cells at normoxia, E^H epithelial cancer cells at hypoxia, H high-level, I intermediate-level, L low-level, M mesenchymal cancer cells. (Source: [41] under CC BY 4.0)

OXPHOS depending on environmental conditions, allowing survival under fluctuating nutrient and oxygen levels [41].

In summary, malignant transformation is a stepwise evolutionary process in which cancer cells progressively acquire the classical and emerging hallmarks of cancer. These changes enhance survival, invasion, metastasis, and therapy resistance, emphasizing the importance of integrating metabolic targeting and immunotherapy in cancer treatment strategies.

11.5.3 Immune Cells Metabolic Reprogramming

It has been demonstrated that various anti- and pro-tumorigenic immune cells have various metabolisms, responding to their specific actions in the TME. This section outlines various metabolisms in the immune cells (Fig. 11.2).

Antitumor immune cells depend on certain metabolic programs that support their cytotoxic and inflammatory functions within the TME. For example, NK cells utilize both glycolysis and oxidative phosphorylation (OXPHOS) to fuel their rapid production of perforin, granzymes, TNF, and IFN-γ during MHC-independent tumor cell killing. Similarly, M1-type macrophages rely predominantly on aerobic glycolysis and the pentose phosphate pathway (PPP) to sustain high rates of pro-inflammatory cytokine production (IL-1β, TNF) and ROS generation. DCs preferentially rely on glycolysis, which supports their antigen processing and migration into lymphoid tissues. Effector T cells, including cytotoxic $CD8^+$ T lymphocytes and Th1 $CD4^+$ cells, are highly glycolytic but also use OXPHOS, PPP, and amino acid metabolism to support clonal expansion, cytokine secretion, and cytotoxicity. In contrast, memory T cells adopt a metabolically conservative phenotype

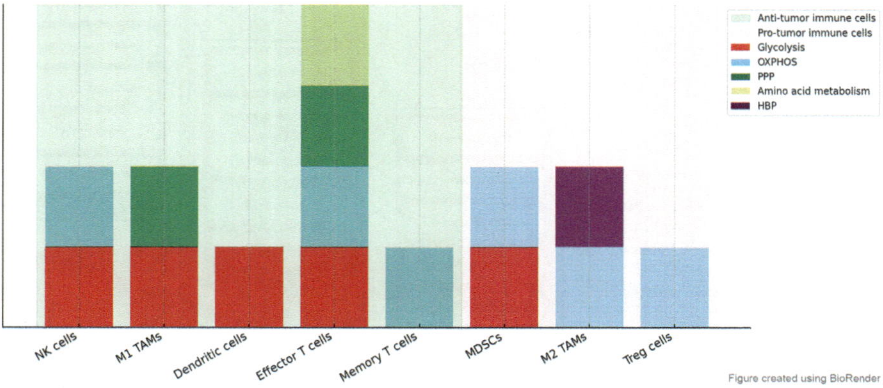

Fig. 11.2 Immunometabolic pathways in anti- versus pro-tumor immune cells within the tumor microenvironment. (Figure created using BioRender)

dominated by OXPHOS, which enables long-term survival, self-renewal, and rapid secondary immune responses. Overall, antitumor immune cells exhibit metabolic flexibility but predominantly utilize glycolysis and mitochondrial respiration to sustain robust anticancer functions in nutrient-limited and hypoxic tumor settings [45].

In contrast, pro-tumor immune cells adopt metabolic strategies that promote immune suppression and support tumor progression. MDSCs concurrently exploit glycolysis and OXPHOS to generate immunosuppressive mediators such as polyamines and kynurenine that inhibit T cell proliferation. Immunosuppressive TAMs rely primarily on OXPHOS and the hexosamine biosynthetic pathway (HBP), a glucose-derived anabolic route that supports tissue remodeling, angiogenesis, and tumor growth through VEGF and IL-10 production. Tregs are also key suppressors of antitumor immunity and depend almost exclusively on OXPHOS, allowing them to survive and function in hypoxic tumor regions. Together, these pro-tumor immune cells create a metabolically hostile environment for cytotoxic lymphocytes, reinforcing tumor immune evasion and resistance to immunotherapy [45].

11.5.4 The Battle for Energy: Mitochondria in Cancer–Immune Interactions

Cancer cells continuously adapt their metabolic landscape to support uncontrolled proliferation, survival under stress, and resistance to immune attack. A pivotal component of this adaptation is their ability to enhance mitochondrial fitness. To secure sufficient bioenergetic and biosynthetic capacity, cancer cells employ multiple strategies to increase both the quantity and quality of their mitochondria, as described below.

One strategy involves acquiring mitochondria from the surrounding TME components. Cancer cells have been shown to import functional mitochondria from tumor-infiltrating neurons [46], adjacent tumor cells [47], and CAFs [48], boosting their oxidative metabolism and survival under stress conditions. Additionally, as noted in Sect. 11.3.5, cancer cells can directly hijack mitochondria from immune cells and export their own damaged mitochondria into immune cells, impairing their metabolic fitness [16, 17]. Furthermore, immune checkpoint signaling, particularly PD-1/PD-L1 engagement, has been shown to suppress mitochondrial function in T cells [49]. Beyond these competitive interactions, cancer cells intrinsically enhance their mitochondrial capacity by upregulating key regulators of mitochondrial biogenesis and dynamics. Transcriptional coactivators such as PGC-1α stimulate mitochondrial generation, while proteins like mitofusin (MFN1/2) promote mitochondrial fusion, improving respiratory efficiency and stress tolerance [50, 51]. Collectively, these mitochondrial strategies allow cancer cells to secure a bioenergetic advantage over immune cells, promoting tumor survival, immune evasion, and therapy resistance.

11.6 Proposed Therapeutic Strategy: Acid-Sensitive Immunomodulatory Nanoliposomes for Targeted Cancer Therapy

Despite significant progress in cancer treatment, therapeutic resistance and immune evasion remain major challenges, largely due to the protective and suppressive nature of the TME. Tumors create a hostile metabolic and immunological barrier, often likened to a fortified "castle," where cancer cells are shielded by immunosuppressive stromal components and acidic conditions. To overcome this challenge, we propose a two-phase nanotherapeutic strategy using pH-sensitive liposomal delivery systems engineered to selectively release their cargo within the acidic TME, thus maximizing tumor specificity while minimizing systemic toxicity.

11.6.1 Phase I: Disruption of the Tumor Protective Barrier

In the first step, we aim to design acid-sensitive liposomes encapsulating chemotherapeutic agents. Due to their engineered sensitivity to low pH, these liposomes remain stable in physiological conditions (pH 7.4) but dissolve selectively in the acidic TME (pH ~6.5). This controlled release enables localized cytotoxicity, effectively disrupting the tumor frontline by eliminating stromal support cells, tumor-associated fibroblasts, and immunosuppressive myeloid cells. By weakening the physical and metabolic defenses of the tumor, this step primes the microenvironment for subsequent immune intervention.

11.6.2 Phase II: Immune Reinforcement at Frontline and Tumor Eradication

Following tumor debulking and stromal disruption, the second stage introduces a series of acid-sensitive immunomodulatory liposomes designed to fortify antitumor immunity. These liposomes will deliver a synergistic combination of: (1) an STING agonist: to activate innate immune signaling and promote robust type I interferon (IFN) responses, enhancing antigen presentation and immune activation; (2) Idebenone: to support mitochondrial OXPHOS in T cells and NK cells, restoring metabolic fitness and preventing immune exhaustion within the TME; (3) an anti-PD-1 antibody: to block inhibitory checkpoint signaling, restoring T-cell recognition and cytotoxicity against cancer cells.

This two-phase strategy integrates precise tumor targeting with immune reactivation, transforming the TME from immunosuppressive to immunologically permissive. By combining chemotherapeutic debulking with metabolic and immune reprogramming, this approach is expected to promote durable antitumor responses and prevent tumor relapse.

11.7 Conclusions

Cancer progression is strongly affected by metabolic changes that help tumor cells survive and escape immune control. In the TME, cancer cells compete with immune cells for energy sources such as glucose and amino acids. By rewiring their metabolism, cancer cells gain a survival advantage while suppressing the function of antitumor immune cells. They also use additional strategies, such as immune checkpoint activation, reduced antigen presentation, and mitochondrial hijacking, to evade immune responses and promote resistance to different therapies. Targeting these metabolic mechanisms has become an important area in cancer research. Therapies that restore the metabolic fitness of T cells and NK cells, or block tumor-specific metabolic pathways, may improve the effectiveness of current immunotherapies. Combining metabolic intervention with immune activation may provide a more powerful and durable treatment strategy for cancer in the future.

References

1. Makowski L, Chaib M, Rathmell JC. Immunometabolism: from basic mechanisms to translation. Immunol Rev. 2020;295(1):5–14. https://doi.org/10.1111/imr.12858.
2. Khodaei T, Inamdar S, Suresh AP, Acharya AP. Drug delivery for metabolism targeted cancer immunotherapy. Adv Drug Deliv Rev. 2022;184:114242. https://doi.org/10.1016/j.addr.2022.114242.
3. Pandya PH, Murray ME, Pollok KE, Renbarger JL. The immune system in cancer pathogenesis: potential therapeutic approaches. J Immunol Res. 2016;2016:4273943. https://doi.org/10.1155/2016/4273943.
4. Boustani J, Grapin M, Laurent P-A, Apetoh L, Mirjolet C. The 6th R of radiobiology: reactivation of anti-tumor immune response. Cancers (Basel). 2019;11(6):860. https://doi.org/10.3390/cancers11060860.
5. Xu Y, Zhang A, Liu A, Hu Q. Clinical analysis of immune reconstitution after chemotherapy in children with acute lymphoblastic leukemia. BMC Pediatr. 2024;24(1):557. https://doi.org/10.1186/s12887-024-05030-4.
6. Koury J, et al. Immunotherapies: exploiting the immune system for cancer treatment. J Immunol Res. 2018;2018:9585614. https://doi.org/10.1155/2018/9585614.
7. Munhoz RR, Postow MA. Recent advances in understanding antitumor immunity. F1000Res. 2016;5:2545. https://doi.org/10.12688/f1000research.9356.1.
8. Taghizadeh-Hesary F. 'Reinforcement' by tumor microenvironment: the seventh 'R' of radiobiology. Int J Radiat Oncol Biol Phys. 2024;119(3):727–33. https://doi.org/10.1016/j.ijrobp.2023.09.027.
9. Ribatti D. Mast cells and resistance to immunotherapy in cancer. Arch Immunol Ther Exp. 2023;71(1):11. https://doi.org/10.1007/s00005-023-00676-x.
10. Ghaffari S, Rezaei N. Eosinophils in the tumor microenvironment: implications for cancer immunotherapy. J Transl Med. 2023;21(1):551. https://doi.org/10.1186/s12967-023-04418-7.
11. Zamani MR, Šácha P. Immune checkpoint inhibitors in cancer therapy: what lies beyond monoclonal antibodies? Med Oncol. 2025;42(7):273. https://doi.org/10.1007/s12032-025-02822-1.
12. He X, Xu C. Immune checkpoint signaling and cancer immunotherapy. Cell Res. 2020;30(8):660–9. https://doi.org/10.1038/s41422-020-0343-4.

13. You L, et al. The role of hypoxia-inducible factor 1 in tumor immune evasion. Med Res Rev. 2021;41(3):1622–43. https://doi.org/10.1002/med.21771.
14. Sun P, Meng L. Emerging roles of class I PI3K inhibitors in modulating tumor microenvironment and immunity. Acta Pharmacol Sin. 2020;41(11):1395–402. https://doi.org/10.1038/s41401-020-00500-8.
15. Chen G, et al. Exosomal PD-L1 contributes to immunosuppression and is associated with anti-PD-1 response. Nature. 2018;560(7718):382–6. https://doi.org/10.1038/s41586-018-0392-8.
16. Saha T, et al. Intercellular nanotubes mediate mitochondrial trafficking between cancer and immune cells. Nat Nanotechnol. 2022;17(1):98–106. https://doi.org/10.1038/s41565-021-01000-4.
17. Ikeda H, et al. Immune evasion through mitochondrial transfer in the tumour microenvironment. Nature. 2025;638(8049):225–36. https://doi.org/10.1038/s41586-024-08439-0.
18. Jiang Y, Li Y, Zhu B. T-cell exhaustion in the tumor microenvironment. Cell Death Dis. 2015;6(6):–e1792. https://doi.org/10.1038/cddis.2015.162.
19. Wu H, et al. Mitochondrial dysfunction promotes the transition of precursor to terminally exhausted T cells through HIF-1α-mediated glycolytic reprogramming. Nat Commun. 2023;14(1):6858. https://doi.org/10.1038/s41467-023-42634-3.
20. Buchbinder EI, Desai A. CTLA-4 and PD-1 pathways: similarities, differences, and implications of their inhibition. Am J Clin Oncol. 2016;39(1):98–106. https://doi.org/10.1097/COC.0000000000000239.
21. Petrelli F, et al. Immune checkpoint inhibitors beyond progression in various solid tumors: a systematic review and pooled analysis. JCM. 2025;14(18):6680. https://doi.org/10.3390/jcm14186680.
22. Du B, Qin J, Lin B, Zhang J, Li D, Liu M. CAR-T therapy in solid tumors. Cancer Cell. 2025;43(4):665–79. https://doi.org/10.1016/j.ccell.2025.03.019.
23. Wang C, Hao P. Therapeutic vaccine strategies in cancer: advances, challenges, and future directions. Clin Cancer Bull. 2025;4(1):10. https://doi.org/10.1007/s44272-025-00039-x.
24. Yarchoan M, et al. Personalized neoantigen vaccine and pembrolizumab in advanced hepatocellular carcinoma: a phase 1/2 trial. Nat Med. 2024;30(4):1044–53. https://doi.org/10.1038/s41591-024-02894-y.
25. Middelburg J, et al. T-cell stimulating vaccines empower CD3 bispecific antibody therapy in solid tumors. Nat Commun. 2024;15(1):48. https://doi.org/10.1038/s41467-023-44308-6.
26. Eggebø MS, et al. TCR-engineered T cells targeting a shared β-catenin mutation eradicate solid tumors. Nat Immunol. 2025;26(10):1726–36. https://doi.org/10.1038/s41590-025-02252-1.
27. Rady M, Mostafa M, Dida G, Sabet F, Abou-Aisha K, Watzl C. Adoptive NK cell therapy in AML: progress and challenges. Clin Exp Med. 2025;25(1):41. https://doi.org/10.1007/s10238-025-01559-5.
28. Shi R, Tang Y-Q, Miao H. Metabolism in tumor microenvironment: implications for cancer immunotherapy. Med Comm (2020). 2020;1(1):47–68. https://doi.org/10.1002/mco2.6.
29. Zeng Y, et al. Advances in the mechanisms of HIF-1α-enhanced tumor glycolysis and its relation to dedifferentiation. Prog Biophys Mol Biol. 2025;197:1–10. https://doi.org/10.1016/j.pbiomolbio.2025.05.003.
30. Devi D, et al. Hypoxia-driven metabolic and molecular reprogramming: from tumor microenvironment to therapeutic interventions. Pathol Res Pract. 2025;276:156271. https://doi.org/10.1016/j.prp.2025.156271.
31. Lee H, Woo SM, Jang H, Kang M, Kim S-Y. Cancer depends on fatty acids for ATP production: a possible link between cancer and obesity. Semin Cancer Biol. 2022;86:347–57. https://doi.org/10.1016/j.semcancer.2022.07.005.
32. Wang Z-H, Peng W-B, Zhang P, Yang X-P, Zhou Q. Lactate in the tumour microenvironment: from immune modulation to therapy. EBioMedicine. 2021;73:103627. https://doi.org/10.1016/j.ebiom.2021.103627.

33. Gatenby RA, Gawlinski ET, Gmitro AF, Kaylor B, Gillies RJ. Acid-mediated tumor invasion: a multidisciplinary study. Cancer Res. 2006;66(10):5216–23. https://doi.org/10.1158/0008-5472.CAN-05-4193.
34. Wojtkowiak JW, Verduzco D, Schramm KJ, Gillies RJ. Drug resistance and cellular adaptation to tumor acidic pH microenvironment. Mol Pharm. 2011;8(6):2032–8. https://doi.org/10.1021/mp200292c.
35. Fiaschi T, et al. Reciprocal metabolic reprogramming through lactate shuttle coordinately influences tumor-stroma interplay. Cancer Res. 2012;72(19):5130–40. https://doi.org/10.1158/0008-5472.CAN-12-1949.
36. Damgaci S, Ibrahim-Hashim A, Enriquez-Navas PM, Pilon-Thomas S, Guvenis A, Gillies RJ. Hypoxia and acidosis: immune suppressors and therapeutic targets. Immunology. 2018;154(3):354–62. https://doi.org/10.1111/imm.12917.
37. Yu Y, et al. Hypoxia upregulates the expression of PD-L1 via NPM1 in breast cancer. J Immunother Cancer. 2025;13(6):e010151. https://doi.org/10.1136/jitc-2024-010151.
38. Chiu DK-C, et al. Hypoxia inducible factor HIF-1 promotes myeloid-derived suppressor cells accumulation through ENTPD2/CD39L1 in hepatocellular carcinoma. Nat Commun. 2017;8(1):517. https://doi.org/10.1038/s41467-017-00530-7.
39. Yan M, et al. Recruitment of regulatory T cells is correlated with hypoxia-induced CXCR4 expression, and is associated with poor prognosis in basal-like breast cancers. Breast Cancer Res. 2011;13(2):R47. https://doi.org/10.1186/bcr2869.
40. Goswami KK, Banerjee S, Bose A, Baral R. Lactic acid in alternative polarization and function of macrophages in tumor microenvironment. Hum Immunol. 2022;83(5):409–17. https://doi.org/10.1016/j.humimm.2022.02.007.
41. Taghizadeh-Hesary F, Ghadyani M, Kashanchi F, Behnam B. Exploring TSGA10 function: a crosstalk or controlling mechanism in the signaling pathway of carcinogenesis? Cancers (Basel). 2024;16(17):3044. https://doi.org/10.3390/cancers16173044.
42. Hanahan D, Weinberg RA. The hallmarks of cancer. Cell. 2000;100(1):57–70. https://doi.org/10.1016/s0092-8674(00)81683-9.
43. Hanahan D, Weinberg RA. Hallmarks of cancer: the next generation. Cell. 2011;144(5):646–74. https://doi.org/10.1016/j.cell.2011.02.013.
44. Hanahan D. Hallmarks of cancer: new dimensions. Cancer Discov. 2022;12(1):31–46. https://doi.org/10.1158/2159-8290.CD-21-1059.
45. Leone RD, Powell JD. Metabolism of immune cells in cancer. Nat Rev Cancer. 2020;20(9):516–31. https://doi.org/10.1038/s41568-020-0273-y.
46. Hoover G, et al. Nerve-to-cancer transfer of mitochondria during cancer metastasis. Nature. 2025;644(8075):252–62. https://doi.org/10.1038/s41586-025-09176-8.
47. Lu J, et al. Tunneling nanotubes promote intercellular mitochondria transfer followed by increased invasiveness in bladder cancer cells. Oncotarget. 2017;8(9):15539–52. https://doi.org/10.18632/oncotarget.14695.
48. Goliwas KF, et al. Mitochondrial transfer from cancer-associated fibroblasts increases migration in aggressive breast cancer. J Cell Sci. 2023;136(14):jcs260419. https://doi.org/10.1242/jcs.260419.
49. Chamoto K, et al. Mitochondrial activation chemicals synergize with surface receptor PD-1 blockade for T cell-dependent antitumor activity. Proc Natl Acad Sci USA. 2017;114(5):E761–70. https://doi.org/10.1073/pnas.1620433114.
50. Andrzejewski S, et al. PGC-1α promotes breast cancer metastasis and confers bioenergetic flexibility against metabolic drugs. Cell Metab. 2017;26(5):778–87.e5. https://doi.org/10.1016/j.cmet.2017.09.006.
51. Purohit PK, Edwards R, Tokatlidis K, Saini N. MiR-195 regulates mitochondrial function by targeting mitofusin-2 in breast cancer cells. RNA Biol. 2019;16(7):918–29. https://doi.org/10.1080/15476286.2019.1600999.

Tools and Technologies for Studying Cancer Metabolism

12

Ayush Madan, Subhajit Mandal, Soukat Chandra, Joy Das, and Biplab Debnath

12.1 Introduction

The study of cancer metabolism is now a viable discipline using which sweeping conclusions can be made about the molecular aspects of cancer development, growth, and resistance to therapy [1]. Compared to normal cells, the cancer cells are highly reprogrammed in metabolism so that they can sustain their proliferating nature, to adjust to the conditions of nutrient depletion as well as cell death pathways. Such changes include a sequence of biochemical events, which incorporate the process of glycolysis up-regulation (Warburg effect), restructuring and maladaptation of metabolic activities of lipids and amino acids, and imbalanced mitochondrion work [2]. It is in this respect that the understanding of the complex metabolic networks that are facilitative of malignant change is therefore of invaluable importance in meeting the need for effective therapeutic treatment and potential diagnostic or prognostic biomarkers. The latest advances in experimental and analytical methods have immensely augmented the opportunities for scrutinizing the metabolism of cancer at varying ranges of organization between subcellular organelles and the whole body [3]. The available technology in the past could not allow the studies that could have been carried out in the field because of the capabilities and the resolution of the technology. The classic biochemical assays are felt

A. Madan
Department of Biotechnology, School of Research and Technology, People's University, Bhopal, Madhya Pradesh, India

S. Mandal
Department of Pharmaceutical Sciences, Faculty of Science and Engineering, Dibrugarh University, Dibrugarh, Assam, India

S. Chandra · B. Debnath (✉)
Department of Pharmaceutical Technology, Bharat Technology, Uluberia, West Bengal, India

J. Das
School of Pharmaceutical Sciences, Lovely Professional University, Phagwara, Punjab, India

S. Ashique et al. (eds.), *Cancer Metabolism*, Cancer Treatment and Research 195, https://doi.org/10.1007/978-3-032-21861-2_12

to be basic but in the majority of situations cannot indicate the dynamic and context-based nature of the metabolic pathways in tumors [4]. High-resolution imaging platforms, stable isotope labeling, high-throughput genomic and transcriptomic technologies and computational modeling technologies have transformed the metabolic research domain [5]. The developments enable an accurate quantification of the fluxes of metabolic processes and real-time imaging of cellular pathway events and the detection of metabolic heterogeneity in sub-populations of tumors and the microenvironment. Selection and optimization of the test objects is one of the key aspects of the process of development of the science of cancer metabolism. The in vitro two-dimensional (2D) cell cultures offer a high level of control over dissection of specific signaling pathways, but do not recapitulate tumor structure as extensively as in vivo [6]. The spatial arrangement, nutrient gradients, and cell-cell interactions within tumors are vastly better represented using three-dimensional (3D) cultures (spheroids and organoids), making these well-positioned to exhibit a better physiological relation [7]. Added to these mechanisms are the high state-of-the-art metabolic assessment tools such as Seahorse XF Analyzer, which may be employed in order to real-time monitor the rate of oxygen consumption as well as the real-time extracellular acidification and, thus, provide dynamic information about the bioenergetics of the cells. The models in vivo are extremely valuable to comprehend the overall complexity of the cancer metabolism within the natural environment. The weighty models to investigate the metabolic dependencies are the application of genetically engineered mouse models (GEMMs) and patient-derived xenografts (PDXs) pertaining to the influence of systemic factors, mealtime, and stromal contributions [8]. These systems would be further reinforced by in vivo isotope tracing in which stable isotopically labeled substrates would be introduced to animals, with which the metabolic fluxes in living beings could be mapped. Such strategies allow bridging the gap between the in vitro and clinical observations. The second technological field that has been disruptive insofar as the research on cancer metabolism is concerned is the field of imaging technologies. Positron emission tomography (PET) can be utilized with any computed tomography (CT) or magnetic resonance imaging (MRI) that makes it possible to visualize metabolic alterations in tumors in a noninvasive manner [9]. Radiolabeled tracers, particularly ^{18}F-fluorodeoxyglucose (FDG), are commonly used for tumor detection, assessment of tumor metabolism, and monitoring therapeutic response, and are often employed as clinical endpoints in imaging studies [10]. The magnetic resonance spectroscopy (MRS) goes a step higher since it gives chemical information about the presence of metabolites in tissues and gives an insight into the biochemical literature of cancer in vivo.

This together with genomic and transcriptomic approaches brings in the add-on of a powerful molecular dimension to the science of metabolism. RNA-seq and single-cell RNA-seq enable studying the metabolic gene expression at large scale in inter- and intratumor heterogeneity [11]. The ability is remarkable, especially in the identification of subpopulations of metabolism that can result in resistance to treatment. Meanwhile, it is now possible to directly control the metabolism enzymes using genome-editing technologies, such as mediated technology referred to as

CRISPR/Cas9, to discover their role in tumor development, invasion, and treatment response [12]. The complexity of cancer metabolism cannot be deconstructed using the limited set of tools, but integrated and coherent analytical methodologies are required, which have the capability to harmonize the different datasets in mechanistic descriptions and coordinate predictions. GEMs and flux balance analysis (FBA) have become part of the basic tools that computational and systems biology tools have provided. The behavior of metabolism networks can be simulated using these models and predicted pathway susceptibilities, and create specific interventions [13]. Redo experimental measures and insert them into computational models to increase prediction of them, which could be applied to research based on hypotheses and guide the creation of treatments. Such a sub-categorization of the organelle-specific metabolic processes is a highly significant dead-end in the field. Co-optation as well as reprogram may each be found in cancer, as the mitochondria, lysosomes, peroxisomes, endoplasmic reticulum, etc., all exhibit a metabolic function that is correlated and diverse [14]. As this is accompanied by the emergence of new processes in subcellular imaging, now with an ability to target the metabolomics and spatial proteomics, it is not only possible to deal with them with the precision never experienced before [15]. These organelle-centric researchers are not merely interested in the perception of the fundamental concepts in tumor biology, but also in identifying potential sources of focused treatment intervention. All these tools and technologies are stirring our understanding of the role that metabolic pathways must play in facilitating cancer hallmarks and what implications these may have on clinical outcomes. The possibility of visualizing metabolic activity between the molecular and organismal scales, with the ability to maintain spatial and temporal resolution, has offered the abilities needed by the scientists to analyze tumor metabolism in a complete set of tools.

Despite such milestones, huge challenges occur. To a great extent, the metabolism of tumors is context and genetic inheritance-sensitive, as well as being micro-environmentally dependent and therapeutic forces-sensitive [16]. Capturing this dynamic complexity requires continual refinement of experimental systems, expansion of computational models, and integration of multi-omics datasets. Emerging technologies promise to address some of these limitations by enabling real-time, spatially resolved, and longitudinal monitoring of metabolic processes in preclinical and clinical settings [17]. This chapter provides a systematic overview of the current tools and technologies employed to study cancer metabolism. Beginning with in vitro techniques, it examines the capabilities and limitations of various culture systems, isotope tracing methods, and metabolic flux analysis (MFA) platforms. It then addresses in vivo models and imaging strategies that bridge laboratory findings to physiological contexts. The discussion extends to genomic and transcriptomic tools for profiling metabolic gene expression, genome-editing approaches for functional interrogation, and computational frameworks for modeling metabolic networks. Special attention is given to methods for organelle-specific metabolism analysis, highlighting emerging opportunities and technical considerations. Finally, the chapter concludes with future perspectives on integrating these diverse methodologies to accelerate translational advances in cancer metabolism research.

12.2 In-Vitro Technologies for Cancer Metabolism Research

In vitro experimental systems form the cornerstone of cancer metabolism research, enabling controlled interrogation of metabolic pathways under defined conditions [18]. These platforms allow precise manipulation of environmental variables, genetic backgrounds, and nutrient availability, thereby facilitating mechanistic studies of metabolic reprogramming in cancer cells. Over the past decade, the scope and sophistication of in vitro technologies have expanded considerably, providing increasingly physiologically relevant models and analytical capabilities. A comparative summary of key in vitro tools, their features, applications, and limitations is provided in Table 12.1.

Table 12.1 Comparative overview of in vitro tools and technologies for studying cancer metabolism

Tool/ model	Key features	Primary applications	Advantages	Limitations	Sources
2D cell cultures	Monolayer growth on flat surfaces; easy to handle	Fundamental metabolic assays, drug screening	High reproducibility, cost-effective, compatible with high-throughput analysis	Lacks tumor architecture and microenvironment	[19, 20]
3D spheroids	Multicellular aggregates with nutrient/ oxygen gradients	Tumor microenvironment modeling, hypoxia studies	Mimics in vivo gradients, more physiologically relevant than 2D	Limited genetic diversity, less standardized	[21]
Organoids	Self-organizing 3D structures from stem cells or tumor tissue	Patient-specific metabolism studies, personalized therapy testing	Maintains genetic/ phenotypic fidelity, models heterogeneity	Requires specialized culture conditions, costly	[22]
Stable isotope tracing	Incorporation of ^{13}C or ^{15}N into substrates	Metabolic flux mapping, pathway quantification	High precision, direct pathway tracking	Requires advanced MS/ NMR instrumentation	[23]
Metabolic flux analysis (MFA)	Computational interpretation of isotope data	Quantitative pathway analysis	Enables identification of metabolic bottlenecks	Dependent on accurate model assumptions	[24]
Seahorse XF analyzer	Real-time OCR and ECAR measurements	Bioenergetic profiling, mitochondrial function analysis	Dynamic, noninvasive, small sample requirement	Limited metabolite coverage, specialized equipment	[25]

12.2.1 Cell Culture Systems

The cell culture models are invaluable in the dissection of metabolic processes in cancer. The traditional 2D monolayer cultures, where cells are cultured on flat glass or plastic surfaces, provide the convenience of manipulation and allow throughput as well as reproducibility. Such models have been instrumental in the explanation of the underlying problems of tumor cell metabolism, including glycolytic changes, mitochondrial changes, and lipid synthesis. However, 2D cultures inherently lack the spatial architecture, nutrient gradient, and cell-cell or cell-extracellular matrix (ECM) that tumors experience, and restrict their use in translation [19].

Such limitations can be mitigated by the 3D culture system (e.g., multicellular spheroids, organoids), which is more effective at recapitulating the tumor microenvironment [20]. The cancer cells are capable of self-assembly into the shape of a spheroid that generates oxygen and nutrient gradients similar to that of a solid tumor and acts as such, triggering metabolism phenotype alterations that cannot be identified in 2D systems [21]. Even more progressive models are organoids, which are generated based on tumor tissues or pluripotent stem cells and maintain major histological and genetic features of the tissue of origin [22]. These systems allow examination of intratumoral metabolic heterogeneity and therapeutic response in a physiologically relevant environment, and therefore, they are of great importance in the context of translational research.

12.2.2 Stable Isotope Tracing

It has been demonstrated that stable isotope tracing is a powerful technique for mapping metabolic fluxes of cancerous cells. By incorporating nonradioactive isotopes like ^{13}C or ^{15}N into some metabolic substrates (e.g., glucose, glutamine, or fatty acids), it could then be followed by mass spectrometry (MS) or NMR spectroscopy in an interconnected manner by examining the isotope or its constituents (i.e., carbon and hydrogen on a specific position of the molecule).

An example is the use of labeled glucose (^{13}C), which can also indicate glycolytic activity, involvement or inactivity of the TCA cycle, and the production of biosynthetic hairpins, whereas the populations of nitrogen-tagged amino acids can be used to map the contribution of nitrogen to nucleotides (and other macromolecules). The method offers direct and quantitative data concerning the use of pathways in different conditions such as oncogene misuse, malnutrition, and pharmaceutical treatment [23, 26].

Isotope tracing variation of MFA that employs computational models to understand the representation of isotopomer distributions to give good quantitative estimates of the activity of a pathway. Foreseen together with perturbation experiments or genetic manipulations, MFA allows the identification of rate-limiting enzymes and possible weak points in the metabolism of cancer cells [24].

12.2.3 Seahorse XF Analyzer

Seahorse XF Analyzer can now become an indispensable component of real-time bioenergetic measurements of the cancer cells in cell mono-culture. Oxygen consumption rate (OCR), which is a surrogate of oxidative phosphorylation occurring in the mitochondria, and extracellular acidification rate (ECAR), which is a measure of glycolytic activity, are also registered by this system. The Seahorse assay entails the specific data of the contribution of the two energy-generating systems relative to the contribution of the other system when specific inhibitors and activators of either of the mitochondrial or glycolytic networks are included [25].

This has been particularly useful in cancer metabolism studies in which functional demand of metabolic plasticity (i.e., cell capacity to interchange oxidative phosphorylation and glycolysis) is necessary in changes in the surrounding environment or in response to therapeutic intervention [27]. Moreover, measurement of parameters of mitochondrial activity, such as the basal respiration, maximum respiratory capacity, ATP-coupled respiration, and proton leak, can be achieved using it. These measurements will play a very crucial role in identifying the ways the cancer cells adapt modes of energy production to ensure that they are well-adapted to high rates of proliferation, apoptosis resistance, and existence in a metabolic environment.

12.3 In Vivo Models and Imaging Technologies

In vivo models can never be substituted in the metabolism study of cancer in the complication of a living being. Referring to in vivo system in comparison to in vitro models, where the experimenter is able to manipulate the exertion on individual variables, in vivo platforms are prone to systemic body responses to physiological elements (nutrient integrity, hormonal equilibrium, immune surveillance, and organ-distinctive microenvironment). Not only do these models confirm hypotheses based on in vitro studies, but they also emerge with a set of emergent metabolic behaviors based on tumor–host interactions.

In recent years, the integration of animal models, in vivo isotope tracing, and advanced metabolic imaging has transformed the ability to study tumor metabolism at organismal, tissue, and even cellular resolution [28]. These complementary approaches allow researchers to monitor metabolic fluxes in real time, map spatial heterogeneity, and quantify the impact of therapeutic interventions under physiologically relevant conditions. An overview of these tools is presented in Table 12.2, and a conceptual workflow integrating them is illustrated in Fig. 12.1.

12.3.1 Animal Models

12.3.1.1 Genetically Engineered Mouse Models

GEMMs represent one of the most physiologically relevant preclinical platforms for studying cancer metabolism. These models employ transgenic or gene-targeting

Table 12.2 Comparative overview of in vivo models and imaging technologies for studying cancer metabolism

Model/ technique	Key features	Primary applications	Advantages	Limitations	Sources
GEMMs	Tissue-specific or inducible oncogene/tumor suppressor manipulation in mice	Mechanistic studies of metabolism in tumor initiation, progression, and metastasis	Physiological relevance, intact immune system, longitudinal studies	Long generation times, cost-intensive, low genetic diversity	[29, 30]
PDXs	Implantation of patient tumor tissue into immunodeficient mice	Translational testing of metabolism-targeted therapies, patient-specific metabolic profiling	Preserves tumor heterogeneity and architecture	No immune system in standard models, variable engraftment	[31]
Humanized PDXs	PDXs with reconstituted human immune system	Immune–metabolic interaction studies	Retains human tumor and immune features	Complex to establish, higher cost	[32]
In-vivo isotope tracing	Systemic infusion of $^{13}C/^{15}N$-labeled substrates	Quantitative nutrient flux mapping, metabolic competition analysis	Captures systemic regulation, real-time metabolic dynamics	Requires invasive sampling, sophisticated analytics	[33]
PET/CT or PET/MRI	Radiotracer-based metabolic imaging	Tumor detection, therapy monitoring, metabolic pathway mapping	High sensitivity, whole-body coverage	Limited spatial resolution, tracer specificity issues	[34, 35]
MRS (conventional)	MR-based metabolite detection	Noninvasive metabolic profiling	No radiation exposure, metabolite-specific	Lower sensitivity, limited metabolite coverage	[35]
Hyperpolarized ^{13}C MRS	Enhanced-signal real-time metabolic imaging	Dynamic reaction monitoring in vivo	High temporal resolution, pathway-specific	Requires specialized hardware, rapid signal decay	[35]

strategies to introduce oncogenic mutations or delete tumor suppressor genes in a tissue-specific and temporally controlled manner, often using Cre-loxP recombination systems [29]. GEMMs faithfully recapitulate the stepwise progression of tumorigenesis within an intact immune system, allowing exploration of

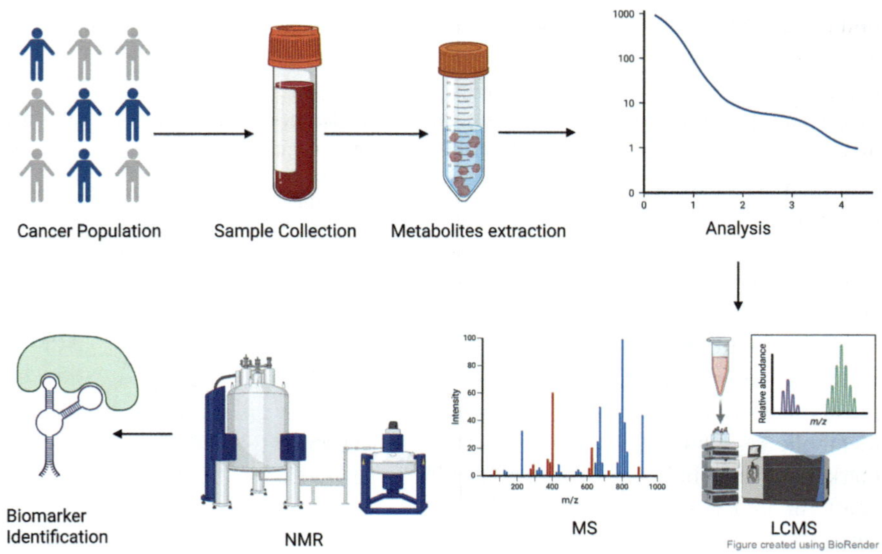

Fig. 12.1 The diagram illustrates the general workflow of metabolomic analysis aimed at identifying biomarkers in a cancer population. The process begins with the selection of cancer patients from whom biological samples, such as blood, urine, or tissue, are collected. These samples undergo metabolite extraction to isolate small biomolecules that reflect the metabolic state of the organism. The extracted metabolites are then analyzed to determine their concentration and structural characteristics, often visualized as signal intensity plots. (Figure created using BioRender)

tumor–immune metabolic crosstalk. They also enable longitudinal studies to assess how metabolic reprogramming evolves during distinct tumor stages, from initiation to metastasis [30]. However, their generation is time-consuming and costly, and the genetic homogeneity of inbred mouse strains may limit extrapolation to genetically diverse human tumors.

12.3.1.2 Patient-Derived Xenografts

PDX models are established by implanting tumor fragments or dissociated cancer cells from patients into immunodeficient mice [31]. This approach preserves the histological architecture, genetic heterogeneity, and many aspects of the metabolic phenotype of the original tumor. PDXs are particularly valuable for testing metabolism-targeted therapies and evaluating interpatient metabolic variability. Nevertheless, the lack of a functional immune system in conventional PDX models limits their ability to model immune–metabolic interactions. Recent developments in humanized PDX models, in which components of the human immune system are reconstituted, are beginning to address this limitation, offering opportunities for immune-oncology metabolism research [32].

12.3.2 In Vivo Isotope Tracing

In vivo isotope tracing extends stable isotope labeling to whole organisms, enabling direct quantification of metabolic fluxes under physiological conditions. In this approach, isotopically labeled substrates such as U-^{13}C-glucose, U-^{13}C-glutamine, or ^{15}N-amino acids are administered via intravenous infusion, intraperitoneal injection, or dietary incorporation. Subsequent MS or NMR analysis of tumors and host tissues provides high-resolution information on nutrient utilization and pathway connectivity [33]. This method allows researchers to:

- Identify nutrient sources preferentially used by tumors in vivo.
- Quantify contributions of glycolysis, the tricarboxylic acid (TCA) cycle, and biosynthetic pathways to tumor biomass.
- Assess metabolic competition between tumor cells and immune or stromal cells.

When combined with pharmacological perturbations, in vivo isotope tracing can reveal on-target and off-target metabolic effects of experimental therapies. It is also increasingly applied in clinical settings using infusion studies in cancer patients, linking preclinical findings to patient-specific metabolic phenotypes.

12.3.3 Imaging Techniques

12.3.3.1 Positron Emission Tomography

PET imaging has become a clinical mainstay for detecting tumors and monitoring treatment responses [34]. The most widely used tracer, ^{18}F-fluorodeoxyglucose (FDG), exploits elevated glucose uptake in cancer cells, but newer tracers, such as ^{18}F-fluoroglutamine (for glutamine metabolism) and ^{11}C-acetate (for lipid synthesis), allow interrogation of additional pathways. When combined with CT or MRI, PET provides both functional and anatomical information, enabling accurate localization of metabolically active tumor regions [35].

12.3.3.2 Magnetic Resonance Spectroscopy

MRS offers noninvasive detection of metabolites such as lactate, choline, creatine, and lipids, without exposure to ionizing radiation [36]. Proton (^{1}H) MRS is most commonly used in oncology, but carbon (^{13}C) and phosphorus (^{31}P) MRS can provide complementary information on specific metabolic pathways. When integrated with hyperpolarized ^{13}C-labeled substrates, MRS can monitor metabolic reactions in real time with exceptional sensitivity [37].

References

1. Bhat GR, Sethi I, Sadida HQ, Rah B, Mir R, Algehainy N, Albalawi IA, Masoodi T, Subbaraj GK, Jamal F, Singh M. Cancer cell plasticity: from cellular, molecular, and genetic mechanisms to tumor heterogeneity and drug resistance. Cancer Metastasis Rev. 2024;43(1):197–228.
2. Thakur R, Kumari N. Targeting metabolic reprogramming: a new frontier in cancer therapy. In: Molecular targets in cancer therapy: understanding cellular pathways for therapeutic interventions. Singapore: Springer Nature Singapore; 2025. p. 201–26.
3. Ruiz-Rodado V, Lita A, Larion M. Advances in measuring cancer cell metabolism with subcellular resolution. Nat Methods. 2022;19(9):1048–63.
4. Danzi F, Pacchiana R, Mafficini A, Scupoli MT, Scarpa A, Donadelli M, Fiore A. To metabolomics and beyond: a technological portfolio to investigate cancer metabolism. Signal Transduct Target Ther. 2023;8(1):137.
5. Zhang H, Lu KH, Ebbini M, Huang P, Lu H, Li L. Mass spectrometry imaging for spatially resolved multi-omics molecular mapping. NPJ Imaging. 2024;2(1):20.
6. Rauner G, Gupta PB, Kuperwasser C. From 2D to 3D and beyond: the evolution and impact of in vitro tumor models in cancer research. Nat Methods. 2025;22:1–2.
7. Shah S, D'Souza GG. Modeling tumor microenvironment complexity in vitro: spheroids as physiologically relevant tumor models and strategies for their analysis. Cells. 2025;14(10):732.
8. Liu Y, Wu W, Cai C, Zhang H, Shen H, Han Y. Patient-derived xenograft models in cancer therapy: technologies and applications. Signal Transduct Target Ther. 2023;8(1):160.
9. Garg P, Singhal G, Horne D, Kulkarni P, Salgia R, Singhal SS. Molecular PET imaging: unlocking the secrets of cancer metabolism. Biochem Pharmacol. 2025;242:117202.
10. Zhu J, Pan F, Cai H, Pan L, Li Y, Li L, Li Y, Wu X, Fan H. Positron emission tomography imaging of lung cancer: an overview of alternative positron emission tomography tracers beyond F18 fluorodeoxyglucose. Front Med. 2022;9:945602.
11. Angius A, Scanu AM, Arru C, Muroni MR, Carru C, Porcu A, Cossu-Rocca P, De Miglio MR. A portrait of intratumoral genomic and transcriptomic heterogeneity at single-cell level in colorectal cancer. Medicina. 2021;57(11):1257.
12. Allemailem KS, Alsahli MA, Almatroudi A, Alrumaihi F, Alkhaleefah FK, Rahmani AH, Khan AA. Current updates of CRISPR/Cas9-mediated genome editing and targeting within tumor cells: an innovative strategy of cancer management. Cancer Commun. 2022;42(12):1257–87.
13. Qiu S, Yang A, Zeng H. Flux balance analysis-based metabolic modeling of microbial secondary metabolism: current status and outlook. PLoS Comput Biol. 2023;19(8):e1011391.
14. Gordaliza-Alaguero I, Cantó C, Zorzano A. Metabolic implications of organelle-mitochondria communication. EMBO Rep. 2019;20(9):e47928. https://doi.org/10.15252/embr.201947928. Epub 2019 Aug 14. PMID: 31418169; PMCID: PMC6726909.
15. Taylor MJ, Lukowski JK, Anderton CR. Spatially resolved mass spectrometry at the single cell: recent innovations in proteomics and metabolomics. J Am Soc Mass Spectrom. 2021;32(4):872–94.
16. Yuan S, Almagro J, Fuchs E. Beyond genetics: driving cancer with the tumour microenvironment behind the wheel. Nat Rev Cancer. 2024;24(4):274–86.
17. Anklam E, Bahl MI, Ball R, Beger RD, Cohen J, Fitzpatrick S, Girard P, Halamoda-Kenzaoui B, Hinton D, Hirose A, Hoeveler A. Emerging technologies and their impact on regulatory science. Exp Biol Med. 2022;247(1):1–75.
18. Martínez-Reyes I, Chandel NS. Cancer metabolism: looking forward. Nat Rev Cancer. 2021;21(10):669–80.
19. Cardoso BD, Castanheira EM, Lanceros-Méndez S, Cardoso VF. Recent advances on cell culture platforms for in vitro drug screening and cell therapies: from conventional to microfluidic strategies. Adv Healthc Mater. 2023;12(18):2202936.
20. Barbosa MA, Xavier CP, Pereira RF, Petrikaitė V, Vasconcelos MH. 3D cell culture models as recapitulators of the tumor microenvironment for the screening of anti-cancer drugs. Cancer. 2021;14(1):190.

21. Ray SK, Mukherjee S. Imitating hypoxia and tumor microenvironment with immune evasion by employing three dimensional in vitro cellular models: impressive tool in drug discovery. Recent Pat Anticancer Drug Discov. 2022;17(1):80–91.
22. Chang CH, Tsai CC, Cheng CF, Chu TY, Chiang CP, Lee YP, Wu CC, Chen JH, Kuo CY, Hsu PC. Tumor organoids: a review of culture methods, applications in cancer research, precision medicine, and drug development. Tzu Chi Med J. 2025:10-4103.
23. Hilovsky D, Hartsell J, Young JD, Liu X. Stable isotope tracing analysis in cancer research: advancements and challenges in identifying dysregulated cancer metabolism and treatment strategies. Meta. 2024;14(6):318.
24. Moiz B, Sriram G, Clyne AM. Interpreting metabolic complexity via isotope-assisted metabolic flux analysis. Trends Biochem Sci. 2023;48(6):553–67.
25. Nikolic A. Chronic stress: tissue-specific impact on energy metabolism and metabolic adaptation. Doctoral dissertation, Dissertation, Düsseldorf, Heinrich-Heine-Universität; (2024).
26. Lackner M, Neef SK, Winter S, Beer-Hammer S, Nürnberg B, Schwab M, Hofmann U, Haag M. Untargeted stable isotope-resolved metabolomics to assess the effect of PI3Kβ inhibition on metabolic pathway activities in a PTEN null breast cancer cell line. Front Mol Biosci. 2022;9:1004602.
27. Caines JK, Barnes DA, Berry MD. The use of seahorse XF assays to interrogate real-time energy metabolism in cancer cell lines. In: Cancer cell biology: methods and protocols. New York: Springer US; 2022. p. 225–34.
28. Xiao Y, Yu TJ, Xu Y, Ding R, Wang YP, Jiang YZ, Shao ZM. Emerging therapies in cancer metabolism. Cell Metab. 2023;35(8):1283–303.
29. Gopinathan A, Morton JP, Jodrell DI, Sansom OJ. GEMMs as preclinical models for testing pancreatic cancer therapies. Dis Model Mech. 2015;8(10):1185–200.
30. Jiang M, Fang H, Tian H. Metabolism of cancer cells and immune cells in the initiation, progression, and metastasis of cancer. Theranostics. 2025;15(1):155.
31. Okada S, Vaeteewoottacharn K, Kariya R. Application of highly immunocompromised mice for the establishment of patient-derived xenograft (PDX) models. Cells. 2019;8(8):889.
32. Verma B, Ritchie M, Mancini M. Development and applications of patient-derived xenograft models in humanized mice for oncology and immune-oncology drug discovery. Curr Protoc Pharm. 2017;78(1):14–41.
33. García-Cañas V, Cifuentes A, Simó C. Applications of advanced omics technologies: from genes to metabolites. Elsevier; 2014.
34. Cintolo JA, Tchou J, Pryma DA. Diagnostic and prognostic application of positron emission tomography in breast imaging: emerging uses and the role of PET in monitoring treatment response. Breast Cancer Res Treat. 2013;138(2):331–46.
35. Pichler BJ, Judenhofer MS, Pfannenberg C. Multimodal imaging approaches: pet/ct and pet/mri. Mol Imaging. 2008;I:109–32.
36. Sharma U, Jagannathan NR. Metabolism of prostate cancer by magnetic resonance spectroscopy (MRS). Biophys Rev. 2020;12(5):1163–73.
37. Golder W. Magnetic resonance spectroscopy in clinical oncology. Oncol Res Treat. 2004;27(3):304–9.

Clinical Trials and Translational Advances in Metabolic Targeting

13

Hariharan Thirumalai Vengateswaran, Mohammad Habeeb, Huay Woon You, and Ciniraj Raveendran

13.1 Introduction

Conventional chemotherapeutic drugs act by blocking key pathways that cause cancer cells to divide rapidly. Although agents that damage DNA and stop mitotic or cellular growth pathways have been extensively examined, conventional chemotherapy drugs do not often target tumor metabolic pathways or broader metabolic dysfunctions observed in various diseases [1]. Significant progress has been made in the field of metabolic clinical trials in recent years. In addition to improving our understanding of metabolic diseases, including cancer, metabolic syndrome, and neurological disorders, these developments have also provided novel approaches to therapy. The connection between oncogene/tumor suppressor mutations and the alterations in metabolic pathways that follow is also an ongoing topic of extensive research [2]. There are recent reports of successfully converting identified metabolic abnormalities in cancer cells and other metabolic pathologies into FDA-approved metabolic inhibitors. In particular, isocitrate dehydrogenase (IDH) mutations that produce d-2-hydroxyglutarate (D2HG) were discovered during the sequencing of brain tumors and acute myeloid leukemia [3].

Based on recent developments, metabolic targeting has provided significant development and improvement in cancer treatment as well as therapeutic promise for metabolic and neurodegenerative diseases [4]. The therapeutic invention of small-molecule inhibitors that selectively block metabolic pathways necessary for

H. T. Vengateswaran · M. Habeeb
Department of Pharmaceutics, Crescent School of Pharmacy, B.S. Abdur Rahman Crescent Institute of Science and Technology, Chennai, India

H. W. You
Pusat PERMATA@Pintar Negara, Universiti Kebangsaan Malaysia, Bangi, Malaysia

C. Raveendran (✉)
Department of Radiation Oncology, Government Medical College Thiruvananthapuram, Thiruvananthapuram, India

S. Ashique et al. (eds.), *Cancer Metabolism*, Cancer Treatment and Research 195, https://doi.org/10.1007/978-3-032-21861-2_13

tumor growth has been a specific field of significant interest. Targeting deficits including glycolysis, glutaminolysis, and lipid metabolism that are indicative of malignant transformation, emerging therapies are increasingly being developed to differentiate between cancerous and normal cells [5]. Combinatorial strategies that combine metabolic inhibitors with immunotherapeutic or chemotherapeutic agents, or with metabolic modulators in diseases like type 2 diabetes and neurodegeneration, may both improve antitumor immunity and limit tumor bioenergetics. The complicated interactions between cancer cells and the immunological milieu, however, make this a challenging task that demands constant development in drug development, patient selection, and metabolic response surveillance [6].

IDH inhibitors, like ivosidenib and enasidenib, have been demonstrated in recent systematic reviews and meta-analyses to provide significant advantages in prognosis and objective responses for individuals with acute myeloid leukemia, cholangiocarcinoma, and various IDH-mutant cancers. By reversing epigenetic dysregulation, blocking the production of the oncometabolite D-2-hydroxyglutarate, and targeting mutant IDH-driven metabolic changes, these agents restore typical cellular differentiation activities. As an example of the transition from the identification of metabolic changes in tumors to the implementation of precision-targeted treatments in clinical practice, IDH inhibitors have a good safety record, which supports them as suggested therapies for IDH-mutant malignancies [7, 8]. This chapter investigates the role of metabolic reprogramming in the pathophysiology of disease and highlights important targets for treatment within modified metabolic pathways. It examines developments in translational research, such as metabolic intervention-focused clinical trials, preclinical models, and the role of artificial intelligence (AI) in personalized treatment. The difficulties in clinical translation and the developing importance of precision medicine in metabolic targeting are further addressed.

13.2 Metabolic Reprogramming in Disease Pathophysiology

13.2.1 Hallmarks of Metabolic Dysregulation

The pathogenesis of many diseases, particularly cancer, obesity, and metabolic syndrome, is associated with metabolic reprogramming. Changes in energy metabolism, reduced mitochondrial function, and modified amino acid and lipid pathways are characteristics of metabolic dysregulation, which together promote the growth of the disease. These metabolic changes produce a cycle of disease amplification by expressing and aggravating cellular breakdown. Targeted metabolomics was employed in a 2025 study by Andrea Di Credico et al. to analyze blood samples across different BMI classes. The results showed specific metabolic dysregulation patterns associated with overweight and obesity. The study specifically revealed that those with higher BMI had considerably greater levels of important metabolites, including branched-chain amino acids (BCAAs; e.g., leucine, isoleucine, valine) and aromatic amino acids (AAAs; e.g., phenylalanine, tyrosine). These increases were strongly related to higher cardiovascular risk, systemic inflammation, and impaired glucose metabolism. The study found that modified heart rate variability (HRV) measures reflected these metabolic fingerprints, indicating the link between disease risk, metabolic inflexibility, and sympathetic overactivity [9]. Similarly, another study on diabetic kidney disease highlights that mitochondrial metabolic reprogramming plays an essential part in the growth of the disease. This study indicates that inflammation, oxidative stress, and eventually fibrosis and renal insufficiency are caused by changes in the metabolism of carbohydrates, lipids, and amino acids in renal cells. Further study is required to determine their long-term effects on the development of disease beyond glucose control. Novel hypoglycemic agents such as SGLT2 inhibitors and GLP-1 agonists indicate potential in delaying pathological conditions by modulating metabolic reprogramming [10].

13.2.2 Glycolysis, Oxidative Phosphorylation, and Glutaminolysis

In many diseases, including cancer and immunological disorders, basic metabolic pathways such as glycolysis, oxidative phosphorylation (OXPHOS), and glutaminolysis experience significant reprogramming. Their dynamic interaction promotes proliferation, regulates treatment resistance, and describes cellular adaptability to stress. Cisplatin-resistant cells decrease glucose uptake while increasing fatty acid metabolism, demonstrating metabolic adaptability, according to a 2023 study on ovarian cancer resistance. By increasing β-oxidation, this reprogramming helps cancer cells withstand the stress caused by chemotherapy. The synergistic suppression of tumor growth by cisplatin and β-oxidation inhibitors suggests that treatment resistance can be overcome by targeting metabolic pathways [11]. Another study on endocrine therapy-resistant breast cancer revealed that certain metastatic cancers have a significant reliance on OXPHOS. In preclinical and patient-derived models, researchers significantly inhibited tumor growth with the mitochondrial complex I inhibitor IACS-010759. OXPHOS dependency is associated with a poor prognosis, based on metabolic profiling, identifying this approach as a metabolic susceptibility for advanced malignancies [12].

13.2.3 Lipid and Amino Acid Metabolism

The metabolism of lipids and amino acids is essential for maintaining cellular energy equilibrium. It is a key factor in the development of cancer and resistance to treatment. These metabolic pathways can be abnormally reprogrammed, allowing tumor cells to continue proliferating rapidly and to adjust to environmental stimuli. Targeting fatty acid uptake by the CD36 receptor has been studied as an effective approach for preventing metastases in malignancies triggered by a high-fat diet. In animal models, researchers discovered that CD36 suppression decreased the extent of metastases, especially when saturated fatty acid-induced stress was observed. Loss of CD36 increased ER stress and lipotoxicity in cancer cells, indicating that anti-CD36 medications and changes in diet or stearoyl-CoA desaturase 1 (SCD1) inhibition may increase anticancer effectiveness. This study shows that altering lipid absorption and metabolism can be therapeutically beneficial for preventing tumor development and overcoming adaptive resistance [13–15].

13.2.4 Role of Metabolism in Immune Cell Function and Tumor Microenvironment

The tumor microenvironment (TME) and immune cell function are significantly influenced by metabolism, which also affects the pathology of cancer and the effectiveness of treatment. Different metabolic adjustments that control their activation, differentiation, and effector roles are exhibited by immune cells such as T cells, dendritic cells, and macrophages.

13.3 Therapeutic Targets in Metabolic Pathways

Targeting metabolic pathways therapeutically has become an ideal approach for treating complicated diseases, including cancer and neurological problems. Metabolic changes that promote disease progression and treatment resistance have broadened because of developments in single-cell technologies, metabolomics, and genomics. The effects of targeting PGC-1α with nanoparticles in bladder cancer have been revealed in a 2025 study by Zhenghua Liu and colleagues. Using liposomal nanoparticles to silence PGC-1α disrupts energy metabolism, particularly by lowering key tricarboxylic acid cycle metabolites and sphingolipids, despite upregulating glycolytic intermediates. This method impairs mitochondrial function and substantially decreases metastasis in vivo, indicating that PGC-1α is an essential translational target in the metabolic regulation of tumor progression. In contrast to chemotherapy, direct intratumoral injection of si-PGC-1α LNP has significant specificity, substantially reducing adverse effects (Fig. 13.1) [16]. Another similar study of radiation-resistant tumor cells exhibits a constant upregulation of carnitine palmitoyl transferase 1A (CPT1A). Inhibition of CPT1A, a crucial enzyme in fatty acid oxidation (FAO), increased radiation sensitivity and inhibited tumor growth by lowering cellular generation of energy and restricting proliferation [17].

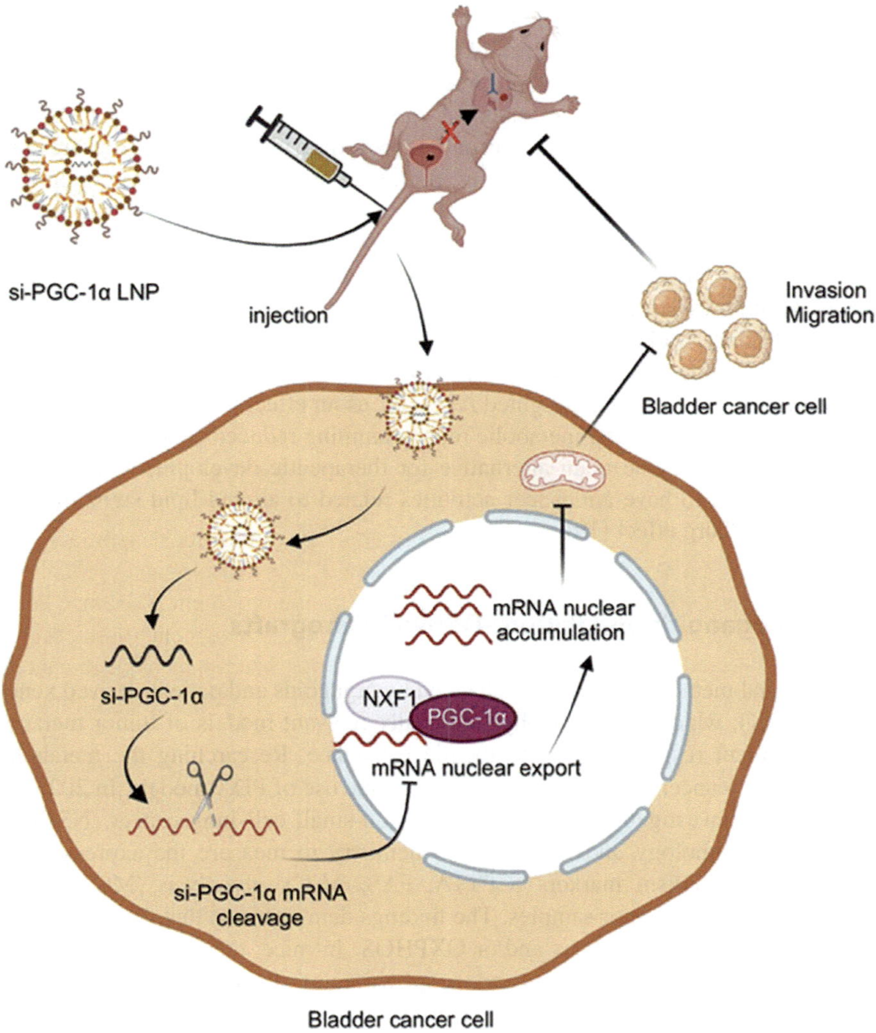

Fig. 13.1 Diagrammatic illustration of the biochemical mechanism of si-PGC-1α LNP inhibiting the regulation of energy metabolism and mitochondrial biology in bladder tumor metastases. (This figure is reproduced from Ref. [16])

13.4 Translational Research and Preclinical Advances

13.4.1 In Vitro and In Vivo Models of Metabolic Targeting

Translational advancements in metabolic targeting have been primarily contributed by in vitro and in vivo models, which facilitate scientists in identifying pathways, optimizing approaches, and forecasting efficacy before clinical trials. In 2025, an investigation examined metabolic vulnerabilities using a genetically modified mouse for acute myeloid leukemia (AML). The investigation revealed a significant dependence on FAO pathways in leukemic stem cells in contrast to their normal counterparts, using in vivo isotopic tracing and metabolic flux analysis. In these models, pharmacological suppression of carnitine palmitoyltransferase 1 (CPT1) inhibited the progression of leukemia and improved survival. These results are confirmed by complementary in vitro tests employing primary AML cells, confirming metabolic targeting of FAO as an effective treatment [18]. Scientists examined the impact of AKR1B1 targeting on metabolic reprogramming in cancer using both in vitro and in vivo models. They demonstrated using cultured tumor cells that AKR1B1 suppression affected lipid and glucose metabolism, which subsequently decreased cancer cell migration and proliferation. Additionally, in vivo studies using animal models showed that AKR1B1 inhibitor therapy considerably inhibited tumor growth. The study highlighted AKR1B1 as an effective target for metabolic interventions, and blocking metabolic reprogramming reduced cancer resistance to treatment. This enzyme is an alternative for therapeutic development, which has been concluded to have anticancer activities related to altered lipid signaling and disrupted Warburg effect [19].

13.4.2 Organoids and Patient-Derived Xenografts

Translational metabolic research is changed by organoids and patient-derived xenografts (PDX), which allow for physiologically relevant models of tumor metabolism, treatment response, and therapeutic resistance. Researching the metabolic foundation of cancer has derived benefits from the use of PDX models. In 2023, an experimental investigation using PDXs for non-small cell lung cancer (NSCLC) used digital pathology and immunohistochemistry to measure the expression of fatty acid metabolism markers (CPT1A, FAS, ACC), glycolysis (MCT4), and OXPHOS (GLS) in tumor samples. The findings demonstrated that the majority of PDXs depended on glycolysis and/or OXPHOS. In mice, there was a correlation between marker expression levels and the growth rates of xenografts, angiogenesis, and tumor cell proliferation [20]. Protease inhibitors were identified as potential drugs in a bile duct cancer study that used patient-derived cancer organoids (PDCOs) to screen for drug sensitivity in vitro. These results were assessed in mouse models that had PDCO transplants, and they showed that the histology and stromal constituents of PDCO xenografts and conventional cell-derived xenografts differed. The complicated differentiation and microenvironment of patient cancers were more accurately represented by the organoid-derived xenografts, confirming their advantage for translational drug development and metabolic therapy assessment [21].

13.4.3 Metabolomics and Transcriptomics in Drug Discovery

Metabolomics and transcriptomics have emerged as key technologies in drug development, transforming the identification of drug targets, metabolic pathways, and disease and treatment responses. Researchers demonstrated metabolomics and transcriptomics by combining them to identify drug action and toxicity pathways. They found that integrating metabolic and transcriptional statistics allowed for accurate mapping of changed pathways and molecular interactions in radiation-exposed mouse models using a multi-omics approach. Their methodology revealed new regulators, including Elovl5 and Fads2, within fatty acid pathways and highlighted amino acid, lipid, carbohydrate, and nucleotide metabolism as major targets affected by radiation. Future research on treatments was impacted by this integration, which made more precise the immediate and downstream impacts of drug action [22]. Neuroblastoma heterogeneity and treatment sensitivity were examined using a combination of transcriptomics and metabolomics. The researchers evaluated the metabolic and gene expression patterns of MYCN-amplified and nonamplified neuroblastoma by examining 96 plasma samples and 52 tumor tissues. In addition to identifying two important biomarkers (elaidic carnitine and C16 sphinganine) for clinical classification and treatment selection, the method exposed several abnormal metabolic pathways. This systematic integration supported metabolomics and transcriptomics as innovative tools in molecular characterization and targeted drug discovery by providing practical insight into molecular mechanisms [23].

13.4.4 CRISPR and Gene Editing for Metabolic Gene Validation

The validation of metabolic genes has been transformed by CRISPR-based gene editing, facilitating unprecedented precision for researching gene function, disease causes, and potential therapeutic targets in metabolic pathways. Huntington's disease model mice were used in a 2024 study that used in vivo CRISPR–Cas9 genome editing to screen for genes that alter the growth of CAG repeats, which is a mutation that causes the condition. Researchers identified these metabolic modifiers as therapeutic targets by observing a distinct modulation of repeat expansion resulting in disease progression by targeting mismatch repair genes (enhancers and suppressors). The results demonstrated effective editing and significant regulation, demonstrating metabolic gene editing might identify novel therapeutic targets in multifaceted combinations of metabolic and neurodegenerative diseases [24]. Using CRISPR/Cas9, researchers modified the CHS2 gene in plant cell lines. A metabolic shift resulted from the developed mutation, which elevated genes involved in stilbenoid formation while suppressing those involved in flavonoid biosynthesis. The work demonstrated that CRISPR/Cas9-induced gene editing changed cellular metabolism, along with disrupting particular metabolic pathways. The direct metabolic effects of specific genetic treatments in this study provide an effective framework for functionally validating metabolic genes [25].

13.5 Clinical Trials in Metabolic Targeting

13.5.1 Cancer

13.5.1.1 Ongoing and Completed Trials (e.g., IDH Inhibitors, Metformin, Glutaminase Inhibitors)

Targeting enzymes and pathways essential to tumor cell survival, metabolic targeting has become an effective cancer treatment method. In patients with grade 2 IDH-mutant gliomas, vorasidenib, an oral brain-penetrant inhibitor of mutant IDH1/2, significantly increased progression-free survival (median PFS 27.7 vs. 11.1 months compared to placebo) with an acceptable safety profile, according to the INDIGO phase 3 trial issued by the Massachusetts Medical Society. This result supports the drug's clinical use and FDA approval [26]. More phase III trials for adjuvant treatment in specific cancers are provided by a phase II translational study that analyzed metformin in nondiabetic patients with advanced-stage epithelial ovarian cancer. The study found a significant decrease in cancer stem-like cells and desirable survival outcomes (median PFS 18 months, OS 57.9 months) with good tolerability [27]. Prodrugs of DON, such as DRP-104, which specifically target tumors and enhance immune cell infiltration, are the glutaminase-related drugs undergoing clinical study. DRP-104 could reverse immunosuppressive TMEs by promoting T cell-mediated antitumor responses and blocking glutamine-dependent nucleotide production. Preclinical and clinical study results indicate that DRP-104 is effective and safe in advanced solid tumors. It is also being studied together with immunotherapies such as durvalumab [28].

13.5.1.2 Combination Therapies with Immunotherapy or Chemotherapy

Combination treatments that combine chemotherapy and immunotherapy have become an effective approach to improve the outcome of cancer treatment. Physicians aim to enhance therapeutic efficacy, overcome resistance, and prolong survival for patients with various malignancies by leveraging the synergistic effects of these techniques. Patients with advanced nonsquamous NSCLC received pembrolizumab (an anti-PD-1 antibody) combined with pemetrexed and carboplatin showed significantly higher improvements in objective response rate (58% vs 33%), median progression-free survival (24.5 vs 9.9 months), and an increase with improved median overall survival (34.5 vs 21.1 months) compared to chemotherapy alone, regardless of PD-L1 expression status. These results correlated with the FDA approving pembrolizumab in combination with chemotherapy as the first-line treatment for this patient population. Patients tolerated the combination well, and those who completed 2 years of pembrolizumab demonstrated exceptionally durable responses [29]. A 2025 study evaluating a triple combination of atezolizumab, paclitaxel, and bevacizumab for unresectable or advanced triple-negative breast cancer found that, highly enriched for PD-L1–negative tumors, the triple combination showed longer median progression-free and survival rates compared to known controls. The benefits of immunotherapy may be enhanced in the PD-L1-positive group by precisely selected combinations [30].

13.5.2 Metabolic Syndrome and Type 2 Diabetes

13.5.2.1 Mitochondrial Modulators, AMPK Activators, and Insulin Sensitizers

Insulin sensitizers, AMPK activators, and mitochondrial modulators are being examined in the treatment against type 2 diabetes and metabolic syndrome. Imeglimin is a first-in-class drug that targets mitochondrial bioenergetics and has advanced through multiple phase III clinical trials. Imeglimin improves β-cell efficiency and insulin sensitivity by modifying mitochondrial complex I activity. According to trials, imeglimin has a manageable safety profile and effectively decreases HbA1c in individuals with type 2 diabetes. Reduced mitochondrial ROS and enhanced FAO are two of its mechanisms, used in lowering insulin resistance and intrahepatic lipid accumulation [31]. Recent research investigated new synthetic direct AMPK-activating drugs, such as PXL770, in comparison to diabetes-related disorders including nonalcoholic fatty liver disease (NAFLD). Even though they show interest in lowering hepatic steatosis and increasing insulin sensitivity, their usage, especially for diabetes, is still in the early stages of research, and further research is being conducted to evaluate their safety and effectiveness in type 2 diabetes [32]. Insulin sensitizers, both old and new, have been studied in trials by Nicholas Shoung and team, with an ongoing focus on customized treatment. Since 2019, metformin, GLP-1 receptor agonists, or short-term insulin therapies have been used in the majority of registered trials to achieve glycemic control and, in certain circumstances, remission. In some studies, newer drugs, such as some GLP-1 receptor agonists (semaglutide), have shown potential for improving blood sugar levels as well as helping people with diabetes and metabolic syndrome lose weight and improve their cardiovascular health [33].

13.5.2.2 Clinical Efficacy and Safety Outcomes

Evaluating clinical efficacy and safety results is important for understanding the exact significance of novel treatments. In the SURPASS study program, tirzepatide, a novel dual GIP/GLP-1 receptor agonist, showed significant weight loss (up to 12.9 kg) and significant improvements in glycemic management (HbA1c drop 1.9–3.0%). In both early and advanced type 2 diabetes, tirzepatide performed better than basal insulin and long-acting GLP-1 agonists. When not combined with insulin or sulfonylureas, the main adverse effects include mild-to-moderate gastrointestinal symptoms (vomiting, nausea), with low rates of hypoglycemia. Regarding ongoing cardiovascular outcome trials, the drug is generally regarded as safe for widespread usage; however, cardiovascular safety data are still being discovered [34].

13.5.3 Neurological Disorders

13.5.3.1 Ketogenic Interventions and Brain Glucose Metabolism

Ketogenic therapies alter the metabolism of glucose in the brain; they are changing the way that neurological disorders are controlled. K.I. Avgerinos and co-researchers examined exogenous ketone ester supplementation in older persons with age-related memory complaints in a recent placebo-controlled crossover study. The idea that increasing brain ketone availability may provide cognitive benefits even without rigorous dietary adherence is supported by the participants' acute boosts in plasma ketone levels and advantages in attention and recollection activities [35]. A modified Mediterranean ketogenic diet changed plasma lipidomic levels in ways that were inversely linked with indicators for Alzheimer's disease, according to a 2025 study by Bryan J. Neth and colleagues. This study revealed an innovative method for dietary management in at-risk groups by demonstrating that ketone-driven alterations in lipid metabolism may be mechanistically connected to modifications in Alzheimer's pathogenesis [36].

13.5.3.2 Clinical Studies on Metabolic Modulators in Alzheimer's and Parkinson's Diseases

Novel approaches to treating Parkinson's and Alzheimer's diseases are being revealed by clinical research on metabolic modulators. Monoclonal antibodies such as aducanumab, lecanemab, and donanemab have been assessed in the latest phase 3 trials (EMERGE, ENGAGE, CLARITY AD, TRAILBLAZER-ALZ 2). These substances mostly remove amyloid plaques, but they have also been demonstrated to have an influence on neuroinflammation and brain glucose metabolism, both of which are important for maintaining metabolic homeostasis. In early-stage Alzheimer's disease patients, donanemab was related to a slower rate of cognitive deterioration (a shift in iADRS score −6.02 vs. −9.27 for placebo in low/medium tau class), and PET imaging confirmed a lower amyloid load. Amyloid imaging abnormalities, which were primarily asymptomatic, were among the adverse effects [37]. Isradipine's potential to change injury through mitochondrial support has been investigated in multicenter phase 3 trials. Isradipine's target in a 36-month trial (NCT02168842) was to reduce mitochondrial stress to prevent the onset of motor symptoms in early Parkinson's disease. The trial showed safety and indicated pertinent secondary outcomes and biomarker alterations, even if it did not yield a substantial slowing of symptoms when compared to a placebo. The primary objectives of EPI-589, an additional mitochondrial redox modulator, are tolerability, alterations in glutathione, an essential antioxidant biomarker, and PD motor symptom results [38].

13.5.4 Rare and Inherited Metabolic Disorders

13.5.4.1 Enzyme Replacement Therapies and Gene Therapy

Novel possibilities for people with rare metabolic abnormalities are being explored by developments in gene therapy and enzyme replacement. Barbara K Burton et al., studied observational data from the 15-year MPS VI Clinical Surveillance Program (CSP), galsulfase ERT improved the six-minute walk test (6MWT), significantly improved pulmonary function (FEV1 and FVC) over 6–7 years, and reduced urinary glycosaminoglycans (uGAGs) by an average of 59.7% after 8 years in 212 patients with mucopolysaccharidosis VI. Particularly, youngsters recovered the most, while even older individuals had their condition stabilize. Adverse effects were primarily associated with the underlying condition rather than the drug itself, and galsulfase was typically well tolerated [39]. AAV-mediated G6PC gene therapy in patients improved growth and metabolic profiles, decreased hepatomegaly, and normalized fasting glucose levels were all displayed by treated individuals, indicating functional metabolic correction and acceptable safety [40].

13.5.4.2 Trials in Disorders Like Phenylketonuria, Mitochondrial Diseases

Examining clinical trials for diseases like mitochondrial disorders and phenylketonuria highlights the complex nature and potential of specialized therapies. Adults with PKU undergoing long-term pegvaliase (PEG-PAL) treatment showed better dietary adherence and sustained blood phenylalanine reductions in a phase 3 clinical program. Compared to typical medical nutrition therapy, patients' blood Phe levels returned to normal more frequently, and the main safety issues were caused by hypersensitivity reactions [41]. The first human experiment of replacing a protein based on mRNA for a mitochondrial FAO problem has been examined by researchers. A novel path in mitochondrial therapy was discovered by intravenous infusions of LNP-encapsulated mRNA, which resulted in temporary but clinically significant elevations in enzyme levels and enhanced indicators of fatty acid metabolism [42].

13.6 Challenges in Clinical Translation

Translating advances in metabolic targeting into clinical practice encounters numerous significant difficulties. Biological variability both inside and among patients affects the predictability of therapy responses and the reliability of biomarkers, as metabolic pathways differ significantly between disease stages and individual biology. Comprehending metabolism within its inherent physiological framework is crucial, although it poses significant technical challenges, hindering the establishment of reliable surrogate markers for therapeutic efficacy [43, 44]. Manufacturing intricacies can impede translation. Advanced formulations, including nanoparticle delivery systems, necessitate reproducible large-scale production with consistent quality—an often challenging and expensive endeavor. The intricacy of dosage forms must be weighed against clinical practicality to guarantee treatments that are both feasible and compliant with regulations. Regulatory, ethical, and economic obstacles introduce further complexities. The elevated expenses associated with multi-omics profiling and tailored therapies may restrict healthcare accessibility, while the necessity for specialized infrastructure and knowledge hinders wider implementation. Safeguarding patient confidentiality and guaranteeing fair trial representation are essential issues to cultivate trust and inclusivity [45, 46]. Moreover, animal models employed in preclinical testing may inadequately represent the variety of human metabolic diseases, hence diminishing the applicability of the findings and elevating translational risk. Meticulous design of preclinical investigations, incorporating diverse models and randomized, blinded techniques, is essential to enhance predictive validity. Ultimately, surmounting these hurdles necessitates interdisciplinary collaboration that amalgamates biology, engineering, clinical sciences, and regulatory knowledge to enhance treatment design, biomarker development, manufacturing, and clinical execution. Holistically addressing these hurdles is essential for the effective transition of precision metabolic medicines from laboratory to clinical use.

13.7 Precision Medicine and Biomarker-Driven Strategies

Precision medicine in metabolic targeting focuses on customizing treatments based on the genetic and metabolic variations among patients, advancing beyond traditional methods to attain enhanced therapeutic results. This technique utilizes multi-omics technologies, encompassing genomes, transcriptomics, proteomics, and metabolomics, to identify critical biomarkers and actionable targets for diseases including cancer, diabetes, and uncommon metabolic disorders. Through the integration of these platforms, doctors can discern distinct patient groupings, enhance pharmacological selections, and more correctly forecast therapy responses, thereby achieving personalized medicine in metabolic disorders. Progress in high-throughput analytics and bioinformatics has enabled the design of personalized interventions and expedited the advancement of next-generation metabolic medicines [47].

13.7.1 Role of Metabolomics and Imaging in Patient Stratification

Metabolomics offers a comprehensive overview of small-molecule metabolites in cells or patient samples, facilitating the identification of metabolic phenotypes linked to disease risk, progression, or therapy response. High-resolution mass spectrometry and nuclear magnetic resonance (NMR) spectroscopy, in conjunction with sophisticated imaging techniques, enable clinicians to stratify patients according to metabolic profiles derived from minimally invasive samples. Imaging techniques such as PET, MRI, and mass spectrometry imaging facilitate real-time, noninvasive monitoring of metabolic alterations in tissues or tumors, hence aiding in early diagnosis, surveillance, and tailored treatment modifications. Validated metabolomic and imaging biomarkers are increasingly pivotal in the design of clinical trials and the selection of patients for targeted therapy [48].

13.7.2 Companion Diagnostics

Companion diagnostics (CDx) are assays created in conjunction with treatments to identify patients who are most likely to benefit from a particular medication, especially in targeted metabolic therapies. These tests generally assess gene mutations, protein expression, or metabolite concentrations that signify the presence or absence of the therapy target or forecast responsiveness. In clinical trials, CDx are crucial for enhancing study populations with individuals who exhibit a high likelihood of responding, hence boosting trial outcomes and facilitating regulatory approval. Integrating CDx into standard care enhances safety profiles, promotes cost-effective treatments, and facilitates real-world outcome monitoring for metabolic interventions [49].

13.7.3 Integration with AI and Machine Learning for Personalized Therapy

Artificial intelligence (AI) and machine learning (ML) are transforming customized metabolic therapy by facilitating unparalleled data integration, predictive analytics, and real-time clinical decision-making for various metabolic illnesses [50]. AI models can analyze and integrate extensive multi-omics datasets, encompassing genomes, transcriptomics, proteomics, and metabolomics, in conjunction with conventional clinical records and imaging data, to generate intricate molecular and metabolic profiles for each patient [51]. AI algorithms may find essential metabolic pathways, uncover novel biomarkers, and categorize patients based on their risk and probable therapeutic response using supervised, unsupervised, and reinforcement learning [52]. AI and ML have facilitated the creation of genome-scale metabolic network models that identify bottlenecks in metabolic processes and propose appropriate interventions, such as gene edits or pharmacological therapies for metabolic reprogramming [53]. In clinical environments, AI-driven solutions are progressively utilized to manage and prevent chronic metabolic disorders, including diabetes, obesity, and metabolic syndrome. These systems facilitate early disease identification, risk assessment, and adaptive therapy modification through the continuous analysis of patient data derived from electronic health records, wearable sensors, and laboratory findings. Transformer-based AI models surpass conventional methods in forecasting disease onset and care delays, hence alleviating undiagnosed disease burden and hospitalizations. Diagnostic and risk-stratification models based on ML, such as XGBoost, random forests, and deep learning classifiers, consistently demonstrate superior accuracy compared to conventional noninvasive testing in metabolic and liver illnesses [54, 55]. In research and drug development, AI-driven metabolomic analysis expedites biomarker identification and informs the optimization of therapeutic targets, enhancing the efficiency of candidate drug screening and the development of CDx [56]. The use of AI in multi-omics and spatial omics facilitates the deconvolution of intricate tissue heterogeneity, which is essential for personalized therapy in oncology and other metabolic-related disorders [57]. Nevertheless, despite these advancements, numerous difficulties persist. To facilitate broader clinical translation, it is essential to address the interpretation and reproducibility of AI-generated outcomes, the necessity for established methodologies, privacy issues, and constraints in data quality. As the domain progresses, persistent endeavors to create transparent, interpretable AI algorithms and guarantee equitable, safe implementation are crucial for achieving the full advantages of AI-driven individualized metabolic therapy [58].

13.8 Future Directions and Emerging Trends

Emerging technologies, including single-cell multi-omics, spatial metabolomics, CRISPR-based gene editing, and next-generation imaging, are breaking new ground in metabolic research and therapy [59]. Increasing integration of systems biology, computational modeling, and real-time patient data via digital health platforms will enable more precise interventions and a shift toward proactive disease management. Collaborative frameworks across disciplines, robust biomarker validation, and adaptive clinical trial designs will be crucial for translating metabolic research insights into effective, individualized therapies for diseases such as cancer, diabetes, and rare metabolic disorders [60].

13.9 Conclusion

Translational advances in metabolic targeting have ushered in a new era of individualized therapy, with promising results in cancer, metabolic syndrome, rare inherited disorders, and neurological diseases. Personalized strategies leveraging multi-omics, CDx, and AI are steadily improving outcomes and safety profiles, moving the healthcare field closer to the realization of precision medicine. Addressing challenges such as metabolic heterogeneity, therapy resistance, and real-world implementation will require continued innovation and interdisciplinary collaboration as the field moves toward truly patient-centered metabolic therapy. The rapid evolution of AI-driven platforms is already accelerating drug discovery, optimizing patient stratification, and enabling dynamic, data-informed clinical decision-making at scale. As breakthroughs in digital health, multi-omics integration, and real-time monitoring converge, the future will see proactive, preventive, and highly personalized interventions become the norm rather than the exception. Ultimately, the successful translation of these innovations into broad clinical practice promises not only to enhance patient outcomes but also to transform global standards of care in metabolic and related diseases through meaningful, equitable advances in precision healthcare.

References

1. Akhenblit PJ, Pagel MD. Recent advances in targeting tumor energy metabolism with tumor acidosis as a biomarker of drug efficacy. J Cancer Sci Ther. 2016;8:20. https://doi.org/10.4172/1948-5956.1000382.
2. Lemberg KM, Gori SS, Tsukamoto T, Rais R, Slusher BS. Clinical development of metabolic inhibitors for oncology. J Clin Invest. 2022;132 https://doi.org/10.1172/JCI148550.
3. Guo C, Pirozzi CJ, Lopez GY, Yan H. Isocitrate dehydrogenase mutations in gliomas: mechanisms, biomarkers and therapeutic target. Curr Opin Neurol. 2011;24:648–52. https://doi.org/10.1097/WCO.0B013E32834CD415.
4. Xiao Y, Yu TJ, Xu Y, Ding R, Wang YP, Jiang YZ, Shao ZM. Emerging therapies in cancer metabolism. Cell Metab. 2023;35:1283–303. https://doi.org/10.1016/J.CMET.2023.07.006.
5. Luo Z, Eichinger KM, Zhang A, Li S. Targeting cancer metabolic pathways for improving chemotherapy and immunotherapy. Cancer Lett. 2023;575:216396. https://doi.org/10.1016/J.CANLET.2023.216396.
6. Muluh TA, Shu X s, Ying Y. Targeting cancer metabolic vulnerabilities for advanced therapeutic efficacy. Biomed Pharmacother. 2023;162:114658. https://doi.org/10.1016/J.BIOPHA.2023.114658.
7. Cai Z, Yang H, Yu Z, Su J, Zhang J, Ye Z, Hu K, Huang T, Zhou H. Efficacy and safety of IDH inhibitors in IDH-mutated cancers: a systematic review and meta-analysis of 4 randomized controlled trials. World J Surg Oncol. 2024;22:1–10. https://doi.org/10.1186/S12957-024-03579-Z/FIGURES/8.
8. Zarei M, Hue JJ, Hajihassani O, Graor HJ, Katayama ES, Loftus AW, Bajor D, Rothermel LD, Vaziri-Gohar A, Winter JM. Clinical development of IDH1 inhibitors for cancer therapy. Cancer Treat Rev. 2022;103 https://doi.org/10.1016/J.CTRV.2021.102334.
9. Di Credico A, Perpetuini D, Izzicupo P, Gaggi G, Rossi C, Merla A, Ghinassi B, Di Baldassarre A, Bucci I. Blood metabolome shows signatures of metabolic dysregulation in obese and overweight subjects that can be predicted by machine learning applied to heart rate variability. Front Mol Biosci. 2025;12:1561987. https://doi.org/10.3389/FMOLB.2025.1561987/BIBTEX.
10. Fan X, Yang M, Lang Y, Lu S, Kong Z, Gao Y, Shen N, Zhang D, Lv Z. Mitochondrial metabolic reprogramming in diabetic kidney disease. Cell Death Dis. 2024;15(6):1–12. https://doi.org/10.1038/s41419-024-06833-0.
11. Tan Y, Li J, Zhao G, Huang KC, Cardenas H, Wang Y, Matei D, Cheng JX. Metabolic reprogramming from glycolysis to fatty acid uptake and beta-oxidation in platinum-resistant cancer cells. Nat Commun. 2022;13(1):1–16. https://doi.org/10.1038/s41467-022-32101-w.
12. El-Botty R, Morriset L, Montaudon E, Tariq Z, Schnitzler A, Bacci M, Lorito N, Sourd L, Huguet L, Dahmani A, Painsec P, Derrien H, Vacher S, Masliah-Planchon J, Raynal V, Baulande S, Larcher T, Vincent-Salomon A, Dutertre G, Cottu P, Gentric G, Mechta-Grigoriou F, Hutton S, Driouch K, Bièche I, Morandi A, Marangoni E. Oxidative phosphorylation is a metabolic vulnerability of endocrine therapy and palbociclib resistant metastatic breast cancers. Nat Commun. 2023;14(1):1–16. https://doi.org/10.1038/s41467-023-40022-5.
13. Terry AR, Hay N. Emerging targets in lipid metabolism for cancer therapy. Trends Pharmacol Sci. 2024;45:537–51. https://doi.org/10.1016/J.TIPS.2024.04.007/ASSET/9660A32F-E5BE-4ACE-8BDC-B541C96F88E4/MAIN.ASSETS/GR5.JPG.
14. Scott JS, Nassar ZD, Swinnen JV, Butler LM. Monounsaturated fatty acids: key regulators of cell viability and intracellular signaling in cancer. Mol Cancer Res. 2022;20:1354–64. https://doi.org/10.1158/1541-7786.MCR-21-1069/704809/AM/MONOUNSATURATED-FATTY-ACIDS-KEY-REGULATORS-OF-CELL.
15. Feng WW, Zuppe HT, Kurokawa M. The role of CD36 in cancer progression and its value as a therapeutic target. Cells. 2023;12:1605. https://doi.org/10.3390/CELLS12121605.
16. Z. Liu, P. Xin, W. Wu, M. Jin, Y. Du, Y. Jiang, T. Liu, H. Zhang, Nanoparticle-mediated targeting of PGC-1α reveals critical metabolic pathways in bladder cancer metastasis, Commun Biol 8 (2025) 1–21. doi:https://doi.org/10.1038/S42003-025-08174-W.

17. Tan Z, Xiao L, Tang M, Bai F, Li J, Li L, Shi F, Li N, Li Y, Du Q, Lu J, Weng X, Yi W, Zhang H, Fan J, Zhou J, Gao Q, Onuchic JN, Bode AM, Luo X, Cao Y. Targeting CPT1A-mediated fatty acid oxidation sensitizes nasopharyngeal carcinoma to radiation therapy. Theranostics. 2018;8:2329–47. https://doi.org/10.7150/THNO.21451.
18. Dreute J, Stengel J, Becher J, van den Borre D, Pfisterer M, Bartkuhn M, Beutgen VM, Ndreshkjana B, Gärtner U, Graumann J, Huck M, Klatt S, Leff C, Farin HF, Nist A, Schmitz R, Stiewe T, Teply-Szymanski J, Wilhelm J, Cabrera-Orefice A, Schmitz ML. Synergistic targeting of cancer cells through simultaneous inhibition of key metabolic enzymes. Cell Death Differ. 2025;2025:1–18. https://doi.org/10.1038/s41418-025-01532-5.
19. Q. Wang, J. Liu, M. Yang, J. Zhou, Y. Li, J. Zheng, H. Jia, S. Yue, Y. Le, Y. Su, W. Ma, N. An, Y. Wang, J. Dong, Targeting AKR1B1 inhibits metabolic reprogramming to reverse systemic therapy resistance in hepatocellular carcinoma, Signal Transduct Target Ther 10 (2025) 1–17. doi:https://doi.org/10.1038/S41392-025-02321-9.
20. Ferrarini F, Zulato E, Moro M, Del Bianco P, Borzi C, Esposito G, Zanin T, Sozzi G, Indraccolo S. Metabolic classification of non-small cell lung cancer patient-derived xenografts by a digital pathology approach: a pilot study. Front Oncol. 2023;13:1070505. https://doi.org/10.3389/FONC.2023.1070505/BIBTEX.
21. Ogawa H, Yoshida K, Hasegawa S, Wada H, Yasui M, Tahara H. Significance of mouse xenograft tumor model using patient-derived cancer organoids for clinical drug development. Front Oncol. 2025;15:1485886. https://doi.org/10.3389/FONC.2025.1485886/BIBTEX.
22. Maan K, Baghel R, Dhariwal S, Sharma A, Bakhshi R, Rana P. Metabolomics and transcriptomics based multi-omics integration reveals radiation-induced altered pathway networking and underlying mechanism. NPJ Syst Biol Appl. 2023;9:1–13. https://doi.org/10.1038/S41540-023-00305-5.
23. Du B, Zhang Y, Zhang P, Zhang M, Yu Z, Li L, Hou L, Wang Q, Zhang X, Zhang W. Joint metabolomics and transcriptomics analysis systematically reveal the impact of MYCN in neuroblastoma. Sci Rep. 2024;14:1–16. https://doi.org/10.1038/S41598-024-71211-X.
24. Mouro Pinto R, Murtha R, Azevedo A, Douglas C, Kovalenko M, Ulloa J, Crescenti S, Burch Z, Oliver E, Kesavan M, Shibata S, Vitalo A, Mota-Silva E, Riggs MJ, Correia K, Elezi E, Demelo B, Carroll JB, Gillis T, Gusella JF, MacDonald ME, Wheeler VC. In vivo CRISPR–Cas9 genome editing in mice identifies genetic modifiers of somatic CAG repeat instability in Huntington's disease. Nat Genetics. 2025;57(2):314–22. https://doi.org/10.1038/s41588-024-02054-5.
25. Lai G, Fu P, He L, Che J, Wang Q, Lai P, Lu J, Lai C. CRISPR/Cas9-mediated CHS2 mutation provides a new insight into resveratrol biosynthesis by causing a metabolic pathway shift from flavonoids to stilbenoids in Vitis davidii cells. Hortic Res. 2025;12 https://doi.org/10.1093/HR/UHAE268.
26. Mellinghoff IK, van den Bent MJ, Blumenthal DT, Touat M, Peters KB, Clarke J, Mendez J, Yust-Katz S, Welsh L, Mason WP, Ducray F, Umemura Y, Nabors B, Holdhoff M, Hottinger AF, Arakawa Y, Sepulveda JM, Wick W, Soffietti R, Perry JR, Giglio P, de la Fuente M, Maher EA, Schoenfeld S, Zhao D, Pandya SS, Steelman L, Hassan I, Wen PY, Cloughesy TF. Vorasidenib in IDH1- or IDH2-mutant low-grade glioma. N Engl J Med. 2023;389:589–601. https://doi.org/10.1056/NEJMOA2304194/SUPPL_FILE/NEJMOA2304194_DATA-SHARING.PDF.
27. Brown JR, Chan DK, Shank JJ, Griffith KA, Fan H, Szulawski R, Yang K, Reynolds RK, Johnston C, McLean K, Uppal S, Liu JR, Cabrera L, Taylor SE, Orr BC, Modugno F, Mehta P, Bregenzer M, Mehta G, Shen H, Coffman LG, Buckanovich RJ. Phase II clinical trial of metformin as a cancer stem cell–targeting agent in ovarian cancer. JCI Insight. 2020;5 https://doi.org/10.1172/JCI.INSIGHT.133247.
28. Moon D, Hauck JS, Jiang X, Quang H, Xu L, Zhang F, Gao X, Wild R, Everitt JI, Macias E, He Y, Huang J. Targeting glutamine dependence with DRP-104 inhibits proliferation and tumor growth of castration-resistant prostate cancer. Prostate. 2024;84:349–57. https://doi.org/10.1002/PROS.24654;CTYPE:STRING:JOURNAL.
29. Awad MM, Gadgeel SM, Borghaei H, Patnaik A, Yang JCH, Powell SF, Gentzler RD, Martins RG, Stevenson JP, Altan M, Jalal SI, Panwalkar A, Gubens M, Sequist LV, Saraf S, Zhao B, Piperdi B, Langer CJ. Long-term overall survival from KEYNOTE-021 cohort G: Pemetrexed

and carboplatin with or without Pembrolizumab as first-line therapy for advanced nonsquamous NSCLC. J Thorac Oncol. 2021;16:162–8. https://doi.org/10.1016/j.jtho.2020.09.015.

30. Gion M, Blancas I, Cortez-Castedo P, Cortés-Salgado A, Marmé F, Blanch S, Morales S, Díaz N, Calvo-Plaza I, Recalde S, Martínez-Bueno A, Ruiz-Borrego M, Llabrés E, Taberner MT, de Laurentiis M, García-Vicente S, Guerrero JA, Boix O, Rodríguez-Morató J, Sampayo-Cordero M, Antonarelli G, Pérez-García JM, Cortés J, Llombart-Cussac A. Atezolizumab plus paclitaxel and bevacizumab as first-line treatment of advanced triple-negative breast cancer: the ATRACTIB phase 2 trial. Nat Med. 2025;31:2746–54. https://doi.org/10.1038/S41591-025-03734-3.
31. Singh AK, Singh A, Singh R, Misra A. Efficacy and safety of imeglimin in type 2 diabetes: a systematic review and meta-analysis of randomized placebo-controlled trials. Diabetes Metab Syndr Clin Res Rev. 2023;17:102710. https://doi.org/10.1016/J.DSX.2023.102710.
32. Cusi K, Alkhouri N, Harrison SA, Fouqueray P, Moller DE, Hallakou-Bozec S, Bolze S, Grouin JM, Jeannin Megnien S, Dubourg J, Ratziu V. Efficacy and safety of PXL770, a direct AMP kinase activator, for the treatment of non-alcoholic fatty liver disease (STAMP-NAFLD): a randomised, double-blind, placebo-controlled, phase 2a study. lancet Gastroenterol Hepatol. 2021;6:889–902. https://doi.org/10.1016/S2468-1253(21)00300-9.
33. N. Shoung, C. Carette, N. Rassy, A. Phan, J.R. Greenfield, F.B. Hu, C. Rives-Lange, S. Czernichow, Registered clinical trials targeting type 2 diabetes remission with pharmacological interventions, Sci Rep 15 (2025) 1–10. doi:https://doi.org/10.1038/S41598-025-00080-9.
34. Sinha R, Papamargaritis D, Sargeant JA, Davies MJ. Efficacy and safety of Tirzepatide in type 2 diabetes and obesity management. J Obes Metab Syndr. 2023;32:25–45. https://doi.org/10.7570/JOMES22067.
35. Avgerinos KI, Mullins RJ, Egan JM, Kapogiannis D. Ketone Ester effects on biomarkers of brain metabolism and cognitive performance in cognitively intact adults ≥55 years old. A study protocol for a double-blinded randomized controlled clinical trial. J Prev Alzheimers Dis. 2022;9:54–66. https://doi.org/10.14283/JPAD.2022.3.
36. Neth BJ, Huynh K, Giles C, Wang T, Mellett NA, Duong T, Blach C, Schimmel L, Register TC, Blennow K, Zetterberg H, Batra R, Schweickart A, Dilmore AH, Martino C, Arnold M, Krumsiek J, Han X, Dorrestein PC, Knight R, Meikle PJ, Craft S, Kaddurah-Daouk R. Consuming a modified Mediterranean ketogenic diet reverses the peripheral lipid signature of Alzheimer's disease in humans. Commun Med. 2025;5(1, 1):–15. https://doi.org/10.1038/s43856-024-00682-w.
37. Huang LK, Kuan YC, Lin HW, Hu CJ. Clinical trials of new drugs for Alzheimer disease: a 2020–2023 update. J Biomed Sci. 2023;30:1–19. https://doi.org/10.1186/S12929-023-00976-6/FIGURES/3.
38. Capriglia F, Burgess T, Bandmann O, Mortiboys H. Clinical trial highlights: modulators of mitochondrial function. J Parkinsons Dis. 2023;13:853–66. https://doi.org/10.3233/JPD-239003;WEBSITE:WEBSITE:SAGE;WGROUP:STRING:PUBLICATION.
39. Burton BK, Harmatz PR, Horvathova V, Lail A, Lampe C, Parini R, Sharma R, Teles EL. Long-term enzyme replacement therapy: findings from the mucopolysaccharidosis VI clinical surveillance program after 15 years follow-up. Mol Genet Metab. 2025;145:109135. https://doi.org/10.1016/J.YMGME.2025.109135.
40. Hwu WL. Gene therapy for ultrarare diseases: a geneticist's perspective. J Biomed Sci. 2024;31:1–13. https://doi.org/10.1186/S12929-024-01070-1/TABLES/3.
41. Harding CO, Longo N, Northrup H, Sacharow S, Singh R, Thomas JA, Vockley J, Zori RT, Bulloch Whitehall K, Lilienstein J, Lindstrom K, Levy DG, Jones S, Burton BK. Pegvaliase for the treatment of phenylketonuria: final results of a long-term phase 3 clinical trial program. Mol Genet Metab Rep. 2024;39:101084. https://doi.org/10.1016/J.YMGMR.2024.101084.
42. Baek R, Coughlan K, Jiang L, Liang M, Ci L, Singh H, Zhang H, Kaushal N, Rajlic IL, Van L, Dimen R, Cavedon A, Yin L, Rice L, Frassetto A, Guey L, Finn P, Martini PGV. Characterizing the mechanism of action for mRNA therapeutics for the treatment of propionic acidemia, methylmalonic acidemia, and phenylketonuria. Nat Commun. 2024, 15(1):–13. https://doi.org/10.1038/s41467-024-47460-9.

43. Vander Heiden MG. Exploiting tumor metabolism: challenges for clinical translation. J Clin Invest. 2013;123:3648. https://doi.org/10.1172/JCI72391.
44. Hua S, de Matos MBC, Metselaar JM, Storm G. Current trends and challenges in the clinical translation of nanoparticulate nanomedicines: pathways for translational development and commercialization. Front Pharmacol. 2018;9:403086. https://doi.org/10.3389/FPHAR.2018.00790/XML.
45. Anaya JM, Herrán M, Pino LE. Challenges and opportunities for precision medicine in developing nations. Expert Rev Precis Med Drug Dev. 2025;10:1–15. https://doi.org/10.1080/23808993.2025.2505796;SUBPAGE:STRING:FULL.
46. Moffitt LR, Karimnia N, Wilson AL, Stephens AN, Ho GY, Bilandzic M. Challenges in implementing comprehensive precision medicine screening for ovarian cancer. Curr Oncol. 2024;31:8023. https://doi.org/10.3390/CURRONCOL31120592.
47. Gao T, Yang L, Zhang Y, Bajinka O, Yuan X. Cancer metabolic reprogramming and precision medicine-current perspective. Front Pharmacol. 2024;15:1450441. https://doi.org/10.3389/FPHAR.2024.1450441/BIBTEX.
48. Gharipour M, Nezafati P, Sadeghian L, Eftekhari A, Rothenberg I, Jahanfar S. Precision medicine and metabolic syndrome. ARYA Atheroscler. 2022;18:1. https://doi.org/10.22122/ARYA.2022.26215.
49. Mankoff DA, Edmonds CE, Farwell MD, Pryma DA. Development of companion diagnostics. Semin Nucl Med. 2016;46:47. https://doi.org/10.1053/J.SEMNUCLMED.2015.09.002.
50. Zhang G, Wang J. Artificial intelligence-driven metabolic engineering is applied to the development of active ingredients in traditional Chinese medicine. BIO Web Conf. 2025;174:03013. https://doi.org/10.1051/BIOCONF/202517403013.
51. Anwar A, Rana S, Pathak P. Artificial intelligence in the management of metabolic disorders: a comprehensive review. J Endocrinol Investig. 2025;48:1525–38. https://doi.org/10.1007/S40618-025-02548-X.
52. Ghosh J, Chaudhury SR, Singh K, Koner S. Application of machine learning algorithm and artificial intelligence in improving metabolic syndrome related complications: a review. Int J Adv Life Sci Res. 2024;7:41–67. https://doi.org/10.31632/IJALSR.2024.V07I02.004.
53. Shao Y, Lv X, Ying S, Guo Q. Artificial intelligence-driven precision medicine: multi-omics and spatial multi-omics approaches in diffuse large B-cell lymphoma (DLBCL). Front Biosci (Landmark Ed). 2024;29 https://doi.org/10.31083/J.FBL2912404.
54. Clarós A, Ciudin A, Muria J, Llull L, Mola JÀ, Pons M, Castán J, Cruz JC, Simó R. A model based on artificial intelligence for the prediction, prevention and patient-centred approach for non-communicable diseases related to metabolic syndrome. Eur J Public Health. 2025;35:642. https://doi.org/10.1093/EURPUB/CKAF098.
55. Pugliese N, Bertazzoni A, Hassan C, Schattenberg JM, Aghemo A. Revolutionizing MASLD: how artificial intelligence is shaping the future of liver care. Cancers (Basel). 2025;17:722. https://doi.org/10.3390/CANCERS17050722.
56. Chi J, Shu J, Li M, Mudappathi R, Jin Y, Lewis F, Boon A, Qin X, Liu L, Gu H. Artificial intelligence in metabolomics: a current review. TrAC Trends Anal Chem. 2024;178:117852. https://doi.org/10.1016/J.TRAC.2024.117852.
57. Balasamy S, Ganapathy D, Nallaswamy D, Sundramoorthy AK. Uracil biomarker for pyrimidine metabolism in OSCC: leveraging AI and machine learning for improved diagnosis. Open Dent J. 2025;19 https://doi.org/10.2174/0118742106360500241226054719.
58. Chen AT, Zhang Y, Zhang J. Artificial intelligence in cardiac metabolism: the next frontier in cardiovascular health. Metab Target Organ Damage. 2025;5(3) https://doi.org/10.20517/MTOD.2024.82.
59. Cai H, Zhang F, Xu F, Yang C. Metabolic reprogramming and therapeutic targeting in non-small cell lung cancer: emerging insights beyond the Warburg effect. Front Oncol. 2025;15:1564226. https://doi.org/10.3389/FONC.2025.1564226/FULL.
60. Tanveer H, Faheem M, Khan AH, Adam MA. Machine learning models for personalized treatment recommendations in diabetes management. Int J Sci Res Manage. 2025;13:2145–54. https://doi.org/10.18535/IJSRM/V13I04.EC03.

Index

S. Ashique et al. (eds.), *Cancer Metabolism*, Cancer Treatment and Research 195, https://doi.org/10.1007/978-3-032-21861-2

D

E

F

GPSR Compliance

The European Union's (EU) General Product Safety Regulation (GPSR) is a set of rules that requires consumer products to be safe and our obligations to ensure this.

If you have any concerns about our products, you can contact us on ProductSafety@springernature.com

In case Publisher is established outside the EU, the EU authorized representative is:

Springer Nature Customer Service Center GmbH
Europaplatz 3
69115 Heidelberg, Germany

Batch number: 10726135

Printed by Printforce, the Netherlands